MW00804217

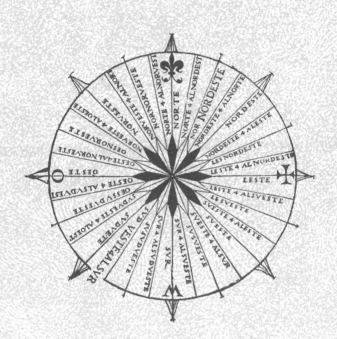

MW00804217

MINISTRY OF CULTURAL AND ENVIRONMENTAL ASSETS

NATIONAL COMMISSION FOR THE CELEBRATION OF THE QUINCENTENNIAL
OF THE DISCOVERY OF AMERICA

NUOVA RACCOLTA COLOMBIANA
ENGLISH EDITION

ISTITUTO POLIGRAFICO E ZECCA DELLO STATO
LIBRERIA DELLO STATO
ROMA

MINISTRY OF CULTURAL AND ENVIRONMENTAL ASSETS

NATIONAL COMMISSION FOR THE CELEBRATION OF THE QUINCENTENNIAL
OF THE DISCOVERY OF AMERICA

NUOVA RACCOLTA COLOMBIANA

THE DISCOVERY OF THE NEW WORLD IN THE WRITINGS OF PETER MARTYR OF ANGHIERA

EDITED BY:

ERNESTO LUNARDI, ELISA MAGIONCALDA, ROSANNA MAZZACANE

Translated into English by

FELIX AZZOLA

Revised by

LUCIANO F. FARINA – The Ohio State University

ISTITUTO POLIGRAFICO E ZECCA DELLO STATO
LIBRERIA DELLO STATO
ROMA

"It is forbidden the reproduction with any proceedings of this work or of some sides of it. As well as the possession and the sale of abusive copies of it. Each abuse will be persecuted by the law 22 may 1993 n. 159".

Originally published as *La Scoperta del Nuovo Mondo Negli Scritti di Pietro Martire D'Anghiera*
Translation © 1992 by Felix Azzola and Luciano F. Farina

© ISTITUTO POLIGRAFICO E ZECCA DELLO STATO - LIBRERIA DELLO STATO

NATIONAL COMMISSION FOR THE CELEBRATION OF THE
QUINCENTENNIAL OF THE DISCOVERY OF AMERICA

Scientific Committee for the Nuova Raccolta Colombiana:

PAOLO EMILIO TAVIANI, president; ALDO AGOSTO; GABRIELLA AIRALDI; OSVALDO BALDACCI; GIUSEPPE BELLINI; ALBERTO BOSCOLO †; FRANCO CARDINI; LUISA D'ARIENZO; GAETANO FERRO; FRANCESCO GIUNTA; ILARIA LUZZANA CARACI; GEO PISTARINO; FRANCESCO SISINNI.

ENGLISH EDITION OF THE «NUOVA RACCOLTA COLOMBIANA»

Published and printed by Istituto Poligrafico e Zecca dello Stato - Libreria dello Stato
Edited and translated by The Ohio State University

Volume Editors:
L.F. FARINA and C.K. ZACHER

Editorial Board:
L. F. FARINA; D. O. FRANTZ; J. B. GABEL; C. D. KLOPP; A. N. MANCINI; C. C. SCHLAM; C. K. ZACHER

INTRODUCTION

The publication of a collection of Peter Martyr of Anghiera's texts in the Nuova Raccolta Colombiana *affords the occasion to read in its Latin original and in translation one of the most important sources of information about Christopher Columbus and the discovery of American lands, which were identified as "New World" by the author himself.*

Up to now there is no English translation of the more than eight hundred letters which make up the Opus Epistolarum [Epistolary], *fifty of which provide precious information about Columbus, the events concerning the Atlantic travels and the Spanish penetration in the new lands at the end of the fifteenth century and the first decades of the sixteenth century.*

Indeed, Peter Martyr, though often quoted in Columbian literature, is an author rarely studied in the original and is one remembered, sometimes unjustifiably, with many reservations.

Some writers of his time, especially Spanish, deny the reliability of Peter Martyr, arguing that he could not know the events of the New World because he had never been there. In truth, he took every care to gather as much information as he could, consulting all those who knew the facts through direct experience, in order to give a scrupulous version, without worrying much if his narrative disagreed with the 'official accounts' sent to the Court, which were often drawn up full of aggrandizements while revealing very little about the conquistadors' arbitrary or criminal behavior.

It must be added that while the pages of the Decades de Orbe Novo *could not be ignored (given the wide circulation which they had achieved in all of Europe, in translations and often in adaptations, Peter Martyr's letters were intentionally forgotten, because, in the climate of the Counter-Reformation, certain explicit reproofs of the actions of the pontiffs, high prelates, and powerful figures could not be divulged.*

Peter Martyr was not a humanist locked away in the literary world; rather, his activity was varied. He dealt with foreign ambassadors on behalf of the Sovereigns and drew up in Latin important diplomatic correspondence. He was an advisor, and even a confidant, to the Sovereigns, although he knew how to maintain his autonomy, clinging to the right to express his opinion.

The humanistic tradition very often led him to look at events not with the detachment of an historian but with sympathy for the sufferings which the ambitions and greed of the mighty cause in defenseless populations, be they from Europe or from the new lands. There is in him a constant yearning for peace, justice and respect for life and human freedom.

His Latin (and he wrote almost exclusively in Latin) is a living language, always precise, full of neologisms derived from the vernaculars and from the lexicon which comes to him from the realities of the New World, a lexicon which through his pages enters into all the European languages.

He was a man of remarkable classical culture, with a preference for scientific texts, which reflected the same intellectual restlessness and need for research which engendered the great venture of Columbus.

He was a friend of the Discoverer and witnessed his triumph and defeat. Faced with the ingratitude of the Crown and the slanders of Columbus's enemies, Peter Martyr withdrew into a bitter silence, interrupting for many years his writings on the New World, but continuing to collect all the information that he could obtain.

There is a singular identity between him and Columbus: both were Italians who had to look for their road to success outside of their country, not disowning but hiding a bit their origins because they found themselves in a context in which belonging to the Spanish nobility was nearly indispensable as a means of avoiding humiliations. Both had the good fortune of meeting an exceptional person, Queen Isabella the Catholic, who protected and helped them. And both reached greatness only to endure ingratitude, hostility, and slander.

Life brought them together and a great friendship arose between them, but their different responsibilities and positions with respect to the Spanish Crown made their contacts less frequent and less close. While they may have disagreed on scientific matters, they always remained supportive of each other.

Peter Martyr's world in terms of geographical spaciousness, but also in terms of human dimension, is indeed one of the most comprehensive provided by his time, because 'man,' in his different behavior, with his potential for virtues and vices, is always at the center of Martyr's attention, always a protagonist on the scene of the world.

Simply reading the texts is certainly not sufficient for a full evaluation of his testimonials. It is necessary to consider more attentively the writer, the historic moment in which he lives, the people who are at the center of the event, and the psychological implications. To reduce Peter Martyr's importance to that of a simple informer is, in our opinion, to forget the personality of the author and therefore the spirit with which he wrote his works, to ignore purposely the cultural turmoil which gave rise to the modern world, extending, in all its dimensions, what up to that time had been a "world" divided in geographic and spiritual areas unknown to each other. What energizes Peter Martyr is his humanistic concern for learning and for placing it in the context of the traditional culture, in his holding men responsible for events always, and in all cases, without seeking other causes (provi-dence or fortune) for their successes or failures.

A first attempt to deepen research on this author was made during the studies of the second "Convegno Internazionale di Studi Americanistici," held in Genoa in 1978. The Conference proceedings published in the volume Pietro Martire d'Anghiera nella storia e nella cultura *(A.I.S.A., Genoa, 1980) form a reliable reference for scholars of this topic.*

In line with the purpose of this volume of the Nuova Raccolta Colombiana, *we have chosen and reproduced the fifty-two letters of the* Opus *which deal with Columbus and the new lands. The texts are presented in their entirety in both the original Latin and the translations, so as to make evident the nature, breadth of interest, and sharpness of observation of the letters, which rarely deal with only one topic.*

For the Decades *the selection is limited to the three books which deal specifically with the travels and the discoveries of Columbus (I 1-7; III 4). What is presented is a critical text based on the collation of the oldest editions, since the originals have not reached us.*

Accompanying the critical edition of the text are some notes with information on the more interesting themes concerning the life of the humanist and his activity as a writer who first made known the New World to all of Europe. The volume closes with basic bibliographical references and indexes of names and places found in the texts and in the notes.

ERNESTO LUNARDI

The introduction to the text, the edition and translation, the summaries preceding the texts, the indexes of the corresponding passages and the critical appendixes are by Elisa Magioncalda and Rosanna Maz-zacane.

The notes are by Ernesto Lunardi.

The selective bibliographical references and the indices of the names and places are by Simonetta Conti.

Revisions and integrations are by Luciano F. Farina.

INTRODUCTION TO THE TEXT

Collating the oldest editions in print, the only evidence in our possession of the *Opus Epistolarum [Epistolary]* and of the *Decades de Orbe Novo* by Peter Martyr of Anghiera, we have observed that they do not present substantial textual variations, but mostly orthographic fluctuations (rather common in humanistic texts) which, in order to facilitate reading, we did not deem it useful to keep. We have, therefore, adopted conventions which, generally, as one will note, are not based solely on the identification of prevalent forms.

Indeed, this latter procedure would not have been meaningful, in our opinion, inasmuch as the present volume proposes only a partial edition; and, at any rate, even in the case of an examination of the entire work, in the absence of the autograph, it would have determined only a relative certainty in the definition of Peter Martyr's 'usus scribendi.' On the other hand, even normalization of the text, introduced out of necessity only in some cases, would not have respected the development process of the language and the Spanish influences undergone by it. Consequently, although the early editions of both the *Opus Epistolarum* and the *Decades de Orbe Novo* are nearly contemporaneous and present orthographic problems at times parallel, given the differing genres of the two works, we have distinguished the conventions adopted in each case.

a) *Opus Epistolarum*

Of the letters gathered in the *Epistolary* that came down to us under the name of Peter Martyr, we have included those specifically pertinent to Christopher Columbus as well as those which provide news on the life of the author, the discoveries, and the new world.

As far as we know, the *Opus Epistolarum*, of which we do not possess any original manuscript, was printed for the first time after the death of the author, in 1530 at Alcalá de Henares, by M. de Eguía, together with the *Legatio Babylonica* and the second edition of the *Decades de Orbe Novo* (see p. 12). The second edition in print, edited by D. Helzevier at Amsterdam, is dated 1670; evident in it is the effort to normalize the text according to accepted seventeenth-century criteria. Such an edition arose from the need to have a text of the *Opus*, because at the beginning of the seventeenth century it was already very difficult to find it even in Spain. Next to these two texts we could place a manuscript of 1657, preserved in the Vatican Library (ms. Barb. Lat. 2117) and until now neglected by scholars, which contains the letters of the 1530 edition without changes in content. It ends with a statement by a notary which declares that the *Opus, de re et fideliter, concordat cum suo originali, de verbo ad verbum* (that is, with the text edited by M. de Eguía). There is a letter of 20 December 1656 to Cardinal Francesco Barberini by Nicolò Ricci, confirming that it is a pure and simple transcription. From this letter it is plausible to assume that the writer was sent to Alcalá with the task of inquiring into "something misquoted and different" from that *Opus* which was "taken and transferred" to Rome for the canonization of Francisco Jimenez de Cisneros, founder of the College of Alcalá. The book with the same heading of the 1530 edition, in "small size," found "with difficulty," was copied and given back. From examining the letters we conclude that, in all probability, the manuscript is a copy of an original similar to the 1530 edition. It shows differences only in the numbering of the letters and insignificant graphic variances such as those related to the use of the intervocalic consonant, usually the s, which is sometimes single, sometimes double.

The text offered here is based on the 1530 edition, of which it essentially reflects the orthography, and takes into consideration the corrections made in the 1670 edition, necessary where the typographical misprints of the first are obvious. The collation of the two editions and the handwritten transcription, distant in time from each other, does not provide useful elements for the reconstruction of the original orthography. And, moreover, the letters, even if addressed *ad dinastas* (as we read in the letter of Nicolò Ricci), that is, to persons in power of the time, seem to be written *currenti calamo* (see Dec. I 10 C², pg. 76: ... *per epistolas raptim scriptas* ...), in a Latin mixed with hispanicisms and with learned literary allusions; it therefore does not seem appropriate to tamper with it, even if with the intent of improving the text. The letters present problems which are not always easily solved, because they are characterized by that psychological immediacy and daily flavor of the lexicon and of structure of phrase which are rather traits more of the epistolography of common people. Therefore, since we could not restore the text to its genuine form, we have tried to restore it in a form agreeable to the reader, establishing orthographic conventions and using as terms of comparison the Latin-Spanish dictionary by Antonio de Nebrija (1492), Peter Martyr's friend and supporter.

Generally, we have normalized the consonants, which are sometimes simple, sometimes double (with the exception of the verb forms derived from the perfect of *reperio*, which maintain a constant spelling), because such alternating use, although practiced by the writers, certainly had an effect on the printer influenced by changes in pronunciation. The clusters *ci* and *ti* and graphic forms such as *ae*=*e*, *oe*=*e*, *i*=*y*, *ch*=*c*, *mq*=*nq*, *ph*=*f*, *th*=*t* and, viceversa, *x*=*xs*, *t*=*ct*, have been retained if they are for the most part used consistently; in isolated cases and in those of graphic fluctuation of the same word, we have adopted whenever possible the form attested by Nebrija; otherwise we proceeded to normalize them. We have accepted those words clearly patterned after the corresponding Spanish terms, such as, for example, *bergantini, caravela, carraca, filateria, francisci, freila*. For geographic names that present alternate spelling for which there is no classical Latin correspondence (e.g., Valladolid, Medina del Campo), we have resorted to the dictionaries of ancient geography (see Bibliography); in other cases of proper and geographic names we have preserved the Latin spelling that is closer to the Spanish or the original (e.g., *carvaialus* from the Spanish Carvajal; *Magallanes* from the Portuguese *magalhaes* [Spanish *magallanes*]; *Portugalia, Portugalenses* from the Spanish Portugal). We preferred to keep the spelling of the adjective *Portugallicus*, which occurs almost consistently in this form, because it might be possible to support the assumption for it of a false etymology from the adjective *Gallicus*.

Before the heading of each letter, in which is indicated only the receiver and the sender omitted (*P.M.A.M.*=*Petrus Martyr Anglerius Mediolanensis*), we provide progressively numbered references to the letters as collated in the texts, with the following abbreviations:

C=1530 edition, M. de Eguía, ed. (*Complutum*=Alcalá de Henares), reprinted anastatically at Graz (*G*) in 1966 (=*C²*; see p. 12);

A=1670 edition, D. Helzevier, ed. (*Amstelodamum*=Amsterdam);

ms.=handwritten copy (*ms. Barb. Lat.* 2117).

In order to justify the chosen reading, we indicated in the appendix (app. I) the mistakes and orthographic variances attested in the editions and in the manuscript.

We have marked with an asterisk the cases in which the chosen form is attested also by the dictionary of Antonio de Nebrija.

We have indicated, on page margins with the sign ‹, those passages that relate to Christopher Columbus and to the New World.

b) *Decades de Orbe Novo*

This partial edition of the books of the *Decades de Orbe Novo* concerning the travels of Columbus is also based, as are the letters, on extant printed editions, since, as we said, up to now, neither the autograph nor any manuscript of Peter Martyr's history have been found.

We have therefore collated the four oldest editions, as follows:

C^1 = 1516 edition, A. de Nebrija, ed. (*Complutum* = Alcalá de Henares) containing the first three *Decades*;

C^2 = 1530 edition, M. de Eguía, ed. (*Complutum* = Alcalá de Henares), reprinted anastatically at Graz (*G*) in 1966, containing the eight *Decades*, the *Legatio Babylonica* and the *Opus Epistolarum* (= *C*, see p. 11);

B = 1533 edition, I. Bebel, ed. (*Basilea* = Basel), reprint of the 1516 edition;

P = 1587 edition, R. Hakluyt, ed. (*Parisii* = Paris), containing the eight *Decades*.

The subsequent, more recent editions were not taken into consideration because they reproduce those earlier ones used in this study. In addition, we cannot take into consideration the Seville edition of 1511, even though it has been collated by us, because it was published without the knowledge of the author (*me inconsulto*: see *Dec.* II 1 C^2, pg. 78 *G*; II 7 C^2, pg. 96 *G*) and, besides, it was incomplete (I 1-10).

Besides the omissions and additions present in the 1511 Seville edition, we have also encountered recurrent graphic and textual variants, most of which disappear in a later edition, that reveal a textual preparation of the work and a not normalized spelling (when normalization is generally common as early as the 1516 edition) closer to that of the Epistolary. In this regard, we have listed in Appendix II only the textual variants (omissions and additions) of this edition, marked with the initial *H* (Seville = *Hispalis*), since they are useful in understanding the genesis of this work; we do not, however, show regular graphic variants which are insignificant, such as, for example, the use of *e* for *ae*, of *ch* and *cc* for *c*, of *ss* for *s*.

As mentioned, the editions examined here present few textual variants, generally irrelevant to the reconstruction of the text that we wanted to restore in a form as close as possible to the original, even when it was to the detriment of a correct classical Latin form. Thus we have retained some typically medieval constructions, such as the consecutive *quod*, the use of *singulus* for *quisque*, or analogical forms such as *illinitas* for *illitas*, *quoto die* for *quotidie*. Remarkable, on the other hand, is the number of spelling fluctuations found even within the same edition and for the same term, fluctuations which led us to establish, as we did in the case of the Epistolary, precise orthographic criteria for the text reconstruction. We wanted to respect as much as possible the graphies of the first two editions (C^1 and C^2) published in Spain, that is, in the linguistic and cultural context in which the author lived (see *Dec.* II 7 C^2, p. 98 *G*: *Latinissimi viri...voloque sciant me Insubrem esse, non Latium et longe a Latio natum, quia Mediolani et longissime vitam egisse, quia in Hispania...*). In particular, we have accepted spellings closer to Spanish for Amerindian words and proper names of the natives, that have come down to us through Spanish (e.g., *Canibales* from the Spanish *Caníbal; cacicus, chi* from the Spanish *cacique*), and some true neologisms with respect to classical Latin, peculiar to the linguistic patrimony of its humanistic author (*caravela* = Spanish *carabela; almirantus* = Spanish *almirante; adelantatus* = Spanish *adelantado*; etc.), occasionally present also in the Epistolary (see *Dec.* VII 7 C^2, p. 230 *G*: *vulgaribus utor vocabulis quando illis caret vetus lingua Latina et liceat quae de novo emergunt novis induere tegminibus, cum id negantium bona venia volo intelligi*).

With regard to the formulation of the dedications of some books of the *Decades* (I 1-6) we have quoted the one confirmed in C^1, leaving out repeated formulas, such as: *Oceanee Decadis P. Martyris Angli Mediol. Consiliarii Regii Prot. Apl. Oceaneae Decadis liber primus...*, common in the editions with variants of no significance.

In general, when C^1 and C^2 record a reading conforming to the classical usage, this lection was accepted independently of the variants registered in *B* and *P*. Even when the norm would not have allowed it, we have retained those spelling forms which are in agreement in the two oldest editions. In the case of different but confirmed spellings of the same term in C^1 and C^2, we have accepted the reading of C^1, the edition which is supposedly closer to Peter Martyr's original (at least for the part with which this study deals).

The graphic fluctuation of the same term, which can be seen in C^1 and C^2, calling for normalization of forms, has led us to accept the more prevalent form for uniformity sake, or in case of undefined prevalent spelling, such as, for example, the compounds (*nãque. namque* ~ *nanque: utrũque* ~ *utrumque. utrunque*, etc.), the form more often found in C^1.

If C^1 and C^2 do not agree and do not present forms attested in classical use, then the followed normalization criterion, usually supported also by *B* and *P*, was to opt for what was more closely faithful to the spelling of classical Latin. Inconsistency of consonantal gemination has been systematically normalized, as done for the *Opus Epistolarum*. The *e* has been always substituted by the better known and more frequently used *ae*, in order to be more familiar to today's reader.

The typographical errors denounced since the 1516 edition (p. 125-126 *C¹*: *Ad lectorem de quibusdam locis leviter depravatis*), have been systematically corrected.

Appendix III lists the mistakes and the spelling and textual variants so that our choice of the adopted reading may be documented for the readers who thus can see the differences among the collated texts.

We have introduced, both in the Epistolary and in the *Decades*, a different system of punctuation and capitalization in order to add clarity to possibly obscure passages or not easily understood. We have highlighted, with italics or bold type, Amerindian words, proper nouns and the names of places of the New World given by Columbus the first time they appear, and terms stressed by Peter Martyr specifically.

For convenience sake, we have indicated next to the Latin text the corresponding pages of the anastatic reprint of Graz at the beginning of each letter and of each book of the *Decades*.

In order not to burden the text with a critical apparatus at the bottom of the page, as is customarily done in critical editions, and to facilitate reading for a non-specialist, we chose to make use of appendices, where one will notice that the differences among the collated editions are mostly in spelling, but, equally interesting, in their evidence for the influence exercised by the spoken over the written language and the already common spelling uncertainties which evidently not even Peter Martyr could avoid. In the apparatus we did not indicate the compounds relative to -*m* and -*n* because they are so frequent: even they appear resolved sometimes in the oldest editions (*C¹*, *C²*), only when documented graphic variants did allow us to restore them and in accordance with the established criteria of the more attested forms.

For a more in-depth analysis of the author's Latin, a very rich and pliable instrument of varying expressive and lexical levels, we refer the reader especially to the comprehensive studies by G. Ponte, M. Damonte and J. Gil-Consuelo Varela (see Bibliography). At the bottom of the Latin text we have added some explanatory notes and have identified some of the more evident classical references following the abbreviations adopted for citations.

Unlike the previous translations, of which we have only a partial one limited to the *Decades* in Italian (see Bibliography), in this study we have attempted, as much as possible, to place alongside the Latin text an [italian] transliteration without altering the complex structure of the sentences, making at times for a syntactically laborious result complemented, however, by the original Latin text for specialists. In order to render the immediacy and the expressive liveliness of the author in an effort to reproduce his style, we have preferred to preserve the alternating use of present and past tenses which we find in the text. The geographic names of the New World have been translated with the corresponding Spanish terms. Only *Hispaniola* (Española) appears in the English text in the same Latin form adopted by Peter Martyr. The term Hispaniola is usually used in English and in other languages and therefore also in the volumes of the *Nuova Raccolta Colombiana* to refer to the entire island which includes the territories of the modern republic of Haiti (French-speaking) and the Dominican Republic.

The text's critical notes, translation, summaries and indexes of the corresponding passages have been divided among the editors as follows (the numbering refers to the first edition): *Opus Epistolarum epp.* 131, 141, 159, 165, 169, 177, 180, 189, 205, 247, 537, 542, 559, 630, 650, 650 bis, 715, 717, 758, 774, 812 (Elisa Magioncalda); epp. 134, 135, 136, 139, 143, 145, 147, 153, 157, 161, 181, 185, 190, 201, 529, 544, 548, 557, 558, 624, 635, 766, 770, 773, 782, 786, 791, 801, 804, 806, 809, 814 (Rosanna Mazzacane). *Decades de Orbe Novo*, books I 1-4, 7 (Rosanna Mazzacane); books I 5-6; III 4 (Elisa Magioncalda).

From the *Opus Epistolarum* [*Epistolary*]

Epp. (the progressive numbering refers to the 1530 edition):

131, 134, 135, 136, 139, 141, 143, 147, 153, 157, 159, 161, 165, 169, 177, 180, 181, 185, 189, 190, 201, 205, 247, 529, 537, 544, 548, 557, 558, 559, 624, 630, 635, 650, 650 bis, 715, 717, 758, 766, 770, 773, 774, 782, 786, 791, 801, 804, 806, 809, 812, 814.

To help the reader better understand the context in which the letters were written we have provided very concise summaries of specific events and facts to which Peter Martyr often refers. We have also included two letters which do not deal with the New World, one autobiographic in content (ep. 247, p. 98), the other treating the Portuguese travels (ep. 185, p. 84) in search of new trade markets, since Portugal played an important role during the time of the Discovery.

To Giovanni Borromeo – 14 May 1493 (ep. 131, p. 35).

Reference to an attempt on the life of Ferdinand the Catholic; return of Christopher Columbus from the antipodes with gold and precious goods; Italian heads of states call Charles VIII into Italy to restore order in the peninsula; mention of the disagreement between Borromeo and Ludovico il Moro; diplomatic efforts of Charles VIII with the powers of the time; invective of Peter Martyr against the Italians, not to accept the French; transfer of Perpignan and of the county of Rossiglione from France to Spain; sorrow of the writer for the situation in Italy.

To the Count of Tendilla and the Archbishop of Granada – 13 September 1493 *(ep.* 134, p. 37).

Insistence of Columbus on obtaining the necessary means to undertake the planned venture; the return of the Navigator; description of the life and the foods of the natives; loss of a ship near the coast of Hispaniola where thirty-eight men, entrusted to the cacique Guarionex, are left to explore; preparations for a bigger fleet.

To Ascanio Sforza – 13 September 1493 *(ep.* 135, p. 39).

Praise of Columbus' venture, accomplished with the patronage of the Catholic Sovereigns; the products of the New World; observations on the behavior of the natives as similar to that of the Europeans in the relationship between winners and losers; delivery of Perpignan to Spain.

To the Archbishop of Braga – 1 October 1493 *(ep.* 136, p. 43).

Discovery of many islands by Columbus; first intuition of a New World; mention of the Portuguese expeditions to the equator; further reference to the transfer of Perpignan to Spain; Charles VIII seeking assistance from Spain to seize the throne of Naples; descent of Charles VIII into Italy headed for Rome.

To Ascanio Sforza – first of November 1493 (*ep.* 139, p. 45).

Reference to a royal document requested by Ascanio Sforza through Garcia Cañas, brother of Ascanio's personal servant, to assert his rights over some possessions given him by Alexander VI; protests of those who up to that time had benefitted from them; announcement of the death of John, king of Portugal; the send off to a fleet, under the leadership of Admiral Columbus, to found a new city in the new lands; allusion to the French invasion of Italy.

To the Archbishop of Granada – 31 January 1494 (*ep.* 141, p. 47).

Appointment of Columbus as Admiral of the ocean sea and honors bestowed upon him by the Sovereigns.

To Giovanni Borromeo – 20 October 1494 (*ep.* 143, p. 49).

Reference to the attempt on the life of King Ferdinand, to the delivery of the Rossiglione county and to the French invasion of Italy; the antipodes discovered by Columbus; restitution of Perpignan to Spain; the Catholic Sovereigns support Charles VIII's conquest of the kingdom of Naples; agreements about the marriages between the heirs of the Sovereigns of Spain and those of Maximilian of Hapsburg (John, son of the Catholic Sovereigns, will marry Marguerite, daughter of Maximilian of Hapsburg, and Philip, son of Maximilian, will marry Juana, daughter of the Catholic Sovereigns); news concerning Columbus and his discoveries and in particular the cannibals; hint at the drafting of the *Decades*.

To the Archbishops of Braga and Pamplona – 31 October 1494 (*ep.* 145, p. 51).

Antonio de Fonseca is chosen by the rulers of Spain as ambassador to Charles VIII; preparation of a fleet in the roadstead of Malaga in order to transport to Naples some soldiers under the command of Gonzalo Fernandez de Aguilar de Córdoba (the *Gran Capitán*); coalition of some Italian states favored by Spain against the French threat; further reference to the marital agreements between the Catholic Sovereigns and Maximilian of Hapsburg; the Admiral is sent to Hispaniola to found a city; exhortation to report the news to Ascanio Sforza, even if he is now a puppet of the French.

To Pomponius Letus – 5 December 1494 (*ep.* 147, p. 55).

Sad words of grief by the writer about the situation in Italy, a country now in ruin; return of the ships from the New World; the islands of the cannibals, description of their customs; Emanuele succeeded John of Portugal with the favor of the Catholic Sovereigns; reference to the attempts to persuade Isabella, daughter of the Catholic Sovereigns and widow of Alfonso, son of John II, king of Portugal, to marry the new King Emanuele.

To Pomponius Letus – 29 December 1494 (*ep.* 153, p. 59).

Joy of Pomponius Letus at the reports on the New World; mention of Ascanio Sforza, previous correspondent of the author; the slaughter of the thirty-eight men left by Columbus at Hispaniola and Columbus's attitude in this circumstance; the activity of Columbus at Hispaniola, founding of a city, astonishment of the natives at the sight of the Spaniards; the shape and geographic position of the island of Hispaniola.

To Pomponius Letus – 10 January 1495 (*ep.* 157, p. 63).

Repetition of the data relative to Hispaniola, mention of the conflicting opinions concerning its coordinates (longitude, latitude), the fertility and the climate of the island, description of the dwellings and beds (hammocks) of the natives.

To the Archbishop of Granada – 15 January 1495 (*ep.* 159, p. 67).

Announcement that Cardinal Pedro Gonzales de Mendoza is dead; possible marriage between Isabella, widow of Alfonso, son of John, king of Portugal, and Emanuele, successor of John, a marriage wanted by the Sovereigns of Spain even against Isabella's will; marriage agreements between Maximilian of Hapsburg and the Sovereigns of Spain for their children; the king of France, Charles VIII, fears this alliance; very brief hint at the reports coming from the New World and the possibility of the conversion of the natives to Christianity.

To Bernardino de Carvajal – 11 June 1495 (*ep.* 161, p. 69).

Appointment of Bernardino as cardinal; mention of former correspondents (Ascanio Sforza, Giovanni Arcimboldi, cardinal of Milan, Diego de Sousa, Alonso Carrillo and Pomponius Letus) interested in the reports on the antipodes; hint at the expedition to the New World; appointment of Francisco Jiménez, after the death of Cardinal Mendoza, as archbishop of Toledo; ambassadors to the Spanish court of Ludovico il Moro after the death of Gian Galeazzo Sforza, and from Venice; convocation of the *Cortes* in Aragon to oppose the expansion plans of Charles VIII.

To Bernardino de Carvajal – 9 August 1495 (*ep.* 165, p. 71).

Exploration of Cuba and Columbus's return to Hispaniola; description of the seas among those lands and of their fauna; Columbus's conviction that those lands are India and part of a continent.

To Bernardino de Carvajal – 5 October 1496 (*ep.* 169, p. 75).

Resolution of the writer to condense many reports in a few lines; mention of the necklaces of pearls brought back by Columbus; description of the land of Paria and customs of its inhabitants; festive reception by the natives; reference to the *Decades'* treatment of these topics; dispatch of ambassadors to the Spanish court to draw up marriage agreements between the children of Maximilian of Hapsburg and those of the Catholic Sovereigns; breaking-up of the *Cortes*; transfer of the court to the city of Alfaro, where it is joined by Queen Isabella; new transfers of the court to the city of Alfaro, where they are joined by the queen Isabella; new transfers of the court to withstand the king of France, Charles VIII, whereas Queen Isabella goes to Laredo to send her daughter Juana to Philip; preparation of a fleet to transfer the troops along the French coasts; the Queen, sad for the departure of her daughter, joins the court in Burgos to await the arrival of the King.

To Pomponius Letus – 13 June 1497 (*ep.* 177, p. 79).

The natives of Hispaniola; contacts of the hermit Ramón Pane with the native chiefs to teach them Spanish religion and customs; beliefs of the natives concerning the origin of the courts and of men's; allusion to the draft of the *Decades*.

To The Cardinal of Holy Cross – 27 July 1497 (*ep.* 180, p. 81).

Praises for Garcia Lopez, brother of the cardinal of Holy Cross, Bernardino de Carvajal, a man of talent and a poet; reports on the beliefs of the natives, especially on a small gourd which gives birth to the sea.

To Pomponius Letus – 1 September 1497 (*ep.* 181, p. 83).

Comparison between the scholarship of Pomponius Letus and that of Carvajal; reference to the previous letter on the origin of the sea and the fish; the discoveries of Columbus in the West and of the Portuguese in the South; landing of the Portuguese at the Cape of Good Hope: guided by natives they reach the regions from which come the spices and finally Calicut; the inhabitants of Calicut, instigated by the merchants of Damascus and Alexandria, clash with the Portuguese, suffering defeat; the writer's excitment in sharing the news on the New World.

To Pomponius Letus – 7 November 1497 (*ep.* 185, p. 87).

The friendship of the Portuguese ambassador at the court of Spain allows Peter Martyr to provide news on the explorations of the Portuguese; Emanuele of Portugal sends a fleet to Calicut; naval clash between the inhabitants of Calicut and the Portuguese; slaughter of the inhabitants of Calicut.

To Pomponius Letus – 18 December 1497 (*ep.* 189, p. 89).

Description of some beliefs and superstitions of the natives about the origin of things and of men. The *boviti*: native physicians and priests; recollection of the Roman mysteries of the sacred shield and of the *Mater Matuta*.

To the Archbishops of Braga and Pamplona – 5 April 1498 (*ep.* 190, p. 93).

Reference to the relationship between Beatrice of Hungary, daughter of Ferdinand I, king of Naples, and her husband Ladislaus II Jagellone, king of Bohemia, and to the subsequent annulment of their marriage granted by Alexander VI; the Sovereigns of Spain, relatives of Beatrice, prefer to ignore the situation and not to send, as perhaps intended earlier, Peter Martyr as intermediary to the Pope; another cult of the natives: the *Zemi*, gods appeased by the *boviti*.

To Pomponius Letus – 4 February 1499 (*ep.* 201, p. 95).

Dissension between the republic of Venice and Ludovico Sforza; new discoveries of the Castilians in the West; the customs of the natives; clashes between the Portuguese, the king of Calicut and the merchants of Damascus; the hostile situation brings damages and troubles to the Venetian merchants.

To Pomponius Letus – 12 May 1499 (*ep.* 205, p. 97).

Reference to the flooding of the Tiber; news about the natives: the *boviti*, physicians and priests; digression of the writer on the natives' interest in medicine.

To Pedro Fajardo [Fagiardo] – 10 August 1502 (*ep.* 247, p. 101).

The genealogy of the Milanese lineage of Anghiera; praise of his family's ancient nobility from which forty kings and the Viscontis might have descended; migration of Peter Martyr's parents to Arona on Lake Maggiore; description of the city and of the lake's rich fishing waters; the writer's joy for the temporary return to his native land and for meeting with old friends.

To Luis Hurtado de Mendoza – 18 December 1513 (*ep.* 529, p. 105).

Description of new lands and rivers discovered by Columbus and the Spaniards; abundance of gold and pearls; vegetation and climate of those regions; founding of two colonies, one in the gulf of Urabá, the other in Veragua; death of Alfonso de Hojeda, Diego de Nicuesa and Juan de La Cosa, assigned to those regions; reference to the forthcoming publication of the *Decades*.

To Luis Hurtado de Mendoza – 23 July 1514 (*ep.* 537, p. 107).

Reports from the New World: Vasco Núñez de Balboa usurps power in Darién, but he is not punished because he discovers new sources of wealth in the discovered territories to which Pedro Arias was appointed; reference to a promise of marriage never carried out between Marguerite, sister of the king of England, Henry VIII, and the king of France, Francis I, opposed by Maximilian I of Hapsburg and Ferdinand the Catholic; mention of an uprising in Hungary, caused by the decision of Hippolitus I of Este, cardinal of Esztergom (*Strigonium*), to earmark for other purposes the sum of money collected for the crusade authorized by the Pontiff Alexander VI against the Turks of Selim I, engaged at that time in a war against the Persian Ismàil of the Sophy dynasty; reference to the situation in the city of Siena afflicted by internal fights and to the hostility of Alexander VI toward that city.

To Luis Hurtado de Mendoza – 31 December 1514 (*ep.* 542, p. 111).

Mention of the battles fought by Sigismond I Senior, king of Poland, against the neighboring nations to the east, with the approval of the Pontiff Julius II; Catherine of Aragon, wife of Henry VIII, had a miscarriage because of the grief brought on by the disagreement between her husband and her father, Ferdinand the Catholic; Giuliano de Medici, duke of Nemours, brother of Leo X (Giovanni de Medici) marries Filiberta, sister of Charles II, duke of Savoy; Giovanni Vespucci is sent to the court of Spain by the pontiff Leo X; unhealthy climate of some regions of Darién, which, however, are abundant in natural resources; clash with the cacique Cemaco; the Swiss side with Maximilian of Hapsburg; clashes between Venetians and Spaniards in the territory of Padua, after the expulsion of Spain's viceroy from Rovigo; travels of Ferdinand the Catholic, afflicted by dropsy, to Medina del Campo, without the court.

To Luis Hurtado de Mendoza – 3 April 1515 (*ep.* 544, p. 113).

Having spent the holy Week at Mejorada, in the convent of the monks of St. Jerome, the King transfers to Olmedo and then to Aranda de Duero; the queen, Germana de Foix (second wife of the King), convenes the *Cortes* at Monzón; the King goes hunting at Ventosilla; uncertainty of Leo X about the alliances to form as a result of the marriage arranged by the brother; the Pope claims the possession of Parma and Piacenza; advantage of the Swiss, winners at Novara (1514) over the French, opposed to those claims; reference to an incident between Henry VIII, king of England, and Francis I, king of France; Charles Brandon, count of Suffolk, carries letters to Francis I of France, to request in marriage the sister of Henry VIII, Mary, widow of the king of France, Louis XII; Francis I, interpreting the letters in his own way, favors marriage between the widow and Brandon; Pedro Arias, governor of Darién, sends Gaspar de Morales to the island sighted by Vasco Nuñez de Balboa; friendly reception of the natives after a clash with the cacique of the place; sale of a pearl the size of a walnut.

To the Marquis of Mondéjar – 16 August 1515 (*ep.* 548, p. 115).

Reference to an out-of-season hard-frost which ruined the vineyards; recollection of the exchange of letters with the father of the receiver, Iñigo Lopez de Mendoza; mention of quarrels with Rome for which Peter Martyr seeks the legal services of Doctor Aguiñiga, native of Orduña; mention of a conflict between Lorenzo de Medici, nephew of Leo X and the Spanish court, and the ambiguous attitude of the Pontiff; reference to the drafting of the *Decades*; antecedents of the battle of Marignano: the condottiere Gian Giacomo Trivulzio incites the young king of France, Francis I, to fight against the Swiss; reference to the fate of Italy at the mercy of the foreigners; mention of the illness of Ferdinand the Catholic and of the arrest of the vice-chancellor of the King.

To the Marquis of Mondéjar – 5 December 1515 (*ep.* 557, p. 119).

Announcement of the death from quartan fever of Gonzalo Fernández de Aguilar de Córdoba, called the *Gran Capitán*, who led two campaigns against the French in Italy, contributing to establishing the Spanish kingdom in Naples; mention of the appreciation of the *Decades* read by the Pontiff during a banquet on 29 September, the day of St. Michael; Gaspar de Morales is dispatched to the island of Rica and the southern sea discovered by Vasco Nuñez de Balboa; friendship, after a clash, with the natives of the island very rich with pearls; mention of the improved climate of Darién.

To the Marquis de Los Velez – 12 December 1515 (*ep.* 558, p. 121).

Arrival of the court at Plasencia, from where the King leaves again to go to the villa of the duke of Alba, Enrique Alvarez de Toledo; Adrian Florensz, dean of the Academy of Louvain, tutor of the future Charles V, nephew of Ferdinand the Catholic and Isabella, is received by the King; the Swiss, although defeated by the French at Marignano (September 1515), continue fighting and encourage emperor Maximilian of Hapsburg to back them; reference to the clashes in the territory of Verona between the Venetian troops and those of William IV, son of Albert IV of Bavaria, nephew of the Emperor; Enrique de Colmenares is sent to the people of Darién to ask for honorary titles; reference to the king's successful huntsmanship.

To Pope Leo X – 26 December 1515 (*ep.* 559, p. 125).

By invitation of Galeazzo Butrigario, ambassador of the Pope, and of Giovanni Corsi, of the Florentine Republic, the writer sends news of the New World to Leo X, intercepted by the emissaries of the king of France, Francis I; forthcoming news will be related to the Pope by Doctor Aguiñiga, Peter Martyr's attorney in Rome; reference to the unsuccessful attempts of Ferdinand the Catholic to obtain special favors from the Pope for the author; Peter Martyr's decision to print the *Decades* and the *Legatio Babylonica* in one volume, also because after the encouragement of the humanist, A. de Nebrija; attitude of submission with regard to the Pope; mention of the poor health of the Catholic King about which the archbishop of Cosenza, Giovanni Ruffo, will report to the Pope.

To the Marquises – 21 July 1518 (*ep.* 624, p. 127).

News of the marriage between Eleanor of Hapsburg, daughter of Philip of Hapsburg and of Juana the Mad, with Emanuele, king of Portugal; the dowry of Eleanor is sent to Flanders with the Portuguese ambassador, through the Sienese banker Galvano, by Guillaume de Croy, who is lord of Chiévres (called Chèvre), tutor of Philip's sons and holder of an important position at court; reports about the cities located south-west of the island of Cuba, called Fernandina, which shows well-developed customs; finding of great quantities of pearls, easy prey of the Flemish and Frenchmen at the court of Charles; the greed of Guillaume de Croy's wife (Marie de Hamal) is underscored.

To the Marquises – 17 September 1518 (*ep.* 630 p. 129).

Mention of the Turkish incursions into Hungary, despite the open desire of the Turkish Selim I and the king of Hungary, Louis II Jagellone, to maintain friendly relations; reference to the belief that in the province of Brescia there existed witches and sorcerers and to incidents connected with this belief; decision to entrust the command of a fleet of five ships headed to the Moluccas to Ferdinand Magellan and to Ruy Faleiro, distinguished astronomer, once both in the service of Emanuele of Portugal, in order to assure the trade in spices; news of the death of the grand chancellor, Jean de Sauvage, lord of Escaubeque, and of his replacement with Mercurino Arborio of Gattinara, once president of the Senate of Burgundy and ambassador of emperor Maximilian of Hapsburg to Ferdinand the Catholic in 1510.

To the Marquises – 30 January 1519 (*ep.* 635, p. 133).

New references to the thefts by the French and the Flemish at the court of Charles and to the greed of Guillaume de Croy's wife; mention of the payment of huge sums of money, in gifts and compensations to the voters by Charles, to support his candidacy; announcement of the death of Maximilian of Hapsburg; shipwreck of some Spanish ships, under the command of Hugo de Moncada, viceroy of Sicily, near the island of Ibiza, which is then ravaged by starving soldiers; the inhabitants of the island dispatch ambassadors to the King.

To the Marquises – 1 December 1519 (*ep.* 650, p. 135).

Request of help in food and arms by messengers coming from the Spanish forts besieged by local people in Africa; reports from the New World on the fertile island of Jamaica, governed by Francisco de Garay, who is getting ready to explore other islands; mission entrusted to Peter Martyr and to Jeronimo Cabanillas in Valencia, because Charles wants the *Cortes* of the kingdom of Valencia to swear allegiance to the king, even if he is not present at the ceremony; inkling of a possible rebellion in Valencia.

To the Marquises – 2 December 1519 (*ep.* 650 bis, p. 137).

Diego Velázquez, progovernor of Cuba, sends soldiers to the new lands under the command of Hernán Cortés, who decides to stay and to found a colony, disregarding orders to the contrary.

To the Grand Chancellor – 6 March 1521 (*ep.* 715, p. 139).

News of the rebellion of the *Comuneros* prompted mostly by the people of Toledo against Charles because of high taxes levied on various cities of Castile, which Peter Martyr does not seem to believe: the intervention of the Grand Chancellor, Mercurino Arborio of Gattinara, to restore order is deemed desirable; return of some ships from Cuba, an island which shows a certain level of civilization.

To the Marquises – 7 March 1521 (*ep.* 717, p. 141).

Proceeding beyond Cuba, the Spaniards discover the city of Tenustitán (Tenochtitlán - ancient name of Mexico City [Teotihuacan]), governed by King Montezuma; description of the city and of the way of life of its inhabitants; reference to more detailed accounts of this topic in the *Decades*.

To the Grand Chancellor – 14 February 1522 (*ep.* 758, p. 145).

Mention of the situation in Spain where the arrival of Arborio of Gattinara is expected, in the hope that he may restore order in the cities of Castile troubled by the rebellion of the *Comuneros*; Játiva, center of the rebellion: in its fort is imprisoned since 1521 the duke Ferdinand of Calabria, accused of a plot against the Catholic King; reports on a clash near the city of Canales between the men of Don Diego de Mendoza and the *Comuneros*; piracy acts by the French Florin against a ship of the Spanish fleet; wreck of the Spanish fleet under the command of Pedro de Bobadilla; reflections of the writer on the loss of the fleet.

To the Archbishop of Cosenza – 14 July 1522 (*ep.* 766, p. 149).

Detailed reports on the siege of Fuentarrabía, a frontier city between France and Spain, freed from French dominion by the Spaniards, under the command of Don Ludovico de La Cueva, son of Alfonso, duke of Albuquerque; Spanish victory at Beovia; attack on the village of Saint Jean de Luz and on Bayonne; the count of Miranda, viceroy of Navarre, occupies and destroys the stronghold of Maya on the Pyrenees, garrisoned by Jacobo Vélez, leader of the faction of the Agramontese of Navarre;

mention of the city of Tenustitán [Teotihuacan] and of King Montezuma; clashes between Montezuma and the Spaniards supported by his enemies: the writer refers to the *Decades* for details.

To the Archbishop of Cosenza – 30 August 1522 (*ep.* 770, p. 153).

Reports of the siege of Rhodes by Solyman [or Suleiman] the Magnificent; Spanish siege of the French Bayonne; further reference to the rebellion of the *Comuneros*: execution of seven leaders at Medina de Campo, and of Pedro Maldonado in the stronghold of Simancas, responsible for having helped the rebels; arrival of emperor Charles V at Valladolid; Ferdinand Magellan dispatched with five ships to the new lands; death of Magellan by the hand of the natives; return of the ship *Victoria* with the survivors, after many hardships.

To the Marquises – 4 November 1522 (*ep.* 773, p. 157).

News about Rome stricken by a grave pestilence; Solyman the Magnificent continues the siege of Rhodes; new clashes between French and Spaniards at Fuentarrabía; Spain's renewed claims to the islands of the spices after Magellan's trip; contrasts with the Portuguese; reference to the *raya* drawn up by Alexander VI; new reference to the return of the ship *Victoria* of the fleet of Magellan; reference to the writing of the fourth *Decade*.

To the Archbishop of Cosenza – 19 November 1522 (*ep.* 774, p. 159).

Edict of Emperor Charles V on the popular uprisings: pardon for the populace and punishment for the leaders, the best known of whom are named; after the death of Emanuele, king of Portugal, Luis Fernandez de Cordoba, count of Cabra, don Alonso Manrique, bishop of Cordoba, and the lawyer Doctor Cabrera are sent to escort back to Spain Eleanor, widow of Emanuele, sister of Charles V; John III of Portugal, who succeeded his father Emanuele, receives only doctor Cabrera; landing of three ships of Hernán Cortés in the Cassiteridi islands (Azores); mention of the treasures of the new lands and of the ventures of the pirate Florin; Juan de Ribera, secretary to Cortés, brings gifts for the Emperor, including a cage with tigers; lack of safety in the ocean because of the presence of pirates; reference to fuller reports in the *Decades*.

To the Archbishop of Cosenza – 11 June 1523 (*ep.* 782, p. 163).

News of the death of the ambassador of Venice Gerolamo Adorno, brother of the doge Antonio; appointment in his place of Cardinal Marino

Caracciolo; conflicts between Spanish soldiers on their way to Perpignan and Belgian officers, resolved by the Emperor in order to avoid worse consequences; pirate Florin renewed attacks on Cortés's ships which bring gifts for the Emperor; description of the goods coming from the treasure of Montezuma, signs of an advanced culture; Henry II of Albret, backed by Francis I of France, does not allow the soldiers of emperor Charles V, on their way to France, to pass through his territory (French, or southern Navarre, that Ferdinand the Catholic had left him after having taken his lands).

To Adrian VI – 13 August 1523 (*ep.* 786, p. 167).

The deanery of Ocaña is granted to Peter Martyr; acknowledgment of the services of Peter Martyr to the Crown during the rebellion of the *Comuneros*; the Pope's encouragement to continue writing the *Decades*; mention of the city of Tenustitán [Teotihuacan]; reference to the position of eminence of Giovanni Ruffo, archbishop of Cosenza.

To the Archbishop of Cosenza – 7 October 1523 (*ep.* 791, p. 169).

Mention of the goods coming from Hispaniola, Cuba and Jamaica; unsuccessful attempt by the grand constable Charles de Bourbon to enter in the city of Fuentarrabía by cunning; occupation of the port of San Sebastián; unsuccessful attempt to besiege Bayonne from the sea; pillage of the city of Capbreton; the writer's reflections on the vicissitudes of fate.

To the Archbishop of Cosenza – 20 June 1524 (*ep.* 801, p. 173).

Letters of Gil Gonzáles from the new lands; Francisco de Garay, governor of Jamaica, wants to found a colony on the Panuco river, against the will of Cortés, conqueror of Mexico; the decision to prepare a new fleet to travel the same route of the ship *Victoria* is postponed by emperor Charles V by request of John III of Portugal who claims those territories for himself; arguments between Castilians and Portuguese in the bordering city of Badajoz; reference to the *raya* drawn up Alexander VI; marriage between Henry III, count of Nassau, who had taken the place of Chièvres at the court, with Mencia de Mendoza; news of a flood in Spain; the French cause troubles along the coasts of Galicia.

To the Archbishop of Cosenza – 3 August 1524 (*ep.* 804, p. 177).

Reference to the ill health of the Emperor; dispatching to the new lands of Estevão Gomes (a Portuguese who participated in the expedition of Magellan only to abandon it and return to Spain); preparation of a fleet for the Moluccas [or Spice Islands]; personal vicissitudes of doctor Vargas; the Germans in Rossiglione; deferential words of Peter Martyr for the Emperor; appointment of the writer as abbot of Jamaica; description of the climate of the island of Jamaica; promises of the writer to tender complete revenues; contrasts between the count of Potenza and Fernando Francisco d' Avalos, marquis of Pescara, at a difficult time for Charles V, engaged against the French who had invaded Rossiglione; renewal of the members on the Council of the Indies: don García de Loaysa, confessor of Charles V, is appointed president; attack of the French pirate Florin on a Portuguese ship returning from the Indies; news of the decision to have Catherine of Hapsburg, sister of Charles V, marry John III of Portugal.

To the Archbishop of Cosenza – 18 November 1524 (*ep.* 806, p. 181).

Recollection of the loving exchange of words between Juana the Mad and her daughter Catherine, promised in marriage to John III of Portugal; reports from the Council of Hispaniola: landing in Cuba of Cristóbal de Olid, entrusted by Cortés with traveling along the coast of Figueras and founding a colony; dispatch of troops by Pedro Arias into the same territory; death of Francisco de Garay at the hands of Cortés, denounced by Olid; death of some bishops, among them Alessandro Geraldini, at Hispaniola; a fleet, on its way to the new lands, having sailed from Sanlúcar de Barrameda, at the mouth of the Guadalquivir, is damaged by a storm, returns and then departs again; reports on the illness of Charles V, who is treated by a Neapolitan masseur with a special ointment; attack of French pirates, who have traveled up the river (Nervión) to Bilbao on a ship built by Jacobo de Vera, headed toward the markets in Belgium.

To the Archbishop of Cosenza – 22 February 1525 (*ep.* 809 p. 187).

Odet de Foix, viscount of Lautrec, in the service of Francis I of France, is summoned by his king; return of three ships from Hispaniola; death of Diego Velázquez, governor of Cuba; death of Francisco de Garay at the hands of Cortés; Peter Martyr's observations on the freedom to be granted to the Indians.

To the Archbishop of Cosenza – 4 March 1525 (*ep.* 812, p. 189).

Ships loaded with treasures coming from New Spain, sent by Cortés, land in the Cassiteridi islands (Azores); dispatch of Rodrigo d'Albornoz as constable, together with Lopique, the writer's pupil; news about the transfer of prelates and of the distribution of assignments.

To the Archbishop of Cosenza – 13 June 1525 (*ep.* 814, p. 191).

Departure of a fleet for the island of Jamaica; description of the island; reference to the *Decades* for more detailed information; founding of two colonies in Jamaica; decision to build a stone church in Seville, Jamaica; dispatch of Juan de Mendigorría as treasurer in Jamaica; clash between Hernán Cortés and Cristóbal de Olid; other admirals head toward the same territories; mention of a possible marriage between Henry VIII, king of England, and a French princess, wished for by the English minister Wolsey, after the repudiation of Catherine of Aragon; news of the death of John of Grandeburg, governor of Valencia, husband of Germana de Foix, former wife of Ferdinand the Catholic; pressure on the part of the *Cortes* to have Charles V marry Catherine of Portugal (or is it rather Isabella of Portugal, daughter of Emanuele?), despite the opposition of the king of Portugal and the king of France; reference to the VII Decade, dedicated to Francesco Maria Sforza, duke of Milan, and taken to the duke by the ambassador Camillo Gillino; resentment of Arborio of Gattinara toward the Emperor.

TEXT AND TRANSLATION

Ioanni Borromeo, aurato equiti

     Si forte quicquam ad vos fama de percusso Rege meo detulerit, ne fallamini, scitote non malivolentia, non invidia potentis cuiuspiam, non ut se quisquam ab iniuria Regibus peculiari nota exolveret, facinus accidisse; iniuriam nanque nulli
5 viventium unquam mei Reges, praeterquam Iudaeis aut Sarracenis, intulisse reperiuntur. Sunt quippe iustissimi, integerrimi, religiosissimi, rectores, non tyranni. Furore ductus tartareo, vesanus quidam, humilis opilio, id patravit. Vivit tamen Rex, evasit apud infernos manes extructum scelus illud. Post paucos
10 inde dies, rediit ab antipodibus occiduis Christophorus quidam Colonus, vir ligur, qui a meis Regibus ad hanc provinciam tria vix impetraverat navigia, quia fabulosa quae dicebat arbitrabantur; rediit, preciosarum multarum rerum, sed auri praecipue, quae suapte natura regiones illae generant, argumenta tulit. Sed
15 aliena omittamus, Comes egregie, omittamus. In Italiam vocantur Galli: quibus colubris agitamini, miselli homines![1] Sentio te domumque tuam a Ludovico dissentire, sed prodesse parum. Stupet nanque iam Ludovicus, amore regni pellectus, nec demersus ebullit ultra. Ex Hispania haec fervent. Ut in
20 Italiam Gallus traducere queat liber exercitum, foedus parat inire cum meis Regibus, quaecunque volunt illis impartiens. Pacem et cum regibus Romanorum et Britanniae Maioris, qui ambo in Gallicos fines armati irruperunt, eadem ratione quaeritant. Veh tibi Italia, bonarum attium genitrix et disciplinae
25 militaris magistra! Si vires tuas cum Gallo commiscueris, si Gallum in tua viscera admiseris, peribis misera, universam dabunt in praedam. Proclamate omnes, rumpite vocibus ilia[2] in immissores. Quodvis malum potius inter vos sustinete, infoelices, quam in errorem tantum praecipites cadere velitis. In
30 Gallia qui Perpinianum et Rosilionis comitatum dedent oratores, iam parantur; assentiri videntur mei Reges. Caeteti collegae, in Galli potentiam coniurati, meorum Regum (ut arbitror)

---

   * See Abbreviations in the note to the text.
   [1] See Cic. *ad Att.* III, 23,5; *ad fam.* XIV 4, 3.
   [2] See Verg. *buc.* VII 26.

To John Borromeo, Knight of the Golden Ram

So that you may not be mistaken, in case rumor has related to you something about the violence suffered by my King, know that what happened is not due to ill-will, not to the envy of some mighty one, not to vengeance by someone for a particular wrong known to my Sovereigns; in fact it appears that my Sovereigns have never done harm to any living person, with the exception of the Jews and the Saracens. Indeed, these rulers are very fair, very upright, and highly religious; they are not tyrants. A madman, driven by a hellish rage, a poor shepherd committed that crime. However, the King is alive; he has escaped this wicked deed devised among the infernal spirits. A few days ago there came back from the western antipodes a certain Christopher Columbus, a Ligurian, who had with difficulty ob- <
tained three vessels for that mission from my Sovereigns, because they thought that what he was saying was full of fantasy; he came back and brought evidence of many precious things, but especially of gold, which these regions yield spontaneously. But let us leave out subjects which do not concern us directly, dear Count, let us leave them out! The Frenchmen are called in to Italy: poor men, how you are afflicted by these snakes! I understand that you and your family are not in agreement with Ludovico, but that helps very little. In fact, Ludovico is by now dulled, seduced by the craving for a kingdom and, overwhelmed, cannot get himself out of it. From Spain we have news of these turmoils. The King of France, in order to be able to transfer with ease the army to Italy, is readying to make an agreement with my Sovereigns, giving them anything they wish. For the same reason they insistently beg for peace, even with the King of the Romans and with the King of Great Britain, both of whom have broken into the French territory fully armed. Woe to you, Italy, mother of fine arts and teacher of military discipline! Were you to mix your forces with the Frenchmen, or accept such Frenchmen in your territory, you will perish, wretched; they will overwhelmingly reduce you to spoils. Cry out, all of you; with your voices hurl yourselves against those who let them in! Among yourselves, unfortunate ones, bear whatever ill rather than voluntarily fall headlong into such a ter-

iudicium sequentur, foedusque una cum Gallo iacturos esse
arbitramur. Haec omnia ut vos liberius a lupis rapacibus, quos,
35 miserae oves, in caulam, ut vos a catellis tueantur, immittitis,
deglutiamini. Vestra res agitur. Eo minore ego dolore conficiar,
quo minus angit aurium sonus, quam oculorum prospectus.
Vale! Cleofae uxori tuae et utriusque natis, meo nomine, salutes
impartitor.

Barchinonae, pridie Idus Maii .M.CCCC.XCIII.

ep. 134 *C* = 133 *A* = 132 *ms.*   *p.* 361 *G*

Comiti Tendillae et Archiepiscopo Granatensi

Attollite mentem sapientissimi duo senescentes, audite novum inventum! Meministis Colonum Ligurem, institisse in
castris apud Reges de percurrendo per occiduos antipodes,
novo terrarum hemispherio; meminisse oportet, quia de re
5 vobiscum aliquando actum est, nec sine vestro, ut arbitror,
consilio rem hic aggressus est. Is rediit incolumis, mira se
reperisse praedicat, aurum aurifodinarum in eis regionibus argumentum ostentat, gossampium[3] aromataque, tum oblonga,
tum teretia, Caucaseo pipere acutiora, detulit, quae simul et
10 coccineas arbores suapte natura tellus parit. Occidentem secutus, a Gadibus milia passuum, uti praedicat, quinque milia, in
plures incidit insulas. Inter eas unam captavit, quam maioris
esse ambitus quam Hispania universa asseverat. Homines reperit
natura contentos, nudos, cibis depastos nativis et pane radicali,

---

[3] From Lat. *gossypium* (See Landino 264: «Trees similar to the cotton tree and
more aromatic than linden [basswood or tulip trees]; but smaller... Jubas writes that
they produce a downy beard used to make linen [flax] cloth»).

36

rible mistake! Ready in France, are now the ambassadors who will hand over Perpignan and the county of Rossiglione; my Sovereigns seem to be in agreement. All the other allies, even if in league against the power of the King of France, will follow (as I think) the opinion of my Sovereigns, and we believe they will form an alliance with the King of France. All these things are happening so that you may be more easily swallowed up by greedy wolves, whom you, miserable sheep, welcome into the fold in order to be protected from puppy dogs. Your welfare is at stake. I will be afflicted by a sorrow as much less in intensity as the hearing of the ears is compared to the sight of the eyes.* Take care. Give my regards to your wife Cleofe and to your children.

Barcelona, 14 May 1493

To the Count of Tendilla and the Archbishop of Granada
(Iñigo López de Mendoza – Hernando de Talavera)

Pay heed, you two who are now elders and very wise; < hear of the new discovery! You will remember that the Ligurian Columbus had put pressure on the Sovereigns, while they were in camp, about a journey to the new hemisphere through the western antipodes; you must remember him, since the topic was sometimes discussed with you, and, not without your support, I believe, did he set about this venture. He has returned safe and sound; claims he has found marvelous things; displays, as evidence, the gold from the mines that are found in those regions; and has brought cotton, spices both long and round in shape and of a fragrance more penetrating than the black pepper of the Caucausus, and those products the earth yields spontaneously, as well as the trees of scarlet color. Having followed the route to the West, he goes on to say, he ran into many islands five thousand Roman miles from Cádiz.

---

* I will suffer much less if I only hear about rather than seeing these evils befall Italy. (Translator's Note)

ex spitamalibus qui-busdam fructetis internodiis plenis, quae
ipsi terra suis contegunt temporibus; ex quorum internodiis
singulis, singuli turgescunt globi, in piri aut cucurbitulae similitudinem. Hos maturos, uti nos rapas et rafanos eruunt, ad
solem siccant, scindunt, terunt in farinam, pinsunt, coquunt,
comedunt. Vocant hos globos *ages*. caetera ex arboribus, ut
plurimum edulia, a nostratibus diversa. Quadrupes nullum insula gignit, praeter immensos lacertos, minime tamen noxios
et cuniculi quoddam parvuli genus, quod nostros mures aemulatur. Reges habet gens haec et alios aliis maiores; fudibus,
arundinibusque adustis praeacutis et arcubus intra se certant.
Viget inter eos, quamvis nudi sint, imperii cupido; uxores
ducunt. Quid colant praeter numen coeli, nondum didicit. Tria
Colono dederatis navigia; in eius insulae littore, illisum super
rupe aquis cooperta, plana, grandius amisit. Cum duobus reliquis minoribus regressus est, octo et triginta viros, qui interea,
dum ipse revertatur ad eos, locorum naturam scrutentur, in
insula reliquit, commendavitque regulo eius provinciae, quam
trivit, nomine *Guadcanarillo*, nudo et illi. Maior paratur classis;
redibit. Quae succedent, per me, si vixero, scietis. Valete!

Barchinonae, Idibus Septembris .M.CCCC.XCIII.

ep. 135 *C* = 134 *A* = 133 *ms.*   *pp.* 361-362 *G*

Ascanio Sfortiae Vicecomiti, cardinali, vicecancellario

Tanta est obsequendi tibi, Princeps illustrissime, mea cupido, ut etiam summis rerum fluctibus implicito, gratum facturum putem, si quae accidunt apud nos tibi significavero. Mira
res: ex eo terrarum orbe, quem sol horarum quattuor et viginti
spatio circuit, ad nostra usque tempora, quod minime te latet,
trita cognitaque dimidia tantum pars, ab Aurea, utpote, Cher-

He landed on one which, he assures us, is wider than all of Spain. He found people contented with nature; naked, they feed on local foods and on a bread of roots drawn from tiny shrubs full of knots, which they cover with earth at the right time; from each of their knots, one by one, swells up a round ball, much like a pear or a gourd. They dig these up when they are ripe, in the same fashion that we pick turnips and radishes; then they dry them in the sun, cut them up, reduce them to flour, crush them and cook them, and finally eat them. They call these round balls *ages*; other fruits from the trees, most of them edible, are different from ours. No four-footed animal is born on the island, except huge lizards, altogether harmless, and a breed of small rabbit which is similar to our mice. These people have kings, some more important than others; they fight among themselves, using slings, spears pointed and ablaze, and bows. The desire for power thrives among them, although they be naked; they marry. He has not yet understood what they worship, besides heaven's deity. You had given Columbus three vessels; on the beach of this island he has lost the larger one, shattered against a flat rock covered by waters. He came back with the two smaller ones; he left thirty-eight men on the island to examine the nature of the region until he returns to them there; and he entrusted them to a man by the name of *Guacanagarí*, who is the chief of a tribe in the territory that he had travelled; he too is naked. A bigger fleet is being readied; he will return. You will know through me what will happen, if I live. Take care.

Barcelona, 13 September 1493

To Cardinal Ascanio Sforza Visconti, Vice Chancellor

The desire to pay my respects to you, most illustrious Prince, is so great that I think I shall please you if I inform you of what happens here, although you are involved in the < most intense of storms. An astonishing event: of that world, around which the sun revolves in the span of twenty-four hours, only half has been travelled and known up to now, that

soneso, ad Gades nostras Hispanas; reliqua vero a cosmographis, pro incognita, relicta est; et si quae mentio facta, ea tenuis
et incerta. Nunc autem, o beatum facinus meorum Regum
10 auspiciis! Quod latuit hactenus a rerum primordio, intelligi
coeptum est. Res sic se habet, adverte, Princeps illustrissime!
Secutus occidentem solem a Gadibus, Christophorus quidam
Colonus, vir Ligur, praebitis illi a meis Regibus tribus navigiis,
perrexit ad antipodes, miliaria supra quinque milia. Tres et
15 triginta continuos dies, coelo tantum contentus et aqua, adnavigant. Terram post haec, e cavea grandioris navis, qua Colonus
ipse vehebatur, speculatores proclamant. Insulas percurrit ab
aequore sex. In ipsarum una, quam Hispania maiorem esse
cuncti, qui sunt illum secuti, rei novitate pellecti, praedicant,
20 in terram descendit; ibi, dies aliquot immoratus, aurum, gossampium, aromata, oblonga, in cinnami formam et in piperis
teretia, arbores coccineas, succinum, colorem glaucum, multa-
rumque rerum apud nos preciosarum copiam, terram illam
suapte natura gignere comperit. Ex quacunque re, in argumen-
25 tum tulit tantillum. Reges habet insula plures, sed nudos, et
cum eis omnes utriusque sexus. Quamvis natura contenta, utpote nuda, solisque arborum cibis et radicali quodam pane gens
illa vescitur; imperii tamen est ambitiosa, seseque invicem arcubus et praeacutis adustis sudibus, mutuis bellis ea cupiditate
30 conficiunt, cogiturque victus regulus victori parere, ac si
"meum ac tuum", veluti inter nos, inter eos versaretur lautique
apparatus ac pecuniarum cumuli desiderarentur: qua nanque re
indigere nudos homines putabis! Caetera quae succedent, si
optare ista Galli permittent, significabo. Fertur Carolum regem,
35 dato iam Perpiniano per Episcopum Albigensem, de illustri
Ambasiae familiae genere, accingere se ut ad vos eat. Dii bene
vertant! Vale atque utinam bene!

Barchinonae, Idibus Septembris .M.CCCC.XCIII.

40

is from the Golden Chersonese to our Spanish Cádiz; this fact is hardly unknown to you; the other half was undocumented by cosmographers because unknown or, if mentioned at all, the reference is insignificant and vague. Yet now, what a successful undertaking, under the auspices of my Sovereigns! That which from the beginning of the world up to now lay hidden is beginning to be revealed. This is the situation: note well, most illustrious Prince! After having followed the westerly route from Cádiz, a certain Ligurian named Christopher Columbus, with three vessels that had been given him by my Sovereigns, reached the antipodes more than five thousand miles away. They sailed for thirty-three consecutive days, only surrounded by water and sky. Later, from the topmast platform of the larger vessel, aboard which Columbus himself was traveling, the look-out men yelled: "land!" From the sea he discovers six islands, one after another. He lands on one of those islands, which all those traveling with him, attracted by the newness of the undertaking, declare to be bigger than Spain. During his stay there for several days, he discovers that the land by its own nature makes available gold, cotton, elongated-shape spices like a cinnamon plant stem but round as a pepper and scarlet-colored trees, amber, grey-green in color, as well as an abundance of many products which we consider precious. He brought back samples of each product as evidence. The island has many chieftans, naked, as are all their inhabitants of both sexes. These naked people, demanding no more of nature, live only off the fruits of trees and on a type of bread made from roots; they seem, however, so ambitious for power that they wear each other out in constant wars out of that ambition, using bows and spears pointed and ablaze; the head of the tribe, if defeated, is forced to submit to the conqueror, as if dominance existed among them, as it does for us, and as if they wished to have solemn pomp and an accumulation of riches: you would think that these naked men needed such things! I will let you know of other events, if the Frenchmen will allow us to hope for this. It is said King Charles is getting ready to come to you after having handed over Perpignan through the Bishop of Alby, who is from the illustrious house of the Amboise family. May the gods be on our side! Take care and hope for the best.

Barcelona, 13 September 1493

Archiepiscopo Bracharensi

Consuevi hactenus de una tantum re scribere, tria tibi nunc est animus significare. Colonus quidam occiduos adnavigavit, ad littus usque Indicum (ut ipse credit) antipodes. Insulas reperit plures; has esse de quibus fit apud cosmographos mentio, extra oceanum orientale, adiacentes Indiae arbitrantur. Nec inficior ego penitus, quamvis spherae magnitudo aliter sentire videatur, neque enim desunt qui parvo tractu a finibus Hispanis distare littus Indicum putent. Utcunque fit, magna se reperisse praedicant. Die his quae dicit, signa tulit, maiora se inventurum pollicetur. Nobis satis quòd latens dimidia orbis pars in luce veniat; et Portugalenses in dies magis ac magis aequinoctiali se circulo subiiciunt. Ita ignota hactenus littora, pervia cuncta efficientur propediem, alter nanque, alterius aemulatione, sese laboribus ac periculis exponit ingentibus. Ad caetera veniamus. Carolus, Francorum rex, quom primum vulneratum fuisse Regem meum intellexit, oblatum misit Perpinianum Rosilionisque comitatum, quem Rex petebat, aviti quondam iuris Aragonici; distulit tamen in Septembrem mensem. Quo tempore oratores destinavit plures, primatum inter eos tenet Episcopus Albiensis de illustri familia de Ambasia, qui, sui regis nomine, Perpinianum reddant, dummodo libere provinciam in Alfonsum, Neapolitanum regem, sumere liceat. Hinc atque hinc multa agitantur, pacis tamen foedera instituuntur, ut amici sint utrique alterutri amicis, inimicique inimicis. Die Neapolitano vero rege ut Carolo regnum petere Neapolitanum armis liceat, si iura ipsius potiora esse constiterit; Perpinianum, his compositis, receperunt. Meis Regibus id adnitentibus, Caesar et rex Anglus, caeteri collegae, ab armis in Gallum discedunt. Restat tertium. Carolus, militibus iam instructis, ad Italiam vocatus a miseris obcaecatis armentis, ut lupus a catellorum latratibus inermibus, ipsa tueatur, iter coepit. Vos mihi credite, Caucaseas rupes, in Italiam casuras et Acroceraunia[4] fulgura imminentia fugite;

---

[4] Ancient's Epirus's Acroceraunian cliffs were so denominated because of their frequent storms. They rise opposite Valona.

To the Archbishop of Braga

(Diego de Sousa)

Up to the present I have usually written about a single topic, but now I intend to inform you of three events. A certain Columbus has sailed toward the western antipodes up to the Indian coasts (so he believes). He has found several islands; they seem to be those which the cosmographers make mention of and are located beyond the eastern ocean, near India. And I do not completely disavow it, although the greatness of the globe would seem to suggest otherwise, and in fact there are people who believe that there is little distance between the Indian Coast and the Spanish borders. However it may be, they are claiming publicly to have made great discoveries. He has brought evidence of what he says and promises to make even greater discoveries. For us it is sufficient that the half of the world which lay hidden is coming to light; the Portuguese too get nearer to the equinoctial circle day by day. And so shores, up to now unknown, will all very soon become accessible, for competition drives these people to great hardships and dangers. But now let us go on with other affairs. Charles, king of the Frenchmen, as soon as he found out that my King had been wounded, offered to hand over Perpignan and the county of Rossiglione which my King was seeking, being one time under the jurisdiction of the Aragonese royalty; however, he postponed the decision until the month of September. At that time, he appointed several ambassadors (pre-eminent among then is the Bishop of Alby of the illustrious family of Amboise), so that they might return Perpignan in the name of their king, provided that he be allowed freely to lead forces from the territory against Alfonso, King of Naples. There is much turmoil all over; however, peace agreements are being established so that each may be friendly to the friends of the other and hostile to his enemies. Actually, concerning the King of Naples, they negotiated that Charles be allowed to conquer the kingdom of Naples with arms, if he can show that his claims to it are superior; on these terms they received back Perpignan. Since my Sovereigns agree with this, the Emperor and the King of England and the other rulers do not oppose

43

nec vobis ignoscetur Hispanis, quom vagari solutis habenis,
35 Galli incipient. Roma illis iter est. Romam deserite; si minus
auscultaveritis, poenitebit, quando poenituisse nil proderit.
Vale!

Barchinonae, Kalendis Octobris .M.CCCC.XCIII.

ep. 139 *C* = 138 *A* = 137 *ms.*   *pp.* 363 *G*

Ascanio cardinali Vicecomiti, vicecancellario

Venit ad nos Garsias Cagnas, Alfonsi Cagnas familiaris
tui cubicularis germanus, cum tuis ad me literis; ut regium
habeat chirographum petit, quo possessores templorum Mar-
chienne ac Teve, Ardales extra urbem Hispalensem, in eius
5 diocesi, et Sancti Romani, intra ipsius urbis menia siti, parro-
chiales, et unius de sex praestimonialibus Antecherae, de veteribus possessionibus eiiciantur, quorum titulos pontifex Alexander ad te transmisit, quom eos ipse cardinalis haberet, quia
sic per praetorium, quod *Rota* dicitur, pontificum, datis exe-
10 quutorialibus decretum est. Multi veniunt de re hac conquestus,
graves agitantur querellae, suspiria gemitusque acerrimi: Teve,
Ardales rector sese torquet qui annum octavum et vigesimum
sese redditus illos, nullo perturbante, possedisse ait. Quid hoc
nunc mali emergat se non intelligere proclamat, iure ipso se
15 liberatum ab onere regressus, quo ab Alexandro premebatur
cardinali, quom primum Pontifex effectus est, minimeque fieri
solitum ut per accessum ad pontificatum idem restet super
beneficiis pondus, vocibus curiam obtundit, supraemam esse
dicens feritatem, si de loco, ubi tot annos sacra ministravit,
20 deiiciatur, se non audito praesertim, et si legibus forte contra
se decernentibus de regressu, iustam solverit, ut aiunt, pensio-
nem, tolli minime debere probat. Hic acrius torquetur, quam
caeteri, qui opimiori fruebatur sacculo. Post nanque stratos
Granatenses, qui regiunculam illam incursionibus iacere incul-

44

the King of France. As for my third topic. Charles has begun the march, with soldiers now ready to fight, after being summoned to Italy by miserable blind herds, so that he may defend them like a wolf from the harmless barking of puppy dogs. Trust me, avoid the cliffs of Caucasus and the threatening lightning bolts of Acroceraunia about to fall on Italy; not even you Spaniards will be spared when the unbridled Frenchmen begin to roam. Rome is their destination. Leave Rome; will you not heed, you will be sorry, when regret will be vain. Take care!

Barcelona, 1 October 1493

To Cardinal Ascanio [Sforza] Visconti, Vice Chancellor

García Canãs, brother of Alfonso Canãs, who is your personal chamber-servant, came to us with your letters for me; he asks to receive a document from the King by which those who administer as pastors the churches of Marchena and Teba and Ardales, outside the city of Seville but within its diocese, and of the parish of San Román, inside the city walls, and of one of six chaplaincies of Antequera, be driven out of their old possessions, whose titles Pope Alexander has passed on to you, since he possessed them when he was cardinal, having thus been decreed by executive order of the pontifical tribunal known as the *Rota*. Many complaints come concerning this matter, and loud laments are raised, sighs and deep groans: the rector of Teba and Ardales, who states that he has enjoyed that income now for the twenty-eighth year without anyone bothering him, is distressed. He cries out that he does not understand why this evil comes up now, and deafens the court repeating that he had been freed from the danger of remotion precisely on account of this right, by which he was pressed into service by Cardinal Alexander as soon as he became Pope, and that it is not at all the custom that the tax over the income remains the same with the accession to the papal throne. He maintains that it would be an extreme cruelty if he were thrown out from the place where for many years he had performed the sacred functions, especially without the chance of being

45

25 tam cogebant, adeo coaluit ut redditus ipsius dragmas attinge-
ret, ducatus dicit vulgus, septingentas. Hoc si homini tollatur,
in desperationem incidat oportet. Supplicabo tamen tuo nomine, tu autem qui petis, et illi qui concessuri sunt, si concesse-
rint, literas, humanum ne sit au immane, aequum an araneae
30 tela viderint. Eadem est aliorum querella, licet non precio par.
Bracharensi Archiepiscopo significetur Ioannem, Portugaliae
regem, qui illum et patruum eius cardinalem erexit, interiisse;
magni quippe animi rex erat! Colonus ille, novi orbis repertor,
architalassus (quem Hispani *admiraldum* vocant) maris Indici,
35 ab occidente, a meis Regibus effectus, cum decem et octo
navium classe milleque armatis et opificibus omnifariam, ad
novam urbem condendam, remissus est animaliaque ac sementes
omnis generis secum affert. Valete, si per Gallos ad vos euntes
licuerit!

In Kalendas Novembris, ex curia, .M.CCCC.XCIII.

ep. 141 *C* = 140 *A* = 139 *ms.*   *pp.* 364 *G*

Archiepiscopo Granatensi

Quae de bellico tumultu accidunt ad illustrem nostrum
Comitem scribo; perturbari nanque huiuscemodi cruentis narrationibus sanctum animum tuum, per supernos orbes continue
incedentem, nequaquam licere arbitror. Colonum, ex ea pro-
5 vincia honorifica redeuntem, Admiraldum oceani maris Rex et
Regina, Barchinonae, erexerunt sedereque illum coram ipsis,
quod est (ut nosti) supraemum apud Reges nostros benivolentiae et honoris, ob res praeclare gestas, tributi argumentum
fecerunt. Dehinc classem illi decem et octo navium munitam,

heard; and even if he has paid the proper tax — as it is claimed —, he is of the opinion, should the laws concerning the tax regression chance to judge against him, he should not be removed. He who was enjoying a fatter purse, grieves more than the others. After the inhabitants of Granada, who with their invasions had forced that small territory to lay fallow, were defeated, it had recovered to such an extent that its revenues reached seven hundred drachmas or, as the people say, ducats. If that is taken away from this man, he will necessarily fall to desperation. I will, however, beg in your name; but you, who do the asking, and those who are to yield such documents — if indeed they do — will decide if it be humane or inhumane and fair or a spider's web. Equally goes for the complaint of the others although not equal in worth. It will be reported to the Archbishop of Braga that John, King of Portugal, who has raised him and his paternal uncle to the dignity of cardinal, has died; he truly was a king of great heart! Columbus (whom the Spaniards call *Admiral*), that discoverer of a new world, appointed by my Sovereigns head of the [west] Indian sea, < has been given a new fleet of eighteen ships, a thousand armed men and workers of all kinds to found a new city as well as animals and seeds of all kinds. Fare well, if at all possible with the upcoming French invasion.

From the court, first day of November 1493

To the Archbishop of Granada
(Hernando de Talavera)

I write to our illustrious Count about those events which are occurring in the tumult of war; for I think that it is not at all proper to upset with such bloody reports your holy spirit and constant advancement into heavenly realms. The King and the Queen, in Barcelona, have raised to the position of Admiral of the ocean sea Columbus, upon his returning from that < glorious venture. They had him seated facing them, which is, among our royalty (as you know), the highest sign of friendship and honor, given for valiant undertakings. Hence he was

10 qua regressus est, sunt impartiti. Magna pollicetur se detecturum ad occiduos antarcticosque antipodes. Nil aliud est quod nunc referri possit; propediem Complutum, quod *Alcalá de Henares* dicitur, proficiscemur. Inde recentiores habebitis literas meas, qui propiores eritis nobis.

Ex Valdoleto, pridie Kalendas Februarii .M.CCCC.XCIIII.

ep. 143 *C* = 142 *A* = 141 *ms.*   *pp.* 365 *G*

Ioanni Borromeo, aurato equiti, civi Mediolanensi, comiti lacus Verbani

Decembri mense anni secundi et nonagesimi quadringentesimo supra millesimum, benignissime Comes, triumphatorem Regem meum fuisse ab insano percussum ruricula, oratoresque destinatos a Gallis fuisse, qui nostrum Rosilionis comitatum,
5 in Galliae Narbonensis visceribus situm, dederent, et Gallos de armis in Italiam ferendis cogitare, per mensem tibi, ut arbitror, Februarium sequentem scriptitavi. Nec minus tibi (ni fallor) latentes hactenus antipodes pcr Christophorum Colonum Ligurem fuisse repertos significavi; ab eo die, quo ad te profec-
10 turus esset nuncius, ad hunc usque, qui alterius anni Decembris est vigesimus, nullus occurrit. Accipito igitur brevibus, quae apud nos eo temporis intervallo, gesta sunt: Perpinianum ad veteres dominos Reges meos, per Septembrem anni tertii cum suo comitatu redactum est; foedus cum Carolo rege initum
15 est. De re autem Neapolitana conventum est, ut aiunt: tunc liceat Carolo armis Neapolim repetere, quando potiora constiterit sua esse quam Alfonsi regis iura. Sumpsit nihilominus, Ludovico Sfortia stimulante, provinciam in Alfonsum Carolus. Icti foederis iam meos Reges poenitet nec ut Alfonsus rex,
20 eorum affinis, discerpatur patientur, si poterunt; per oratorem, Carolum monent ut abstineat, donec quid iuris discernatur. Pergit tamen Carolus, apertius ista, quam nos cernitis; a vobis igitur ista nos expectamus. Nos autem impraesentiarum duplices excitamus hymeneos. Unicum habet Maximilianus, Romanorum
25 rex, marem filium Philippum, unicum et mei Reges, Ioannem;

48

given a fortified fleet of eighteen ships with which he went back. He promises to make great discoveries around the Western and Antarctic antipodes. There is nothing else to report now; we will leave soon for *Complutum*, which is called *Alcalá de Henares*. From there you will receive more up-to-date letters from me, since you will be closer to us.

Valladolid, 31 January 1494

To John (Giovanni) Borromeo, Knight of the Golden Ram, Citizen of Milan, Count of lake Verbano

I wrote to you, very kind Count, the following [1493] February, I believe, to tell you that in the month of December of 1492 my triumphant King was struck by an insane peasant and that ambassadors had been dispatched by the French to hand over our County of Rossiglione, located in the heart of Narbonese Gaul, and that the Frenchmen were considering taking up arms into Italy. No less have I informed you, if I am not mistaken, that the antipodes, up to this time unknown, have been discovered, thanks to the Ligurian Christopher Columbus; from that day on, since the messenger set < out to come to you, up to today, the twentieth of December of the following year, no courier has presented himself. Therefore, hear briefly what went on here during that span of time: Perpignan has been given back with its county to its previous lords, my Sovereigns, during the month of September, 1493; an agreement has been entered into with King Charles. Concerning the Neapolitan question, on the other hand, here is the understanding as it is reported: Charles is to be allowed to take back Naples with arms, only when he will have shown that his rights are better than those of King Alfonso. Nevertheless, Charles, upon the urging of Ludovico Sforza, has taken up the governance of the provincial territory against Alfonso. My Sovereigns already regret the agreement reached and, if they will be able to, will not allow King Alfonso, their relative, to be ruined; through an ambassador, they warn Charles to

nubiles uterque filias alterne filiis despondent. Ita vinculo adnectuntur invicem duplici. Mira in dies magis ac magis ab orbe novo, per Colonum eum Ligurem Praefectum maritimum, ob res bene gestas a meis Regibus effectum, afferuntur. Auri copia
30 ingens in terrae superficie reperitur. Percurrisse inquit se, ab *Hispaniola* rotati orbis ad occidentem tantum terrae, ut Auream fere Chersonesum ab oriente cogniti orbis termini ultimi attigerit; duas tantum horas de quattuor et viginti, quibus sol ambiens perlabitur, universum se putat reliquisse. Homines
35 reperit humana carne depastos (*Canibales* vocat vicinia eorum) et hos nudos veluti universa est gens illa. Libros coepi de tantae rei invento perscribere. Si dabitur vivere, nil memoratu dignum praetermittam; qualescunque decussi evadent, illorum ad te mittetur exemplar. Praebebo saltem viris doctis, magna scribere
40 aggredientibus ingens ac novum materiae pelagus. Valete!

Ex oppido Compluto in Oretania, quod dicitur *Alcalá*, .xiii. Kalendas Novembris .M.CCCC.XCIIII.

ep. 145 *C* = 144 *A* = 143 *ms.*   *pp.* 366 *G*

Bracharensi et Pampilonensi Antistitibus

Quae in Italia gerantur, vos aptius (quia factis propiores) assequimini. A nobis haec habetote. Antonius Fonseca vir equestris ordinis et armis clarus, ad Carolum destinatus est orator, qui eum moneat ne, priusquam de iure inter ipsum et Alfonsum
5 regem Neapolitanum decernatur, ulterius procedat. Fert in mandatis Antonius Fonseca ut Carolo capitulum id sonans ostendat,

50

abstain, until his rights are determined. Nevertheless, Charles goes forward; you see these things more clearly than we do; therefore we wait to hear from you. At this time we encourage a double wedding. Maximilian, King of the Romans, has an only male son, Philip, and my Sovereigns also have an only child, John; they both promise their unmarried daughters to each other's son. In this way they are bound to each other by a double bond. Each day more and more extraordinary news is brought from the new world, thanks to that Ligurian Columbus, made Admiral by my Sovereigns for his successful < undertakings. A great quantity of gold is found on the surface of that land. He claims to have covered so great a distance by traveling from *Hispaniola* in a westerly direction of the revolving earth, that he has almost touched the Golden Chersonese, the last boundary of the world known to the east; he believes the only land left to cross are those countries which the sun lights up during the last two hours of its revolution. He finds people who eat human flesh (their neighbors call them *Cannibals*) and who are also naked, the way everyone else is there. I have begun to write books on this discovery, which is of such great importance. Were I to live long enough, I will not leave out anything worthy of note; a copy will be sent to you of any book that, once drafted, will come out. I will offer, at least to learned men preparing to write about important subjects, a great and new sea of material. Fare well.

From the city of *Complutum* in Oretania, which is called Alcalá, 20 October 1494

To the archbishops of Braga and Pamplona
(Diego De Sousa – Alonso Carrillo)

You (being nearer to the facts) understand better what is happening in Italy. From us, learn this. Antonio de Fonseca, a knight famous also for his ability in arms, has been dispatched as an ambassador to Charles, so that he may warn him not to proceed any further before a decision is reached on his legal claims and Alfonso's, King of Naples. Fonseca is

antequam ipsius oculos (si detractaverit) pacti veteris chirographum laceret, atque indicat inimicitias. Instruitur et in statione Malacensi classis, qua militum quidam numerus, Gonsalo
10 Fernando Aquilario, Cordubensi duce, Neapolim transportetur. Parte alia, quod forte nondum attigit vestras aures: nostri Reges, per Ioannem Emanuelem, Ianuenses, per Alfonsum a Silva, Ludovicum Sfortiam, in Carolum, ni provinciam deserat, concitare nituntur. Periculum imminens utrisque opponunt:
15 si Carolus Neapolitanum regnum possederit, reliquum se usurpaturum facile ostendunt; Venetis, quoque, ut suis et ipsi rebus consulant suadere faciunt, quid a victoribus Gallis possint expectare animadvertant; itidem et Alexandro Pontifici Summo, Hispano viro, dici imperant. Dum ista Mars ventilat, ex Ger-
20 mania per tabellarios allatum est prope conclusum esse ut Margaritam, unicam Maximiliani filiam, Ioanni nostro principi, tot regnorum haeredi, Maximilianus ipse despondeat dedentque illi mei Reges in nurum Ioannam ex quattuor quas habent filias, secundam. De nuper autem ab occidente hemispherii antipodum
25 rebus repertis haec audite. Idem Colonus Praefectus maritimus cum decem et octo navium classe, ut in ea insula, *Hispaniola* ab ipso vocitata, ubi pedem fixerat, civitatem condere studeret, missus est, caeteraque ut ulteriora littora percurreret, classis partem maiorem remisit. Mira referuntur. Haec ut conscribam
30 nuncii celeritas non patitur, nec iam sapida fore arbitror, quia non recentia: Methymnae nanque agebamus, cum ea classis advecta est. Quid novi aliud referam, non occurrit. Ascanio, meo nomine, si divertere a Gallis, qui eius ad Italiae perniciem implicant animum, aliquando licuerit, ista dicetis, quandoqui-
35 dem estis illi familiares. Et valete!

Compluti, pridie Kalendas Novembris .M.CCCC.XCIIII.

52

charged with showing Charles the contents of that chapter, before tearing up in front of his eyes (if he refuses) the original document of the old agreement, before charles declares war. A fleet is also being prepared in the port of Malaga, with which a certain number of soldiers, under the command of Gonzales Fernández de Aguilar, of Cordoba, will be transported to Naples. About another topic, news of which perhaps has not yet reached your ears: our Sovereigns are trying to stir up against Charles, if he does not leave the territory, the Genoese through João Emanuele and Ludovico Sforza through Alfonso de Silva. They describe to both of them the impending danger: if Charles takes possession of the kingdom of Naples, it shows how easily he will usurp the rest; they also convince the Venetians to protect their goods themselves, and to consider what they could expect from the victorious Frenchmen; similarly they give orders that the Supreme Pontiff Alexander, a Spaniard, be informed. While Mars ventilates these matters, through couriers news was brought from Germany that an agreement had almost been reached that Maximilian promises in marriage Marguerite, his only daughter, to our Prince John, heir to many kingdoms, and that my Sovereigns would give him, as daughter-in-law, Juana, their second daughter of four. Listen also to this news about the latest discoveries West of the hemisphere's antipodes. Admiral Columbus himself has been sent with a fleet of eighteen ships to seek to found a city on that < island, called by him *Hispaniola*, where he had set foot, and he has sent back the major part of the fleet in order to explore other shores farther away. Other marvelous things are related as well. The haste of the messenger does not allow me to write down all these things; besides, I do not think they will now be as delightful, since they are no longer recent: in fact we were in Medina when that fleet arrived. Nothing else new to report occurs to me. You will relate this to Ascanio on my behalf, since you are his close friends, in case it would ever be possible to distance him from the Frenchmen, who profoundly influence his thinking, to the detriment of Italy. Fare well!

Alcalá de Henares, 31 October 1494

Pomponio Laeto, viro insigni, amico

    Mirari te dicis, Pomponi, quod in tanta Italia e pertur-
batione neminem videas quem Italiae, pro Italia, tanquam
patria cadente, misereat. Quo tempore bonis ac fortibus viris
quondam imperii dignitatem et rerum rei publicae gloriam
5 Roma deserebat, haudquaquam satis multi cives boni ac for-
tes reperiebantur, qui vero dissidiis studerent, ad rei publicae perniciem tenderent illamque vexarent, violarent, pertur-
barent evertereque conarentur, innumeri. Quid miraberis igitur hac nostra, Sirio Cane infecta, tempestate, qua nullus
10 non tyrannus Italas regat habenas, si rabidis videas affectibus, spumas ad interitum mandere rabidos homines, alios in
dammas excitando molossos, alios dissimulando formidine
percussos, vertere terga, alios sibi, non rei publicae Italae
consulendo? Nulla vis animi iam, nulla maiorum ad liberta-
15 tem tuendam Italiamque ab exteris conservandam cura, nulla
fortitudo, caeci omnes, nemine excepto, suum dedecus, suam
ruinam, non vident, aut si conspiciunt, suum tamen patiuntur incommodum aequo animo, dum vicinorum prius animas
perturbent, prostrent, suffocent. Inter has Italiae procellas
20 magis in dies ac magis, alas protendit Hispania, imperium
auget, gloriam nomenque suum ad antipodes porriget.
A Bracharensi et Pampilonensi Praesulibus quaerito quae ad
illos, de nuper altero ab occidente hemispherio reperto, scripserim, tuque illis haec super addita referto, quom eos ha-
25 beas, quia sunt amatores bonarum artium, in amicorum numero. Ex navibus decem et octo, quas a meis Regibus ipsi
Colono (*Almirante*, ut aiunt Hispani) Praefecto maritimo da-
tas, ad secundam navigationem, ad eos memini me scripsisse, duodecim rediere. Suapte natura referunt, qui ab eo hac-
30 tenus orbe latenti redeunt, tellurem illam, coccineas, ingentes
silvas, gossampium atque alia multa apud nos preciosa enutrire, sed, praeter caetera, non parvam auri copiam. Proh
mirum, Pomponi! In terrae superficie globos reperiunt au-
reos, rudes, nativos, tanti ponderis ut pudeat fateri. Uncia-
35 rum ducentarum quinquaginta nonnullos reperere, multo
maiores se reperturos sperant, uti nostris insinuant nutibus
incolae, quom noverint nostros aurum magnifacere. Nec fuisse

54

To my Distinguished Friend Pomponius Letus

Pomponius, during such a confusing time for Italy, you express your amazement in seeing no one, who has pity on Italy, for Italy as a country in ruins. In past times, when Rome reserved the dignity of office and the glory of public affairs to capable and valiant men, there could not be found sufficient numbers of citizens capable and valiant whereas countless indeed were those who favored disagreements, aimed at the destruction of the state trough attacks, damages, disturbances, and attempts to overturn it. Why, then, are you so puzzled at our times, that, under the sinister influence of the Dog-star Sirius, show Italy to be esclusively in tyrants' hands [?]; do you not see savage men driven by unrestrained feelings froth at their mouth to the point of destruction, either turning their backs, enraging their molossine hounds against fallow deer, or pretending not to be struck by fear when they are controlled by it and, finally, those merely concerned with their own wellbeing and none for the condition of Italy? There is no inner strength left, no concern about defending the freedom of the ancestors and keeping Italy from foreign hands, no courage; everyone, without exception, is blinded; they do not see their disgrace, their ruin, or, if they do, they nevertheless bear their own calamities with resignation, witnessing first the degrading and then the destruction and suffocation of their neighbors. In the midst of such troubling events — ever increasing in Italy —, Spain stretches its wings, enlarges its possessions and extends its glory and its name to the antipodes. Ask the Arch- < bishops of Braga and Pamplona for the news I have written them concerning the other hemisphere, recently discovered to the west, and report these additional items to them, since, being admirers of the beautiful arts, you hold their friendship. Of the eighteen ships given by my Sovereigns to the Admiral Columbus himself (*Almirante*, as the Spaniards call him) for a second trip, twelve have returned, from what I remember writing. Those who come back from that world, hitherto uncharted, relate that the land produces spontaneously huge scarlet-colored forests, cotton and many other things we regard as precious, and, above everything else, an abundance of gold.

Lestrigones[5] vel Poliphemos, humanis carnibus depastos, dubites adverte et cave ne, horrore, tibi insurgant aristae.[6] Quom
40 ex Fortunatis (quas volunt aliqui *Canarias*) movetur ad *Hispaniolam* (hoc nanque nomine insulam, in qua pedem figunt, appellant) proras aliquantulum si verterint ad meridiem, in insulas inciditur innumeras, ferorum hominum, quos vocant *Canibales* sive *Caribes*. Hi, quamvis nudi, bellatores sunt egregii,
45 arcubus et clava maxime valent, lintres habent uniligneos, multicapaces (*canoas* vocant), quibus ad vicinas insulas mitium hominum, traiiciunt turmatim. Pagos incolarum adoriuntur; quos capiunt homines, comedunt recentes; pueros castrant, uti nos pullos, grandiores pinguioresque effectos iugulant, comedun-
50 tque. Argumento nostris id fuit: quod, applicantibus se navigiis, insolita mole navium territi, domos Canibales deseruere, ad montanaque ac densa nemora profugere, ingressi domos Canibalium, nostri, quas habent ex trabibus erectis constructas, sphericas, appensas trabibus sale concoctas hominum pernas,
55 ut nos suillas solemus, et nuper occisi iuvenis caput, adhuc sanguine aspersum, atque in ollis elixandas, anserinis et psittacinis permixtas, eius iuvenis partes et verubus assandas, igni appositas, alias reperere. Una navi Canibalicam reginam, comitatam filio sexque aliis viris, deprehensam venatu redeuntem,
60 apprehenderunt. Ex incolis neminem consequi potuerunt, triginta utriusque sexus tamen ex his, quos veluti in stabulis comedendas vitulas servabant, ad nostros profugere, quos ex vicinis insulis raptaverant. Ab his multa didicere, quae aliquando habebis. Dic Praesulibus istis, meo nomine, salutes Asca-
65 nioque ipsi, si a lachrymando Gallorum commercio invenerint aliquando explicitum, easdem si velint impartiantur. Nescio an Bracharensis, qui Portugalius est, ignoret Ioannem regem Portugaliae obiisse coronatumque fuisse non Georgium, quem Rex voluisset, regis spurium, sed Emanuelem, Regis sororium et
70 eundem alias affinem, Bisei ducem, meis Regibus illi, quia recta ad eum attinebat, faventibus. Huic mei Reges Elisabetham primogenitam et Ioannis, Portugaliae regis, unico filio, qui, equi lapsu, dum in castris Granatensibus sederemus, interiit,

---

[5] Population of giants who ate human flesh, living in Sicily according to some mythologists, or far away in the West according to others. Homer's *Odyssey* recounts Ulisses' landing on their shores during his adventurous return from Troy.

[6] See Pers. III 115.

What a marvel, Pomponius! On the surface of the land they find raw nuggets of gold, in its natural state, so heavy that one would doubt the reports. They have found some of 250 ounces; they hope to find some much bigger, as the natives through gestures, lead our men to expect realizing we value gold highly. Be careful not to doubt they were Laestrigonians or cyclops who fed on human flesh, and take care not to let your hair bristle in horror! When from the Fortunate islands (which some want to call the *Canaries*) one moves toward *Hispaniola* (that is how they call the island on which they landed), by turning the prow a bit to the south, you run across many islands of savage men, whom they call *Cannibals* or *Caribs*. These men, although naked, are excellent fighters, showing great dexterity with the bow and club, have vessels carved from a single piece of wood, quite roomy (they call them canoes), with which they cross over, in groups, to neighboring islands inhabited by gentler men. They attack the villages of the natives, eat the younger men they capture and castrate young boys, like we do chickens, so that, grown bigger and fatter, they can be slaughtered and eaten. The following was proof for our men: when the ships approached them, the Cannibals, frightened by their unusual size, left their houses and took refuge on the mountains, in the thick woods; and our men, having entered their huts built with straight logs and round in shape, found salted human legs, hanging from beams as we are accustomed to do with pigs, and the head of a young man recently killed, still wet with blood, and parts of his body mixed in with goose and boiled parrot meat, ready to be in pots, as well as other parts near the fire ready to be roasted on the spits. They captured the queen of the Cannibals, along with her son and six men, caught by surprise while coming back in a boat from hunting. They could not reach any of the inhabitants; thirty prisoners, however, of both sexes, of those abducted from nearby islands and kept in stables like calves to be eaten, sought refuge with our men. They obtained from them much information which sooner or later you will know. Give my regards to the Prelates which, if they wish, they can share with Ascanio himself, if they ever find him not busy with the deplorable dealings with the Frenchmen. I do not know if the Archbishop of Braga, who is a Portuguese, is unaware that John, King of Portugal, died and that George,

viduam despondere vellent, atque id magis cupit Emanuel, sed
75 ipsa virum se velle alium recusat cognoscere, renuit secundas
nuptias, ad hanc usque diem vinci nequaquam potest. Quae
solebam ad Ascanium, dum liber viveret, ad vos, nunc, alterne
scribam. Vale iam, cave ne quibus, inter istas procellosas cautes,
ictibus concutiare!

Compluti in Oretania, Nonis Decembris .M.CCCC.XCIIII.

ep. 153 C = 152 A = 151 *ms.*   *pp.* 370-371 G

Pomponio Laeto viro insigni doctrina, amico

Prae laetitia prosiliisse te vixque a lachrymis prae gaudio
temperasse, quando literas aspexisti meas, quibus de antipodum
orbe latenti hactenus, te certiorem feci, mi suavissime Pomponi,
insinuasti. Ex tuis ipse literis colligo quid senseris; sensisti
5 autem tantique rem fecisti, quanti virum summa doctrina insi-
gnitum decuit: quis nanque cibus sublimibus prestari potest
ingeniis isto suavior, quod condimentum gratius? A me facio
coniecturam. Beari sentio spiritus meos, quando, accitos allo-
quor prudentes aliquos, ex his qui ab ea redeunt provincia.
10 Implicent animos, pecuniarum cumulis augendis, miseri avari,
libidinibus obscoeni! Nostras nos mentes, postquam Deo pleni
aliquandiu fuerimus, contemplando, huiuscemodi rerum notitia
demulceamus. Habebis ista igitur, Pomponi, modo liceat per
Bracharensem Pampilonensemque meos Praesules, ad quos scri-
15 bere ista soleo, postquam desii ad Ascanium, quem procellis
undique circunseptum variis, animum curis gravibus habere
pessundatum video. Ad rem veniamus. Prima navigatione, Colonus maris Indici Praefectus (dicitur Hispanice *Almirantus*) in
Hispaniola octo et triginta viros, in Guadcanarilli regis et ipsi

his natural son, has not been crowned as the king would have wanted, but that Emanuele, the Duke of Viseu, related to the King on his sister's side and in other ways, was chosen with the support of my Sovereigns, because the crown belonged to him by right. My Sovereigns would want to promise in marriage to him their first-born, Isabella, widow of the only son of John, King of Portugal, who died by falling off his horse while we were in the camp of Granada. This is what Emanuele would like as well, but she refuses a second husband, does not want to meet him, turns down a second marriage, and, up to this day, she cannot be convinced otherwise. Now I will write to you, alternatively, the things which I used to write to Ascanio as long as he was independent. Fare well now and be careful to avoid being struck unexpectedly by any rock in these storms.

Alcalá in Oretania, 5 December 1494

To my Friend Pomponius Letus, a Man of Extraordinary Knowledge

My dearest Pomponius, you have let me know that your heart leapt forth with joy and that you barely kept from crying for gladness, when you saw the letter in which I informed you of the world's antipodes that up to now had remained hidden. From your letters I try to perceive how you felt; you have understood and appreciated the event, as much as was fitting for a man endowed with great learning: indeed, what more delicious nourishment than this could be offered to lofty minds, what condiment more pleasing? I can guess it on my own. I feel my heart rejoice, when, having invited them in, I converse with some learned men of those who have come back from that land with knowledge. Let the miserable greedy ones, be lost in their concern for ever-increasing piles of money and dishonest cravings! We instead delight our minds with the news of such events, after having filled ourselves in contemplation of God for a long time. You may Pomponius, learn more about this, therefore, through my archbishops of Braga and Pamplona, to whom I am used to write about these events since I stopped writing to Ascanio, whom I see surrounded by

20 nudo provincia, reliquerat, qui telluris illius naturam, dum ipse
rediret, explorarent. Hos reperit omnes, quom rediit, trucidatos
et aggeres, quos ad habitaculum illis et tutelam condiderat,
aequatis solo fossis, discerptos combustosque. Guadcanarillus,
qui, nostris adventantibus, profugerat, tandem repertus coac-
25 tusque de viris, in eius custodia relictis, rationem reddere,
Caunaboam, regem montium eundemque potentissimum, ipsius
regnum armis invasisse, quod nostros suscepisset nostrosque,
eo invito, lachrymis etiam obortis,[7] et de Caunaboa conquerens
(uti per signa colligere fas fuerat) trucidasse innuebat. Rem
30 dissimulare Colonus ipse Almirantus satius duxit, ne insularum
animos perturbaret; in alia tempora huius admissi sceleris vin-
dictam statuit differre. Qui rediere cum duodecim illis navibus,
quas supra memoravi, mira de regionis illius ubertate, de spe
reperiendorum operum, de aeris temperie, quamvis sint proximi
35 tropico Cancri (nam aequa est illis fere diei toto anno nox), de
aurea illorum icolarum aetate, de moribus referunt. Urbem
condere Colonus, uti ad me nuper scripsit, nostras sementes
iacere, animalia nutrire nostratia incipit. Quid iam mirabimur,
Saturnos, Cereres et Triptolemos[8] nova inventa hominibus
40 praebuisse? Quid Foenices ut Sidona, ut Tyrum conderent, quid
Tyrios ipsos, ut alias regiones inhabitarent, ad alienas terras
migrasse novasque urbes erexisse, novos populos formasse?
Miratur gens illa tubarum tympanorumque sonitus, machina-
rum stupet tonitruis, equorum gressu, cursu, ornatu, mussitat,
45 haeret ab omni rerum nostratium aspectu, attonita pendet ore
aperto. Ex coelo missam gentem[9] hanc putant, sed tunc pro
diis colere nostros coeperunt, quando captos ex itinere septem
Canibales cum eorum regina (qui eos comedunt) truculentos
ostenderunt, vinctos etiam horrore summo cum pavore vide-
50 bant. Aversa illos facie spectabant. Hispaniola haec insula folii
castaneae formam aemulatur; aiunt e septentrione arcticum
elevari polum gradibus sex et viginti, a meridie vero unum et

---

[7] See Verg. *Aen.* XI 41.

[8] Mythical King of Eleusis [near Athens], a hero tied to the worship of Demeter
[Ceres's daughter] in the Eleusinian mysteries. On account of having been hospitably
received, Demeter — out of gratitude — instructed Triptolemos in the art of agriculture
and presented him with a winged oxen-[snakes]-drawn chariot. He is occasionally found
seated in Hades next to Pluto's infernal judges.

[9] See Liv. X 8, 10; Tib. I 3, 90; Plin. *nat. hist.* XXVI 13.

various storms from all sides and burdened down by heavy worries. And now, let us consider the facts. Columbus, Admiral of the Indian sea (called in Spanish *Almirante*), had left < thirty-eight men in his first stop at Hispaniola, in the territory of chief (*Guaccanarillo*) Guacanagarí — who was naked — so that they would explore the features of that land, until his return. When he returned, he found them all slain and the forts, which he had built for their habitation and defense, destroyed and burned, with the ditch mounds leveled to the ground. Guacanagarí, who had fled upon the arrival of our men, was finally found and forced to give an account of the men left in his charge. He led them to understand, with much complaint and tears, that (*Caunaboa*) Caonabó, king of the mountains and most powerful chief, had invaded his kingdom with arms because he had received our men, and had them slain against Guacanagarí's will (as one could gather from his gesturing). Even Admiral Columbus himself thought it better to ignore the deed so as to not upset the inhabitants of the islands; he decided to postpone to another occasion seeking vengeance for the crime committed. Those who have returned with the twelve ships I mentioned above, tell wonderful things about the fertility of that region, the hope for success and, the climate, although so close to the Tropic of Cancer (in fact for them night is almost as long as day all year round) and about the golden age of those inhabitants and their customs. Columbus did begin to found a city, as he wrote me not too long ago, and to plant our seeds and raise animals from our country. Why should we be astonished that Saturn, Ceres and Triptolemos offered men new resources? [should we wonder] That the Phoenicians, in order to found Sydon and Tyre, and the Tyrians themselves, in order to inhabit other regions, migrated to foreign lands, built new cities and formed new nations? The natives are amazed at the sound of trumpets and kettle-drums; they are astounded by the thunder of war machines, by the stepping and running of the horses and their trappings; they whisper; they stand still and in astonishment, their mouth hanging open, intrigued by every aspect of our possessions. They believe that our people are sent from heaven, but they started to worship them as gods when they saw in Spanish hands seven ferocious Cannibals (those who eat them) captured during the trip with their queen; even seeing the cannibals

61

5

viginti, ab oriente ad occidentem produci inquiunt et elongari
sphericae longitudinis gradus decem novem. A Gadibus, per
55 occiduum, distat gradus, ut aiunt, qui accurate rem dimetiuntur
novem et quadraginta. Haec pauca nunc habeto, habiturus
aliquando plura. Et vale! Scribo ista, non quando accidunt,
sed quando a te de mea evocantur officina.

.iiii. Kalendas Ianuarii .M.CCCC.XCIIII.

ep. 157 C = 156 A = 155 ms.   pp. 373 G

Pomponio Laeto, viro singulari doctrina, amico delecto

Vis, Pomponi mi charissime, ut latius, ut capacioribus tibi
tabellis minuta quaeque de novo orbe recitem; non detrecto
mandata tua, vir insignis, sed eo pedibus in iussa tua. Vis
locorum tractus, vis longitudinis et latitudinis gradus, vis ter-
5 rarum et gentium naturam. De his omnibus, non multis ante
diebus, ad te scripsi, sed, cum (uti video) intercepta fuerit
epistola, aut forte, si portum attigit, cum haec tua ad te dimit-
teretur, nondum tibi fuerat in portu porrecta, brevibus pauca
repetam. Scripsi longitudinem eius esse graduum polarium de-
10 cimum nonum, latitudinem, quanto distare aiunt a Gadibus,
per longitudinem orientalem, gradus quadraginta novem, non
recta tamen penitus ad occidentem: elevatur enim Gaditanis
polus gradus nondum sex et triginta, insularibus vero illis unum
et viginti a meridie, a septentrione vero sex et viginti. Varii
15 tamen de gradibus varia sentiunt, stellae polaris motum errorem
istum arbitror enutrire: sunt nanque qui tollant quique augeant
rationem utranque. Terrae illius natura fortunatur uberrime.
Quantum preciosis rebus abundet scripsi alias. Radicali patriae
illius pane vesci malunt nostri, quam tritico, quod sapidi sit
20 gustus, faciliusque stomacho concoquatur: utrunque sunt experti. Aiunt a nocte toto anno parum discrepare diem, nec
spherae ratio adversatur; nec vigere ibi calores immensos, nec
ulla frigora inquiunt. Id arbitror accidere propter imbres, quos

bound, they showed horror mixed with great fear, their faces with hostile stares. This island of Hispaniola bears the shape of a chestnut leaf; they say the arctic pole is 26° N and 21° S and they also say that from East to West the variance is of 19° of spheric longitude. 49° degrees West is Cádiz, as claimed by those who measure distances accurately. Be satisfied for now with these few things; some day you will learn more. Be well! I write you these things not when they happen but when you request them from my office.

29 December 1494

To Pomponius Letus, a Man of Extraordinary Knowledge and Dearest Friend

My dearest Pomponius, you would like me to tell you more extensively and in longer letters every single detail < about the new world; I obey your wishes, distinguished man and follow your commands. You would like me to tell you about the position of the islands, degrees of longitude and latitude, the nature of the land and of their inhabitants. About all these things I wrote to you not too many days ago, but since (I realize) the letter was intercepted or, if perchance it did arrive, was not yet delivered when your letter was sent off, I will repeat briefly the few things I have said. I have written that its location is 19° longitude in reference to the pole; the latitude is 49°, which it is claimed to be the same distance from Cádiz by longitude to the East, however not in a straight line all the way to the West: in fact, for the inhabitants of Cádiz, the pole is not quite 36° above, whereas for the islanders it is 21° S and 26° N. However, concerning the degrees, there are as many opinions as there are people; I think that the movement of the polestar causes this mistake: in fact there are those who increase and those who decrease such calculation. The nature of that land is prosperous and very fertile. I have written on other occasions of how much that land abounds in precious things. Our men prefer to feed on their root bread rather than eat

aiunt cadere creberrimos; aliter enim, cum sint aequatori pro-
25 ximi, aestuarent acriter. Arbores esse aiunt proceras, altissimas,
herbas in pratis ita densas altasque enutriri, ut pedibus aut equo
nequaquam ad iter illas findere possint; armentaque ibi nostratia
nasci corpulentiora, maioraque multo evadere, propter pinguio-
ra pascua, referuntur. Hortensia sataque reliqua, ad illos allata,
30 mira temporis brevitate, coalescunt: cucurbitae, melones, cucumeres, caeteraque huiuscemodi, a iacto semine, intra diem
sextum et trigesimum, comeduntur, lactucae, rafani, boragines
caeteraque id genus olera, intra quindecimum. Ex vitium sa-
tione, secundo anno se aiunt suaves uvas collegisse; cannas, ex
35 quibus saccarum extorquetur, intra diem vigesimum, prodire
cubitales praedicant. Uterque sexus universa in insula nudus
agit, praeter corruptas mulieres, quae femoralibus quibusdam
gossampinis pudenda tantum contegunt. Suos habet quaeque
provincia reges. Domos habent sphericas, ex diversis trabibus
40 constructas, palmarum foliis, aut quarundam herbarum textura
contextas, a pluvia tutissimas; trabium fixarum terrae, ita coeunt
cuspides, ut castrenses aemulentur papiliones. Ferro carent, ex
fluvialibus quibusdam lapidibus fabrilia formant instrumenta,
lectos habent pensiles gossampinis quibusdam lodicibus ad
45 trabes deductis, funibus lodici alligatis; funes ex gossampio vel
herbis quibusdam sparto tenacioribus contorquent. Vocor ad
curiam disceditque tabellarius. Ignosce, si sum brevis et propterea obscurus. Vale!

Compluti in Oretania, quarto Idus Ianuarii .M.CCCC.XCV.

our wheat bread, because it is tastier and it is more easily digested by the stomach: they have tried both. They say that, throughout the year, the day differs very little from the night and this does not go against the principle of the sphericity of the earth; they state that there is neither unbearable heat nor cold. I believe that this is so because of the rains, which are reported to be very abundant; otherwise there would be an unbearable heat, since they are so close to the equator. They say that the trees there are very high, and the grass in the fields grows so thick and tall that they, when trying to find a passage, cannot cleave it by foot or by horse; and here our cattle are reported to be born much fatter and to grow much bigger, because of richer pastures. The vegetables and other plantings taken over there take root in an unusually short amount of time: gourds, melons, cucumbers, and other similar produce are eaten within thirty-six days from the time of sowing; lettuce, radishes, borage and other greens of this kind, within fifteen. From the planting of vines they say they have picked sweet grapes after a year; they also state that canes, from which sugar is extracted, grow one cubit tall in twenty days. Persons of both sexes are naked throughout the island, with the exception of disgraced women, who cover only their private parts with some cotton cloths. Each province has its own chieftain. Their huts have a round shape and are built with various beams, with palm leaves, or are connected together by webbing threads of grass of some kind, quite rain proof; they lean together the tips of the poles dug in the ground, so as to resemble the tents of military camps. They lack iron, and they shape work tools from some river stones; they have hanging cotton blankets beds hooked to the poles with ropes tied to the blanket; they twist ropes of cotton or of some other grass stronger than esparto. I have been called to the court and the courier is leaving. Forgive me if I am short and therefore unclear. Fare well!

Alcalá in Oretania, 10 January 1495

Archiepiscopo Granatensi

Nolci ad Comitem ista, quae nunc referam, scribere, ne subitus illum dolor conficeret. Accitum collegam tuum, priusquam adventent aliorum literae, quae sunt in itinere, (si illum amas) solator, circumito. Communem esse sortem hanc mo-
5 riendi et necessariam disputato. Aequo animo ferenda, quae suo natura trahit ordine, praedicato. Sapientis esse accommodare se necessitati, suadeto, sed quorsum tendas cave intelligat, donec aperiendi quid velis tempus esse duxeris. Periit patruus eius, Petrus ille Gonsalus, Mendotiae domus splendor et lucida
10 fax, periit, quem universa colebat Hispania, quem exteri etiam principes venerabantur, quem ordo cardineus collegam sibi esse gloriabatur. Haec ad te, mi antistes, sed amaram hanc viciam induxisse tibi nauseam sentio, triticeum aliquid suave expectas. Aequum est, candida columba, aures praebeto! Helisabetha,
15 Regum primogenita, ex haerede regni Portugaliae vidua, quam parentes cupiunt inire nuptias cum Emanuele (post Ioannis regis mortem) Portugaliae rege, recusat. Cedet tamen aliquando, instant nanque iusti parentes. Cum Maximiliano, Romanorum rege, duplice propediem astringemur vinculo: filiam nanque
20 ipsius filio unico dabimus uxorem eiusque unicam nostro principi adiungendam accipiemus. Nollet Gallus, rem disturbare per mille ambitus intendit; tantam nanque potentiam grandi sibi fore periculo, a longe videt, sed frustra laborat: est fere in tuto res. Ex antipodibus in dies, magis ac magis, grandia refe-
25 runtur. Praetermitto de opibus, quae tibi sunt parvae curae. Ad Christianam religionem hominum ventura multa milia speramus, et cum hoc suavi postico margine coenae valeto!

Compluti, propediem hinc discedemus ut Burgos Proficiscamur, xviii Kalendas Februarii .M.CCCC.XCV.

To the Archbishop of Granada
(Hernando de Talavera)

I did not want to write to the Count the news which I am about to report, for fear that a sudden sorrow would strike him. Send for your colleague to stand by and comfort him (if you love him), before the letters of other people, which have been mailed, arrive. Discuss with him how common and basic is this fate of death. Point out that we must bear with resignation what happens in the natural order of events. Persuade him that it is a sign of wisdom to accept the inevitable, but be careful that he not understand what you are driving at, until you feel that the time has come to reveal what you want. His paternal uncle, Pedro Gonzáles, died, the splendor or bright star of the house of Mendoza, he whom all of Spain worshipped, and was respected even by foreign princes and whom the college of cardinals boasted to have as member. I share these things with you, my dear prelate, but I realize that this bitter herb has brought you nausea, whereas you await some baked sweet. Fair enough, innocent beloved; listen! Isabella, first-born of our Sovereigns, widow of the heir of the kingdom of Portugal, refuses to enter into marriage with Emanuele, King of Portugal (after the death of King John), although her parents very much want it. She will, however, eventually yield, because her parents, justly so, insist. Very soon we will be bound together by a double bond with Maximilian, King of the Romans: in fact, we will give our daughter as wife to his only son and we will receive his only daughter in marriage to our prince. The French king would not like this and aims at preventing it with a thousand schemes; for he foresees that such great power will be for him a great danger; but he labors in vain: the matter is practically settled. From the antipodes, each day, more and more < wonderful news is reported. I will omit the reports about the riches, which are of little concern to you. Let us hope that many thousands of people may join the Christian religion, and with this sweet dinner-end, fare well.

Alcalá de Henares, we will leave soon to go to Burgos, 15 January 1495

Bernardino Carvaialo cardinali, ex Placentia Hispana

Rubro te galero Alexander sextus Pontifex Maximus insignivit (uti scribis); aequum nobis visum est, ut iam tandem ex eius manibus tale aliquid prodiret, ut scilicet virum aliquem, ratione dictante, senatui admisceret cardineo, quandoquidem
5 appetitu urgente multos erexit, quos tacebo. Gaudebimus nobis tibique gratulabimur, si eundem servaveris in nos animum, ex alto, quem quom ex nobis unus eras pollicebaris. Velles ut tibi quae accidunt in Hispania significarem: nollem cuiquam iniuriam facere. Ascanio ista quondam et, dum vixit, Arcimboldo,
10 cardinali Mediolanensi, scribebam; cum uterque mihi deesset, morte ita volente alter, alter a seipso, postquam in Italiam Gallos vexit, abdicatus, extorris, stupidus, ad alterius generis heroem Pomponium Laetum, cuius ego literas non minoris facio quam centum fortunae illecebras, et ad Bracharensem
15 Pampilonensemque Antistites, quia, dum essem in curia, discipulos mittebam, quae de antipodibus ferebantur. Illa nunc tibi quae supravenient, donec habere te in curia regia procuratorem aliquem sentiam, scriptitabo, hac lege tamen ut horum nemo praetermittat quin per te, de his quae scripsero, fiat certior.
20 Quae ad illos hactenus scripsi, ab eis exigito; nauseam nanque mihi summam incitat, idem velle repetere. Habe igitur quae subsequentur de his nuper inventis. Caetera, quae surgunt in Hispania, tam parvi sunt momenti, ut nec illa scribere ego velim, nec deceat aures tuas, rumoribus aut inanibus vel pusillis,
25 fatigare. Diversi navium ductores ad diversa alterius hemispherii littora missi sunt. Quae reportabunt, per me, si vixero, intelliges. Quid agitemus, velles (uti scribis) intelligere. Advertito: magnus ille cardinalis Mendotius, qui te caeteris praeposuit apud nostros Reges, ut iste ruber galerus, a Pontifice petendus,
30 tuo capiti imponeretur (uti nosti), mense Ianuario concessit ad Superos. Eo vita functo, Burgos, urbem in Castella Veteri, tetendimus. Franciscum Ximenez, cucullatum ordinis crepidalis, Reginae, ut vulgus, confessorem, ad eam antisteam, ut te scire arbitror, designarunt. Aiunt homines esse virum, si non literis,
35 morum tamen sanctitate egregium; re ipsa, qui sit, nondum intelligo: versatus est enim hactenus parum in cutia, quae mutare solet interiorem hominem. Advenientes a Ludovico Sfortia,

To Cardinal Bernardino de Carvajal, from Placentia Hispana

Pope Alexander VI has conferred on you (as you write) the red hat; it seemed right to us that such a gesture would finally come from his hands, that he should admit a "man" to the College of Cardinals at the behest of reason, especially since he raised many, whom I will not mention, at the prompting of greed. We will be happy for ourselves and will congratulate you, if you, now in a lofty position, will preserve toward us the same spirit that you promised when you were one of us. You would like me to inform you of what is happening in Spain: I would not want to offend anyone. I used to write this news to Ascanio and, as long as he was alive, to Arcimboldi, Cardinal of Milan; when both failed me, the first by natural death and the other by voluntary surrender, being stunned and wandering after bringing the French into Italy, I started to send news coming from the antipodes to Pomponius Letus, a different kind of hero, whose letters I value no less than a hundred unexpected flatteries; and to the Bishops of Braga and Pamplona, because they were my pupils while I was at the court. Now I will write regularly future news to you, as long as I know that you have someone at the royal court who can be your agent but on one condition, that through you none of these men be left uninformed of the things I will write about. Ask them what I have written up to now, for I detest having to repeat the same things. Know then the consequences of these recent discoveries. The other events taking place in Spain are of so little importance that neither do I want to write about nor is it proper to tire your ears with empty and petty gossip. Various captains of ships have been sent to diverse shores of the other hemisphere. You will know from me, if I live, what they will report back. You would like to understand (as you wrote) how we are faring. < Pay attention: that great Cardinal Mendoza, who, in front of our Sovereigns, chose you over others so that the red hat, which must be requested from the pope (as you know), be placed over your head, passed away during the month of January. After his death, we came to Burgos, a city of Old Castile. As I think you know, they have nominated for that prelature Francisco Jiménez, friar of a Mendicant Order, who is known as the confessor of

duce Mediolani, post nepotis interitum, et a Venetis oratores
nostri Reges honorifice susce perunt; dein, ut Galli saevientis
40 cogitatibus occurrant, quoad fieri poterit, in Aragoniam, ad
habendos in illis regnis regi haereditariis conventus, a quibus
pecunias et arma exigant, in Gallos perrexerunt. Hic nunc
agimus; comitia quotidie fatigant Aragonica, ut postmodum
caetetis, Valentinis utpote ac Laletanis, inhaereant. Propediem
45 haec perficientur, bono nanque sunt erga Regem animo. Ad
reliqua properabimus. Urget nanque Gallus ferox et nostros
fines, qua sumus illi in Narbonensi provincia finitimi, per suos
milites perturbare intendit. Tu vale!

Ex Caesareaugusta, .iii. Idus Iunii .M.CCCC.XCV.

ep. 165 *C* = 164 *A* = 163 *ms.*   *p.* 377 *G*

Bernardino, cardinali Hispano generoso

Facturum te participem eorum quae scripsero ad meum
heroem Pomponium Laetum et Bracharensem ac Pampilonen-
sem Antistites, auditores quondam meos, e quorum faucibus
tu, quia potentior es, cibum arripis, fuisti pollicitus; vidisse te
5 scribis quae ad illos missa sunt de orbe novo. Alias igitur oras
atque alia littora percurramus. Ex Hispaniola, quam Admirantus
ipse Colonus, tanti autor inventi, *Ophiram* Salomonis aurifodi-
nam putat, in aliam ad occidentem provinciam traiecit, cuius
initium ab ultimo Hispaniolae angulo tractu distat exiguo:
10 septuaginta nanque milia passuum, inquit, cuneata est haec
regio, quam vocant incolae *Cubam*. Latus meridionale huius
terrae Colonus arripit; ad occidentem septuaginta se continuos
dies naturales per eius terrae littora navigasse ad me scripsit.
Reversus nanque est ad Hispaniolam, ibique pedem fixit, et

70

the Queen. The people say that he is a man distinguished for holiness of life, if not for his learning; in fact I do not yet understand what kind of man he is. Up to now he has been engaged very little at court, which usually changes the human heart. Our Sovereigns have welcomed with honor the ambassadors coming from Ludovico Sforza, duke of Milan, after the death of his nephew, and from the Venetians; then, in order to contrast the plans of the raging French king, as long as it can be done, they went into Aragon to convene an assembly of the *Cortes* inherited by the King, so as to exact from them money and arms to be used against the French. Now here we are, working very hard every day to convince the *Cortes* of Aragon so that hereafter they may show solidarity with the others of Valencia and Catalonia. Soon these matters will be resolved, because they are favorably disposed toward the King. We will hasten to the rest. The fierce Frenchman chases us indeed and aims at disturbing with his soldiers our territories in the province of Narbonne where these borders touch. Be well!

From Saragossa, 11 June 1495

To Bernardine, Generous Spanish Cardinal
(Bernardino De Carvajal)

You have promised that you will share what I wrote with my hero, Pomponius Letus, and with the Archbishops of Braga and Pamplona, once my pupils, from whose mouths you, since you are more powerful, take the food away; you write that you have seen the letters which have been sent to them con- < cerning the new world. Let us cover, therefore, other shores and other coasts. From Hispaniola, which Columbus himself, the author of this great discovery, considers to be *Ophir*, the gold mine of Solomon. He went on to another region West of it, a short distance from the extreme corner of Hispaniola: he says this land, which the inhabitants call *Cuba*, is like a wedge extending for 70 miles. Columbus possession of the south side of this land; he took wrote me that he ha sailed in a westerly direction for seventy straight days along shore of that land.

nuncios ad Reges de suo regressu destinavit. Curvari ad meridiem eius littora terrae plurimum scripsit, ita ut se proximum aliquando reperiret aequinoctio. A laeva innumeras se vidisse insulas narrabat; huius magnae telluris littoribus in mare advertit cadere flumina multiformia, frigida haec, illa calidissima, dulcia plaeraque, alia saporis alterius. In plaerisque piscium ingentem copiam, alibi ulla conchilia, ex quibus uniones abraduntur, invenit; per maria se transisse inquit, testudinibus scuta maioribus fere condensata. Per vadosa lacteque albiora alia perque torrentes inter insularum angustias gurgites, iter se fecisse dicit. Per etiam turbida coenosaque alia praedicat. Per inferiorem nobis terrae ambitum maiorem se ignoti orbis partem percurrisse putat, nec existimat se duas integras ad Auream Chersonesum, orientalis termini metam, oras solares reliquisse. Nosti enim, reverendissime Purpurate, cum doctrinae omne genus optime calleas, pro incognito hactenus fuisse relictum, quicquid a Gadibus nostris ad Auream Chersonesum, per inferius hemispherium trahitur. Hanc ergo terram Admirantus iste se humano generi praebuisse, quia latentem invenerit sua industria suoque labore gloriatur. Indiae Gangetidis continentem eam esse plagam contendit; nec Aristoteles,[10] qui in libro *De coelo et mundo* non longo intervallo distare a littoribus Hispaniae Indiam, Senecaque ac nonnulli ut admirer patiuntur. Falcatis portubus regionem hanc essc fultissimam dicit, et internis grandibus animalibus plenam esse illorum vestigia, quae descendentibus cernere erat, indicabant, in mari vero stantibus, horrendi per noctem auditi mugitus magnam esse plagam testabantur. Per suos interpretes insulares, quorum idioma proximum erat huius terrae idiomatibus, nullo in loco desinere terram didicit: pro ccrto igitur habet esse continentem. Nudos tamen et reperit eos incolas, veluti insulares diximus. Paucis in locis ne moraretur, discursu tantum, ex praecepto Regum, contentus, rediit in Hispaniolam, unde se propediem ad Reges venturum, ut late rationem de inventis reddat, pollicetur. Cum amicis ista meis conferantur. Et vale!

Tortosiae, .v. Idus Augusti .M.CCCC.XCV.

---

[10] See *Dec.* I 1, p. 216.

He then went back to Hispaniola, stopped there and dispatched ambassadors to the Sovereigns to inform them of his return. He wrote that the coasts of that land bend so deeply south that at times he was very close to the equator. He reported to have seen to the left a huge number of islands; he observed that from the coasts of this great land various rivers flow into the sea, some cold, some very hot, most of them with fresh water, others of different taste. In most of them he found an enormous abundance of fish, elsewhere some large pearls-bearing shells. He says that he has crossed turtle-filled seas with the largest shells. He relates that he has journeyed across some shallow waters whiter than milk and across swirling gulfs as he ran the narrows between islands. He claims to have crossed turbid waters and others that were marshy. He thinks that he has traveled through a major part of the unknown world, in the hemisphere below us, and does not think to have been more than two whole hours of sun away from the Golden Chersonese's easternmost limit. You are aware, most reverend Cardinal, being superbly versed in every kind of learning, that up to now the whole territory from our Cádiz to the Golden Chersonese along the lower hemisphere, was neglected because unknown. And so this Admiral now is proud of having offered this land to humankind, because through his industry and effort, he has discovered what had lain hidden. He asserts with confidence that that region is the continent of India of the Ganges; neither Aristotle, who in the book *De Coelo et Mundo* holds that India is only a short distance from the coasts of Spain, nor Seneca or some others allow me to be amazed. He says these territories are much protected by sickle-shaped ports and their hinterland full of huge animals as proven by footprints, visible to those who landed and by horrible bellowing heard at night by those who remained at sea, an indication it was an immense region. He learned through his native interpreters, whose tongue was very much like the languages of this earth, that in no place did the land break off: he holds, then, for certain, that it is a continent. He finds those inhabitants to be also naked, as we have said of the islanders. Satisfied with only brief inspection, being instructed by our Sovereigns not to stay too long in a few places, he went back to Hispaniola, whence he promises to return shortly to Spain in order

Bernardino Carvaialo cardinali

Brevi compendio multa complecti angustoque tibi fasciculo Calidonias stringere silvas[11] intendo. Quae hactenus scripsi
colligito, quae impraesentiarum emergunt, habeto. Ex orbe
novo attulit Admirantus noster Colonus, ab oris quibusdam,
5 quas percurrit, ad meridiem, ad gradum ab aequinoctio sextum,
unionum orientalium serta plaeraque; putat regiones has esse
Cubae contiguas et adhaerentes. Ita quod utraeque sint Indiae
Gangetidis continens ipsum, dies et per haec littora navigavit
plures, nec finem aut termini ullum se vidisse argumentum
10 fatetur. *Pariam* ipse tractum hunc appellari ab incolis dicit,
populis refertissimam; habitatores carnibus conchilium, e quibus
uniones abradunt, cum reliquis cibis vescuntur. Plaerisque in
locis gossampinis femoralibus pudibunda contegunt, alibi cucurbitula includunt, alicubi funiculo praeputium, reducto nervo,
15 ligant, ad mictum tantum aut coitum solvunt; caeterum et ipsi
nudi. Fuit magno nostris argumento terram eam esse continentem, quod animalibus passim nostratibus eorum plena sint
nemora, cervis, utpote apris, et id genus reliquis et ex avibus,
ansetibus, anatibus, pavonibus, sed non versicoloribus. A foe-
20 minis parum discrepare mares aiunt. Sagaces sunt incolae venatores: quodvis animal sagittis facile transfigunt. Spinteribus,
tintinnabulis, calculis vitreis et huiuscemodi artis institoriae
mercibus, uniones alacres permutant, quorum se copiam ingentem collecturos, si reversuros se promiserint, innuebant.
25 Haec latius in libris, quos, de his tantum inventis, scribo; ad
alia nunc deveniamus. Superioribus diebus Dertosiae agebamus,
quom a Maximiliano, Romanorum rege, et Philippo eius filio
Burgundo, Flandriae comite, venerunt oratores, ab utroque in

---

[11] See Plin. *nat. hist.* IV 102; Flor. III 10, 18.

to report extensively to his Sovereigns on the new discoveries. Please communicate this news to my friends. Fare well!

Tortosa, 9 August 1495

To Cardinal Bernardino de Carvajal

I intend to say many things quite succinctly and to enclose for you, in one small bundle, the forests of Caledonia [Scotland]. Think of all the things that I have written you up to now, and focus on those now emerging. Our Admiral Columbus brought from the new world's shores which he traveled Southward, six degrees from the equator, great many necklaces < of oriental pearls; he thinks that these regions are contiguous and border Cuba. And so, since both would be of the same continent as India of the Ganges, he sailed on for many days also along these shores and confesses of not seeing either the end nor any clue of the end of this land. He himself says that this very populous region is called *Paria* by the natives; the inhabitants eat the meat of the shells after the pearls are scraped off, besides other foods. In most places they cover their genitals with cotton thigh-pieces; in some places, they cover them with a small gourd; in others, they tie the flaccid penis's foreskin with a string, only to untie it for urination or sexual intercourse; they, too, are otherwise naked. For our men the following was significant proof that the land is a continent: everywhere the woods were full of native animals, such as deer as well as wild boars and other animals of that kind, and teeming with birds, geese, ducks, peacocks, but not of many colors. They say that males and females thus differ little. These natives are reported to be keen hunters capable of striking easily any animal with arrows. They willingly exchange their pearls for bracelets, bells, glass beads and similar traders' merchandise, promising by gestures to gather a great quantity of pearls, if our men promised to return. These things are more amply explained in the books which I am writing exclusively on these discoveries. And now let us go on to other things. In the last few days came at Tortosa, ambassadors from Maximilian, King

mandatis ferentes ut Ioannam, secundogenitam, ad Philippum
mittamus uxorem accipiamusque Margaritam, unicam Maximiliani filiam et Philippo sororem, Ioanni unico nostrorum Regum mari filio, tot regnorum haeredi, copulandam. Foedera coniugalia iacta sunt, discesserunt oratores. Reges autem comitia, quae Dertosiae pro Laletania, haec est Catalonia, et alterne in Sancto Matthaeo, a Dertosia parum distanti oppido, pro regno Valentino, celebrabantur, dissolvunt. Alfarum oppidum, in Castellae finibus situm, Navarrae, quae partim Vasconia, partim Cantabria est, finitimum, adeunt. Ibi, qualiter decuit, Navarrae reginam, ad Reges nostros adventantem, suscipiunt (in huius reginae dotem Navarrae regnum cedit). Paucos ibi dies commorata, magnis donata muneribus, remittitur. Inde nos Almazanum oppidum petimus, unde in Laletaniam, Girundam urbem, Gallis finitimam, ut Caroli regis, qui in Gallia Narbonensi magnum contra Perpinianum parabat exercitum, cogitatibus Rex obviaret, proficiscitur. Regina vero Lauretum Cantabrium ad oceanum, portuosum oppidum, Ioannam filiam ad sponsum missura, subtristis ob mariti a se discessum, graditur. Classis ingens qua duae erant onerariae naves Genuenses (quas appellant *carracas*) [12] octoque supra centum aliae caveatae instruitur, ut aiunt; hominum decem milia armatorum, quia per Gallica littora factuti erant iter, ex Cantabris et Vasconibus montanis deliguntur. Duas cum filia noctes in mari Regina exegit. Undecimo tandem Kalendas Septembris anni .M.CCCC.XCVI. vela dant. Filiam aliquantulum collachrymata, quam se nunquam ultra visuram existimat, Burgos urbem ditissimam (quia mercatoria sit) graditur in interna, ibi nunc agimus. Rex, in Gallorum fronte praesidiis locatis, ad uxorem, uti pollicetur, propediem revertetur; expectatur summo cum desiderio. Tu vale!

Data Burgis, tertio Nonas Octobris .M.CCCC.XCVI.

---

[12] Medieval Latin term, see Sp. *carraca*.

of the Romans, and from his son, Philip of Burgundy, Count of Flanders to convey their joint proposal that we send the second-born Juana in marriage to Philip and receive Margaret, the only daughter of Maximilian, Philip's sister, in marriage to John, our Sovereigns' only son and heir to many kingdoms. The marriage agreements were drawn up and the ambassadors have left. Next the Sovereigns dissolve the assemblies, which were being held at Tortosa for *Laletania*, that is Catalonia, and alternatively at San Mateo, a short distance from the city of Tortosa, for the kingdom of Valencia. They go to the city of Alfaro, located in the territory of Castile but bordering on the region of Navarre, which is partly in Gascony and partly in Cantabria. Here in a fitting way, they receive the Queen of Navarre who was coming to meet them (the kingdom of Navarre was given in dowry to this queen). After stopping a few days there, she is sent back, with many rewarding gifts. Then we went to the city of Almazán, from where the King departs for the city of Gerona in Catalonia, bordering with France, so as to oppose the plans of King Charles, who was preparing a great army in Narbonese Gaul against Perpignan. The Queen, instead, quite sad at the departure of her husband, goes to Laredo in Cantabria, a port city on the ocean, intending to send off their daughter Juana to her husband. A great fleet was assembled including, as they say, two merchant ships from Genoa (known as carracks [arabic word, *caracca* i.e. large ship]) and one-hundred-eight other ships with maintop; ten thousand armed soldiers are chosen from the region of Cantabria and the mountains of Gascony, who are going to march along the French coasts. The Queen spent two nights at sea with her daughter, finally on 22 August 1496 they set sail. She cried a while for her daughter, whom she thinks she will not see anymore then headed for the very rich city of Burgos, (a commercial city), far from the constline, where we are now. The King, promised to return in a few days to his wife after setting up military posts on the French border; he is awaited with great eagerness. Fare well!

Given at Burgos, 5 October 1496

Pomponio suo, de superstitionibus insularum

Erige aures, Pomponi mi suavissime! Legisti, ut arbitror, quaecunque ab initio orbis ad nostra usque tempora, de dissonis et veris cerimoniis coelestium scripta sunt. Ne te ultra iactes cuncta vidisse, auscultato quae nostri insulares Hispaniolae,
5 nudi homines, referant; apud eos diu nostri versati sunt, priusquam an aliud colerent quam coeli numen potuerint intelligere. Nunc autem, cum familiarius apud primores ex Praefecti maritimi Coloni praecepto, Ramonus quidam heremitanus (ut vulgus inquit) conversatus fuerit, ut nostro ritu regulos erudiret
10 nostrosque mores illos edoceret, mire, apud plaerosque observari antra duo cognovit, e quorum profundis specubus solem ac lunam prodiisse puerascunt, veroque verius id esse autumant. Apud alios cucurbitulam summo esse in precio quandam, quoniam ex ea scaturivisse mare cum sua piscium multitudine
15 fabulantur. Ex cuius profluxu terram illam, quae continens erat, innumeras aiunt, quas videre fas est effectas esse insulas, cum ex illa prodeuntium aquarum alluvie valles implerentur, locaque obruerentur, cum suis gentibus et animalibus passim. Magnificiunt alii monilia quaedam, ex auricalco[13], quae affigunt pectori
20 reges, quia data quondam referunt insulari principi primatio, a formosa foemina, ad quam principem eum in profundo maris visam inquiunt, ut cum ea coiret descendisse. De hominum autem origine, pulchrum est audire quid balbutiant. E duobus nanque aliis specubus ortos praedicant. Multa praetermitto, ne
25 me in veteribus his aviis implicem; ex libris, quos de his tantum inventis formo, aliquando cognosces. Nunc vale!

Methymnae Campi, Idibus Iunii .M.CCCC.XCVII.

---

[13] Copper and zinc alloy, sparkling like gold (*see* Cic. *de off.* III 92; Hor. *ars* 202; Verg. *Aen.* XII 87; Paul. Fest. 8, 15 ff. L.; Isid. XVI 20,3).

To my Friend Pomponius, about the Superstitions of the Islands

Open your ears, my dearest Pomponius! You have read, I think, what has been written from the beginning of the world up to our days about discordant and true rituals of heavenly beings. So that you may not further boast to have seen everything, listen to what our naked natives of Hispaniola, report; < our men lived among them for a long time before they could understand if they worshipped any other divinity other than the god of heaven. Now, however, a certain Ramón, a hermit (as the people say), had rather friendly dealings with their leaders by order of Admiral Columbus, so as to instruct the chiefs about our rituals and teach them our customs; he came to know that most of them hold in high respect, astonishingly, two deep gorges, from which they believe, in a child-like manner, the sun and moon have risen, and they assert that this is truer than the truth. Others have the greatest regard for a small gourd, because from it, in the tale they tell, the sea with its great abundance of fish gushed out. From its gushing, they say that the earth, which was a continent, turned into the many islands now visible because the overflowing waters filled up the valleys and the places with their populations and animals that drowned out everywhere. Others hold in great esteem certain necklaces of orichalch, which the kings wear on their chest, claiming to have been once received by a head prince of the island from a beautiful woman in the deep sea. That prince, upon seeing her dove down to stay with her. Curious as well is to hear what they chatter about the origin of mankind, for they claim they were born from two other hollows. I omit many things, so as not to become entangled with these old misleading stories; some time, you will read them in the books I am preparing exclusively on these discoveries. Fare well for now!

Medina del Campo, 13 June 1497

Cardinali Sanctae Crucis

Garsias Lupus frater tuus, ad nos in curiam nuper venit; vir est egregius, clarus ingenio: si Latinas is literas fuisset assequutus, Maroni forte palmam de manibus eruisset. Rithmos componit, idiomate patrio, sapidissimos, gravi succo sententia-
5 rumque pondere praegnantes. Placuit novisse hominem, non minoris illum facio ob suaemet naturae dotes, quam quod tibi frater est; nec me ipse abiicit, tum quia videt me tibi deditissimum esse, tum etiam quia, quaecunque prodeunt ex eius officina, sui ingeni viribus decussa, mihi ostendit, id sibi nec
10 offuisse sentit. Ad haec scripsi quaedam ad Pomponium, ob eius virtutes heroem meum, de ridiculis insularum superstitionibus. Scio tibi ea relaturum, ast quid maris illa creatrix cucurbitula importet, accipito productius. *Naiba* regulus insularis, quondam *Adamati* filii, quem immatura mors praeripuit, cineres
15 cucurbitula inclusit, mirabolano arbori, ne terra macularentur, appendit. Is fertur, post aliquot menses filii desiderio motus, cucurbitulam affixam aperuisse, ut filii cineres conspiceret. Abscede, purpurate Princeps, ne te deglutiant aequorea monstra! Exiit illico, cum magno aquarum gurgite, balenarum et ingen-
20 tium piscium magna copia, qua data sunt mari piscium semina. Quattuor dein iuvenes puerascunt ex eodem partu fratres gemellos, cupiditate piscium et rei fama commotos, cucurbitulam, absente Naiba regulo, deprompsisse, ut eius porticulam ad emittendos pisces aperirent, sed, ex tempore superveniente Nai-
25 ba, prae stupore cucurbitulam solvisse de manibus et confregisse. Cave ne te obruant! Exquilias conscende, si Romae es, ne suffoceris adventante diluvio: Ex cucurbitulae scissuris maria scaturiunt illa quae continentes hactenus eos tractus omnes aquarum per ima montium profluxu insulas effecerunt, quas
30 cernere licet innumeras. Ita et ortum habuisse e cucurbitula mare et ex continenti divisam in partes varias patriam nostri perpolite narrant insulares. I nunc et tibi persuade te cuncta hactenus scivisse; deerat aliquid (uti video). Vale!

Methymnae Campi, .vi. Kalendas Augusti .M.CCCC.XCVII.

To the Cardinal of Holy Cross
(Bernardino de Carvajal)

Your brother, Garcia López, came to us recently at the court; he is a most distinguished man, renowned for his intelligence: had he devoted himself to the study of Latin, he perhaps would have taken the palm from Virgil's hands. He composes most pleasing verses in the native language filled with serious content and profound meaning. I am pleased to have known him, and I do not consider him less for his own natural talents than for being your brother; and he does not think of me less, because he realizes that I am very devoted to you and also because he shows me anything that comes out of his office, that is, the fruit of his intellectual strength, and he does not think that this has caused him any harm. Besides this, I wrote some news to Pomponius, my hero on account < of his virtues, concerning the ridiculous superstitions of the islands. I know that he will report these things to you, but hear more extensively what causes this little gourd to generate the sea. Once upon a time *Naiba*, a native chief, enclosed in a little gourd the ashes of his son *Adamato*, whose premature death had taken away; he hung it on a myrobolan tree, so as to avoid contamination from the ground. After a few months, moved by the longing for his son, he is said, to have opened the hanging gourd to take a look af his son's ashes. Keep at safe distance Cardinal Prince, so that the sea monsters do not swallow you! From the gourd came gushing out, with great swirls of water, huge numbers of whales and big fish, the seeds of fish entrusted to the sea. Then they tell, in a child-like manner, that four twin brothers, excited by their eager desire for fish and the importance of the event, stole the little gourd, while chief Naiba was absent, so as to open the little door and let more fish out; with Naiba coming back unexpectedly and caught by surprise, they let the little gourd slip from their hands and break. Be careful not to drown! Climb up the Esquiline, if you are in Rome, so as to avoid the impending flood! From the cracks of the little gourd sprang forth those seas which with the flowing rivers below the mountains, changed all those previously continental lands, into the dis-

Pomponio Laeto

Aequa lance est animus, clare Pomponi, eruditionem tuam
cum nostri purpurati Carvaiali forte metiri. Unam ad eum
nuper epistolam scripsi, de vero maris ortu et genere piscium
producto in immensum e cucurbitula Naibae; aliam accipito
5 (quia de zona torrida circuloque aequinoctiali) calidiorem. Quid
Castellana gens, Coloni Liguris ductu, ab occidente repererit,
satis ample lateque me scripsisse existimo; meridie tibi caeterisque viris sapientibus Portugalenses maximi littorum novorum
investigatores impartiuntur. Hi tantum scrutati tantumque cum
10 ingenti discrimine pervagati sunt, ut non minus iam ultra aequinoctium, amisso arctico, ad antarcticum processerint, quam
distet ab arctico nostri maris fretum exiguum, quod Calpe
dirimit ab Abila. Hoc omnes, uno ore, asseverant: Praxum isti
promontorium omniaque magni Atlantis latera, omnes in mare
15 prodeuntes ab Atlante cubitos, paulatim, singulis annis procedentes, superarunt, sed ipsius tamen nunquam littora deserere
ausi, donec ad ultimum iam quoddam cornu, quod ipsi *Bonae
Sperantiae Caput* vocant, appulsi sunt. Tunc ab incolis, eorum
tractuum peritissimis nautis, directi relinquere terram atque
20 altum capere ausi sunt per medias quasdam, paucis bene notas
sirtes vadosas; proras ad orientem inde vertentes, ast in laevam
a septentrione paulisper, in eas tandem regiones devenerunt,
e quibus ad nos hactenus aromata allata sunt omnia. Callecutum, intra aequinoctium, ad nos gradus, veluti Meroe, duode-
25 cim per incolas navium gubernatores, tandem ducuntur. Est
Callecutus civitas, lapideis domibus constructa, ingens, earum
regionum grandius emporium, ad quam ex Alexandria et universa Egipto Damascoque et reliqua Siria mercatores semper

covered countless islands. Thus, our natives narrate elegantly how the sea took its origin from a little gourd and how their land, once a continent, was divided into various parts. Now go and be sure that you have known everything up to now; something was missing (as I see). Fare well!

Medina del Campo, 27 July 1497

To Pomponius Letus

Distinguished Pomponius, I had the idea of measuring on an accurate scale your erudition and that of our Cardinal Carvajal. I recently wrote him a letter on the true origin of the sea and the innumerable generation of fish from the little gourd < of Naiba; hear now another one, even "hotter" (since it concerns the torrid zone and the equinoctial circle). I believe I have written rather fully and extensively on what the Castilians found in the West, under their Ligurian leader Columbus; the Portuguese show themselves, to you and other wise people, to be the best discoverers of new shores in the South. They have explored vast territories and wandered, at great danger, to the point of leaving the arctic, and advancind into the antarctic, for no less a distance beyond the equator than the arctic is from the narrow strait of our sea separating Calpe from Abyla. Everyone fully agrees that this is true: these men went past the *Prasum* promontory and in all direction of the great Atlas, advancing little by little, year by year and along the whole distance from Atlas to the sea, without, however, ever daring to leave its coasts, until they finally made the last edge of land they themselves call *Cape of Good Hope*. Then, guided by the natives, most experienced sailors of those regions, they dared leave and push forward into high sea, amid the African coastal shallows known only to few; turning then the prows to the East, but a little to the left from the north, they finally reached those regions from where, up to now, all spices have been brought to us. At last, they were led by the native pilots of the ships to Calicut, 12° below the equator, with respect to us. Calicut is a big city with stone houses like Meroe; it is

confluxerunt, ut ad nos inde odoras merces aromataque, nostras
30 lascivas pecunias, nostrosque proventus habituri, importent.
Laeti Portugalenses tantae rei invento, cum Callecuteo rege
percutiunt foedus. In terram descendunt, domos locant, ut
commercia et ipsi cum Callecuteis ineant, ast invidia, comune
humani generis venenum, cito scidit amicitiam: Damasceni
35 nanque et Alexandrini mercatores, incommodum ingens sibi
affuturum ex Portugalensium commercio olfaciunt, sollicitant
in Portugalenses Callecuteum populum qui, exorto tumultu,
etiam invito rege, domum, quam inhabitabant, ex insperato,
adoriuntur. Expugnant ad unum. Quinquaginta viros, quos in
40 terra reperere, trucidant; non penitus inulti, quia ex navibus
nostris, tormentis plaerasque naves ipsorum concussas, obrue-
runt. Ne metam epistolarem transgrediar, paucis his te volo
esse contentum, Pomponi; caeteraque acta sunt, atque ea non
pauca, significabo alias. Mira intelliges, quia nova, nolo te una
45 coena saturare. Satis sit tibi fuisse lautissimam, nolis et uberrimam. Quid nanque lautius tibi prestare possum, mi Pomponi,
quam id significare, quod natura ad nostram hanc usque tempestatem, qua nos eramus nascituri, servavit incognitum? Sua-
vibus nos his cibis, dulcibus nos dapibus depascit, quibus, si
50 non ieiuna penitus, famelica tamen antiquitas dies exegit suos.
Utrosque posthac antipodes, occiduos scilicet atque antarcticos,
ut suam quisque domum cognoscemus. Inhient alii divitiis,
inhient et titulorum sollicitudinibus alii, mi Pomponi, nos autem nostris ingeniis has escas praebeamus! Et vale!

Methymnae Campi, Kalendis Septembris .M.CCCC.XCVII.

the largest market of those regions, a place the merchants have always flocked to from Alexandria, the whole of Egypt, Damascus and the rest of Syria, in order to import from there aromatic goods and spices for us, and obtain our wanton money and income. Happy for such an important discovery, the Portuguese strike an agreement with the King of Calicut. They settle in rented houses to begin their trading with the inhabitants of Calicut; but envy, the widespread poison of the human race, quickly breaks up their friendly relation: merchants from Damascus and Alexandria fearing the ensuing enormous trade disadvantage with the Portuguese, stirred against them the people of Calicut, who, massively rebelled even against the will of the king, unexpectedly attacking the Portuguese quarters. The ferocity of the assault is total: fifty men were found on the ground slaughtered; however, the dead are fully vindicated because most of their ships were sunk by mortars fired from our ships. So as to avoid being overly long, I want you, Pomponius, to be satisfied with this short letter; other events have occurred and those (and they are not few) I will let you know another time. You will get to know extraordinary things because they are new; I do not wish to satiate you with a single serving. Be glad it was a very fine meal; do not wish it also to be overabundant. What greater delicacy could I offer you Pomponius, than to reveal what nature has kept undisclosed up to this period of time, in which we were destined to be born? Nature spoils us with these delicious items, delightful banquets whereas all of antiquity, if not entirely starved, was nevertheless fasting all along its days. From here on we will be acquainted with both the western as well as the antarctic antipodes, as much as we are familiar with our homes. Let others covet riches, or aspire to worrisome honorific titles; as for us, dear Pomponius, let us indulge our minds with intellectual pleasures! Fare well!

Medina del Campo, 1 September 1497

Pomponio Laeto, viro insigni

Utrunque tropicum torridamve zonam et aequinoctialem circulum Portugalenses (nobis clausos hactenus) immo et multorum iudicio inaccessos aperuerunt, uti superioribus diebus ad te scripsi. Conquiro ista diligentissime, mi Pomponi, atque
5 examussim, neque mihi deest, ad ea enucleanda, copia satis commoda; sum nanque Portugallico, qui hic assidet, oratori familiaris amicus, veniuntque plaerunque non pauci ex his, qui tractus illos adnavigant. Brevi compendio haec habeto; texere longam historiam ociosis relinquo viris atque his eloquentibus.
10 Perturbatus animo Emanuel, rex Portugaliae, de suorum internicie, tria et viginti navigia acribus munita tormentis virisque bello aptissimis instructa, ubi talia sensit accidisse, destinavit. *Caravelas* appellant. Id genus navium, nota iam Afra littora, sui Atlantis ingentes costas, vasta illa tot maria, innumeras insulas
15 praeterlabuntur, Rubri maris ostia, sinus Persici patentes portas, exuperant, regionem, captant tandem, ast priusquam Callecutum adeant, Cochini et Canenoti duos in eis littoribus reges, Callecuteo infensissimos, quos ibi prima navigatione, stricto foedere, in amicitiam sumpserant, conquirunt; de inferendis Callecuteo
20 regi, quacunque daretur, incommodis, conveniunt, sese reficiunt, ad arma parant. Ex Cochini et Canenori navibus plaerasque sumpserunt Portugalenses, ut aliquanto maior classis fieret. Callecutei classem apparant ingentem, nostri portum adeunt Callecuteum: sese illi non modo tueri intendunt, sed Portu
25 gallicam impetunt cum summo furore classem, eam penitus deleturi, si quiverint. Concurrunt igitur, durum ineunt certamen. Miseranda clades exoritur, vincitur tandem, quamvis amplius ducentarum navium Callecutea classis, quoniam eorum tormentis parum Portugallicis navibus oberant, quia lentis et
30 nullo furore emissis. Sunt Callecutei parum armati, sive quia nequeunt ob ingentes calores id armorum pondus sufferre, sive quod arma non assequantur. Capitur eorum praetoria navis; capiuntur et aliae plaeraeque, classis reliqua dispersa, vi nanque tormentorum, vicinis inspicientibus, multas ex eorum navibus
35 in profundum miserant. In Assyriorum et Alexandrinorum mercatorias naves indidere stragem inauditam. Non his contenti Portugalenses, ex adverso, in terram descenderunt, duasque

To Pomponius Letus, Distinguished Man

As I have written you previously, the Portuguese opened the way to both tropics, the torrid zone and to the equinoctial circle (up to now inaccessible to us), that were commonly recognized indeed as unapproachable. My Pomponius, I inquire into these facts with much care and precision, given the opportunity I have to follow the details being a family friend of the Portuguese ambassador who lives here and thanks to the frequent visits here by not a few of those who travel to those regions. Know these facts concisely; I leave to men with time to waste and love for endless talking the task of weaving a long narration. Emanuele, King of Portugal, upon finding out what actually happened and troubled by the massacre of his men, dispatched twenty-three ships, reinforced with powerful mortars and equipped with men well-suited for battle. They call them *caravels.* This type of ship sails along the already known African shores, the coasts of Atlas's massive range across vast seas, past innumerable islands and beyond the ports of the Red Sea, the open gates of the Persian gulf, finally reaching, but before landing in Calicut, the regions of Cochin and Cannanore; on shore, they search for two kings very hostile to that of Calicut, whom they had befriended during their first trip here; they agree on the kind of trouble to bring against the King of Calicut wherever possible; they rest and prepare for fighting. The Portuguese took most of the ships from Cochin and Cannanore, so as to increase their fleet. The people of Calicut prepare a large fleet; our men reach the Calicut port where the defenders actually mount an attack on the Portuguese fleet with the greatest rage, and evident intention of completely destroying it, if possible. They engage each other, and begin a rough battle. A deplorable defeat looms, but then victory prevails notwithstanding the fact that the fleet of Calicut had more than two hundred ships there; the reason being that their mortars, slow and without force, caused little damage to the Portuguese ships. The inhabitants of Calicut are not well armed, either because they cannot bear the weight of the arms, under the intense heat, or because they did not procure enough weapons. Their flagship is seized with most of the other ships

Callecuteae ditionis urbes magnas combussisse ingentesque Callecuteorum copias, manu exigua, profligasse feruntur. Direptio
40 facta, parentatum est interemptorum sanguini satis abunde. Est haec gens, mi Pomponi, ut aiunt, seminuda, fere invalida, quia intra Cancri tropicum iaceat, duodecim habens, uti alias me significasse arbitror, arctici nostri poli gradus elevatos, uti Meroe; nostro tamen more domos habent lapidibus constructas,
45 pecunias amant, voluntque pro pipere caeterisque aromatibus, quae ipsi assequuntur, a se ipsis et a finitimis, veluti ad nundinas concurrentibus, auri ducatos, et si queunt, Venetos; merces alias abiiciunt. Scribo ista ad te, mi Pomponi, quando cadunt in mentem, non quando eveniunt; propterea tu illa capito,
50 quando mittuntur et esto his contentus, quia parvo labore fatigor.

Compluti, .vii. Idus Novembris .M.CCCC.XCVII.

ep. 189 *C* = 189 *A* = 187 *ms.*   *p.* 388 G

Pomponio Laeto

Scribis, Pomponi amantissime, vidisse te quae de superstitionibus insularium exaraverim, conquereris de brevitate, quae obscuras reddit narrationes, quid de cucurbitula quadam velim te non intelligere inquis, cupereque te scribis quid illi de hominum
5 origine lepidissime senserunt, quo pacto ex cucurbitulae in terram collapsae rimulis, mare velint scaturisse. Succenseto nostro Carvaialo, ad quem ista scripsi productius! Is referet, habes ultionem prae manibus, modo velis, eadem illa mensura metitor, qua tibi demensus est[14]. Quae de homine garriant, ne

---

[14] See Vulgate, Lk 6, 38; Mt. 7, 2.

as well, while the rest of the fleet is dispersed because the power of the mortars had sunk many of their ships, under the eyes of neighbors. Incredible damage also involved the transport ships of the Assyrians and those from Alexandria. Not satisfied with this, the Portuguese landed on the opposite side and, it is claimed, they burned two great cities under the jurisdiction of Calicut, besides defeating with a small contingent huge armies of Calicutians. What a plunder; the blood of those who had been slain was thus abundantly avenged. These people, dear Pomponius, are half-naked, as they say, lacking any strength almost, because they live near the tropic of Cancer; as I think to have stated previously, their position falls 12° from the arctic pole, exactly like Meroe; however, they have houses built with stones, as we do, love money and want, in exchange for pepper and other spices which they grow and obtain from the nearby areas to then assemble them there like in a market, gold ducats or, if possible, Venetian Ducats; they refuse other merchandise. Dear Pomponius, I write these reports to you when they come to mind, not as they happen; and, therefore, accept them, when they are sent to you, and be satisfied with them, because I tire easily.

Alcalá de Henares, 7 November 1497

To Pomponius Letus

Dearest Pomponius, you write that you have seen what I have written about the natives' superstitions and complain about my conciseness that renders the reports obscure; you say that you do not understand what I mean by talking about a small gourd, adding that you wish to learn what they so charmingly thought about the origin of mankind, namely, how they conceived the sea to have sprung from the cracks of a small gourd fallen to the earth. Be angry with our Carvajal, to whom I wrote about these things more extensively! He should tell you; revenge is in your hands; if you should like, use that same measure he used with you: do not share with him the natives' thinking about man. They deem that in their

10 feceris participem. Duo esse ingentia in eorum montibus antra
fabulantur, praeter illa e quibus solem et lunam prodiisse puerascunt, in quibus ab initio rerum genus omne hominum lati-
tavit. In utriusque antri foribus alternos semper insedisse duces,
ne quisquam egrederetur insaniunt. Idque pro archano habent
15 sacro. Sed annorum tandem prolapsis curriculis, ipsis ducibus
noctu insulam pervagare audentibus, quaerendarum dapum causa, sole deprehensos, nunc hos, nunc illos (intueri nanque solem
illis minime licebat), in diversa mutatos, in mirabolanos arbores,
ut puta, in saxaque, plaerasque in res alias; efficit tamen longa
20 dies (quod obducta fronte graviterque, tanquam sacrum, oblo-
quuntur), ut multi, licet sole deprehensi, sese servarent, ne
verterentur; sed hos aiunt, relictis matribus, eduxisse parvulos
infantes ulnisque illos cum per diversa portarent, in cuiusdam
fluminis ripa, inspectatis aquis, *toa*, *toa*, emisso vagitu, infantes
25 proclamasse, quod ipsorum lingua significare *mamma*, *mamma*
volunt, et in ranas mutatos asseverant. Inde vocem illam ranis
fuisse haereditariam. Quo modo deinde procederent hi homines,
sine uxorum commercio, interrogati, animalia quaedam per
mirabolanos serpentia, foeminas aemulantia, se vidisse balbu-
30 tiunt a longe, plaeraque illorum, insectando, licet duriuscule,
quia lubrica, anguillae more, apprehenderunt. Tunc, et cum
muliebri natura carerent, admota inguinibus ave pico, vi per
femora, manibus quorundam callosas habentium palmas, foe-
mineam illis fossore pico naturam effecisse. Ita, eia Pomponi,
35 eia, cervicem excute! In uxores sibi foeminas has susceperunt
boni viri atque inde genus hominum prodiisse volunt; praedicant, instant, contendunt id dirum ac nefarium tantae rei sacra-
menta, nusquam, praeterquam regibus aut *bovitis*, quos habent
pro medicis et sacerdotibus, patefacere. Solum id inventum
40 apud Romanos, de sacro ancili,[15] atque Matutae[16] archanis
existimabas? Sunt et alii magnarum rerum inventores, Pomponi,

---

[15] According to legend, a shield was believed to have fallen from heaven at the
time when Numa Pompilius was king of Rome. To ensure its preservation against it
being stolen, he ordered eleven exact copies made which he entrusted to the Salii
[priests]. The latters' duty twice a year, in early spring and fall i.e. at the beginning and
at the end of the war season, was to carry it in their festal processions. (Paul. Fest. 117,
14-15 L.; Ov. *fasti* III 259 ff.; Liv. I 20; Verg. *Aen.* VIII 663 ff.; Liv. I 20).

[16] *Mater Matuta* was a quite ancient Latin goddess of matutine light (Lucr. V 656;
Ov. *fasti* VI 479, 545 ff.; Cic. *Tusc.* I 12, 28; *de nat. deor.* III 19, 48), venerated in
classical times, above all, as the protectress of fertility.

mountains there are two huge caves, beside those gorges which they naively describe as the birth places of the sun and the moon, in which in the very beginning the whole of humankind lay hidden. They rave about how the chiefs took turns guarding the openings of each cave so that no one would wander out. And they hold this to be a sacred mystery. But one time after a number of years, these leaders themselves, having dared to rove about the island at night in search of food, were allegedly caught by the sun (for they were not at all allowed to look at the sun) and variously changed into either myrobolan trees or rocks and many other things; however, the long day caused many to be spared such mutation (they narrate this with a grave and intimidating look befitting a sacred mystery); but, the story continues by describing how they — leaving the mothers behind — stole the young children and carried them in their arms in different directions, up to the banks of a river where the whining little ones, upon seeing the waters cried out *"toa, toa,"* which in their language means "mommy, mommy," before being transformed into frogs. From that moment on, it is claimed the frogs inherited their cry. Asked how these men could live without female partners, their speech stumbling they relate how they saw from far away animals sliding along the myrobolan trees and resembling women: chased and caught most of them, albeit with difficulty because they were as slippery as eels. Realizing then, these creatures lacked the female organs, the men with the roughest palms applied to their groins a woodpecker near the thigh-bone and shaped them into females thanks to a pecking woodpecker. So, Pomponius, you may now shake your head! Deserving men took these women as their wives, and thus maintain that so the human race originated; they assert with insistence and maintain that it would be forbidden and impious to reveal this truthful mystery to anyone but the kings and the *boviti*, the latter being paramount to doctors and priests. Did you naively think that the right to believe in the *mater matuta* mysteries and the sacred shield was exclusively Roman? Others too, Pomponius, are inventors of great "deeds" that the people may not be allowed to celebrate with music but on holidays.

Alcalá de Henares, 18 December 1497

licet tamen omnia populo diebus festus per rithmos ista conci-
nere, alias minime.

Compluti, .xv. Kalendas Ianuarii .M.CCCC.XCVII.

ep. 190 *C* = 190 *A* = 188 *ms.*   *p.* 389 *G*

Bracharensi et Pampilonensi praesulibus

Non minus mihi quam infoelici Beatrici infaustus advenit
nuncius. Is ab oratoribus nostris, qui isthic assident, apud
Summum Pontificem, rettulit fore supervacaneum ad hanc rem
oratores in Pannoniam destinare; detrectaturum nanque Regem,
5 Beatricis sponsum, quaecunque proponantur, scribunt oratores,
quia illi fixum animo est, nolle iugali thalamo Beatricem reginam adiicere. Inclinari etiam ad Regis postulata pontificem
Alexandrum inquiunt; malunt propterea mei Reges alterum
e duobus, quam utrunque perpeti: durum illis est sanguinem
10 suum repudiatum iri (est nanque Regi propinqua Beatrix, quia
Fernandi primi filia), ast durius, post naufragium, pcrdcrc ct
naulum,[17] demptum nanque de ipsorum autoritate plurimum
putarent, si eorum petita negligerentur. Ne igitur ignominiam
aliam perferant, satius esse ducunt rem dissimulare. Quare
15 sublatum est mihi iter laboriosum, sed iniquo id animo fero,
quia summam mihi erat delectationem pariturum. Me autem
accitum Reges serena fronte gratulabundi fere, quod tantus mihi
labor sublatus fuisset, grave mihi fore putantes compellarunt;
sed falluntur, nil nanque maluissem. Egre quidem haec fero,
20 quia dempta mihi spes, quae surrexerat, vos veteres amicos
visendi. Sed, ne frustra sumpsisse calamum videar, haec pauca
de nostris insularibus habetote, quae nostro Pomponio referatis,
si vobis ille aperit, quae ad eum scribo. Novum genus est apud
eos latriae repertum; vidistis aliquando parietibus depictos le-
25 mures cornutos, dentatos caudatosque, manibus aduncis atque,

[17] See Iuv. VIII 97.

92

To the Archbishops of Braga and Pamplona
(Diego De Sousa – Alonso Carrillo)

The messenger came with unfortunate news for both, me and unhappy Beatrice. On behalf of our ambassadors stationed at the court of the Supreme Pontiff, he related how useless it would be to purposefully send ambassadors to Hungary, for — the ambassadors write — the king promised in marriage to Beatrice refuses all proposals being adamantly resolved not to marry Queen Beatrice. Also, they say that Pope Alexander has yielded to the requests of the King. Therefore, my Sovereigns prefer to bear one of the two evils rather than both: it is hard for them to have their own blood rejected (for Beatrice is related to our King, being the daughter of Ferdinand I), but it would be harsher if, after the shipwreck, they were to lose the freight as well, and they would indeed deem very grave any taking away from their authority, were their requests ignored. In order not to endure then another disgrace, they reckon it is better to pretend not to know. Therefore, I have been spared a very laborious journey; yet, I bear this with heavy heart for it could have been for me a great delight. Whereas the Sovereigns summoned me and appeared relieved for me, almost congratulating me because such a hardship was avoided, I believe their thinking that it would have been heavy toil for me was indeed wrong, for nothing would have pleased me more. The regret I bear is born of my lost hope now of seeing you, my old friends, and which encouraged me all along. However, so that I may not seem to have taken up a pen in vain, here is some news about our natives, which you may relate to our Pomponius, if he shares with you what I write him. Among < them a new kind of cult has been discovered; you have, at

ore aperto, ad deterrendos homines. Ex gossampio intexto gossampioque fulcta construunt simulacra, huiuscemodi lemures ad unguem imitantia; noctu nanque ipsis apparent, in illosque quibus aguntur errores inducunt. *Zemes* appellant haec simula-
30 cra, a quibus se pluvias, si pluvia indigent, dies lucidos, si solem volunt, impetrare fabulantur; a Zemibus iratis tonitrua mitti ac fulgura et grandines putant. Inducunturque a bovitis, quos pro sacerdotibus habent ac sanctis viris, meritis Zemes placare muneribus. Masculos habent ex his ac foeminas; coire
35 masculos aliquando cum regum uxoribus credunt nascique infantes ex illis, vario regum filiis quodam per cervicem sparso tumore. Insensi iam mihi estis et molesti, qui uno velitis spiritu, quaecunque hoc nostro orbe novo emicant, cognoscere; stringite aliquantulum guttur! Et valete!

Compluti, Nonis Aprilis .M.CCCC.XCVIII.

ep. 201 C = 202 A = 199 ms.   *p. 394 G*

Pomponio Laeto, viro eruditissimo

Agimus Occaniae, Pomponi charissime, insigni a Toleto milia passuum viginti municipio; aquarum defluxibus pene submergimur. Sciamus quidnam apud vos humectantia operentur sidera, quaeve sit sapientum sententia et vulgi opinio de
5 iterum surgente murmure ac strepitu Transalpinorum armorum in Italiam? Fibrae mihi gelascunt absenti, ob amorem patriae; quid vos facietis, qui scintillanti iam igni proximiores estis? Dissidium istud, inhiantis imperio rei publicae Venetae et Ludovici Sfortiae, sui hostis potentiam trepidantis, vos trahent
10 omnes in praeceps (ni fallor). Omen Dieus avertat![18] Ab orbe autem novo quid habeatur, petis. Solem secuti nostri Castellani

---

[18] See Cic. *Phil.* IV 4; XI 5.

times, seen painted on walls toothed deities with horns and tail, hooked hands and mouth wide open to frighten people. They make up, to perfection, dumies out of woven cotton supported by thread and which reproduced such monsters; by coming alive for them at night the natives are induced into those false beliefs which keep them entrapped. They call these representation *Zemi*, from whom, they rave about the chance to obtain, through worship, rain, if they need rain, or sunshine, if they want the sun; they believe that thunder, lightning and hail are sent by angered *Zemi* that could be placated by the *boviti*, whom they regard as priests and holy men, with worthy gifts. There are male and female *Zemi*; they think that the males at times visit with the wives of the kings generating children with a distinctive protuberance of some dimension on their neck. By now I hate and detest those of you who wish to know in a single breath, whatever worthwhile thing happens in this new world of ours; control your greed for knowledge a little! Fare well!

Alcalá de Henares, 5 April 1498

To Pomponius Letus, Man of the Greatest Knowledge

We are at Ocaña, my dear Pomponius, a famous small town, 20 miles from Toledo; we are almost flooded by rainfalls. Could we know why, near you, the stars that bring rain are never active and what is the thought of the learned as well as the opinion of the people concerning the ongoing rumbling and crash of a Transalpine [french] army against Italy? Although far away, every fiber of my body stiffens up as I love my country; what will you do, you who are by now so close to the sparkling fire of the arms? That strife between the Republic of Venice, longing for supremacy, and Ludovico Sforza, who fears the power of his enemy, will lead (if I am not mistaken) to a general downfall. May God avert this omen. You go on to ask what news we have from the new world. < Our Castilians, following the sun, advance more and more

ad occidentem magis ac magis in dies progrieduntur. Nudos
omnes sola plaerisque in locis cucurbitula, in modum braculae,
qua membrum ac genitalia includuntur, contentos reperiunt
15 incolas. Alii praeputium, deducto nervo, alligant funiculo, quem
nisi mictus aut coitus gratia solvunt; integra tamen et alii
gossampina femoralia gestant. Aurum gemmasque, sed praecipue uniones multis in locis reperiunt. Portugalenses vero, suum
secuti transaequinoctium aliamque Arcton, aromatum commer-
20 cia prosequuntur. Callecutensem regem Alexandrinosque ac
Damascenos mercatores ad medullas extenuant. Quotquot illorum navigia ab alto prospectant, impetunt capiuntque aut vi
tormentorum submergunt. Soldano Babilonico magnum ex hac
re incommodum proventorum putamus, nec Venetis lucrum
25 pariet, ut multi opinantur. Ex Soldani nanque emporiis et Nili
ostiis sunt a Venetorum abavis proventus, quibus ad eam opum
devenere potentiam, qua nunc pollent, quibusve brachia protendere (uti nosti) maioribus ipsorum licuit, ut plurimum asportati. Siderum cursus aemulatur haec nostra curia, Pomponi:
30 perpetuo nanque in motu est.
Alias propediem terras (uti fertur) visemus. Vale!

Occaniae, pridie Nonas Februarii .M.CCCC.XCIX.

ep. 205 *C* = 206 *A* = 206 *ms.*   *p.* 396 *G*

Pomponio Laeto

Scribis, Pomponi, Tibrim alveos suos adeo superasse, ut
universam fere Urbem inundaverit metasque a maioribus hactenus, ad eius incrementum signatas, cubito amplius transiliisse,
futurae alicuius calamitatis proximae praesagio, antiqui ascribe-
5 bant. Id nos floccifacere iubemur, Deus tamen bene vertat! Ut
sedent animos inter se concordesque sint Itali principes optandum est. De insularibus nostris oceaneis novi aliquid velles:
accipe quod nuper mihi de illis relatum est. Non arbitror decidisse tibi e memoria quae ad te scripsi superioribus diebus de
10 bovitis, qui et medici sunt et sacerdotes; didicerunt nostri

every day into the West. They find all the natives to be naked in most places, with only a little gourd, worn as a loincloth to enclose their genitals. Others, instead, tie the flaccid organ's foreskin with a string, which is loosened to urinate or have intercourse; others still wear thigh-pieces of pure cotton. In many places, they find gold and jewels, most of all pearls. The Portuguese on the other hand, pursuing their trans-equatorial route and destiny continue the spice trade! They annihilate the ruler of Calicut and the merchants from Alexandria and Damascus. All ships sighted by the Portuguese from high up are attacked and either captured or sunk with the power of the mortars. We think this situation carries a loss to the Sultan of Babylon and that it will not be as profitable either for the Venetians, as many believe. In fact, from the markets of the Sultan and from the delta of the Nile came the profits as early as the time of the forefathers of the Venetians; and with that income they achieved an abundance of means now apparent in their power and which enabled said ancestors extend their influence (as you know), since their profits were so huge. This court of ours imitates the course of the stars, Pomponius, for it is constantly moving about. Very soon (as reports have it) we will visit other regions. Fare well!

Ocana, 4 February 1499

To Pomponius Letus

Pomponius, you write that the Tiber has risen so far above its banks that it almost flooded all of Rome and that in the antiquity it was considered an omen of some impending calamity, if the river surpassed by more than a cubit its high-rise limit up to then recorded by their forefathers. We are told not to take this seriously: God may still be looking on us with favor! The thing to wish for is that Italian rulers resolve their animosities and reach an agreement. You now might like to know something new about our natives across < the ocean: listen to what has been recently reported to me

posthaec regibus illis esse curae ut a bovitis in arte medica instituantur, veluti legimus quondam priscos reges et sapientes exoptasse: scis nanque (nec te id praeterire putandum est), Egiptios Persasque, medicos simul et sacerdotes fuisse, reges
15 plures ac duces egregios, Saporem[19], ut puta, Medorum Mitridatemque, duarum et viginti linguarum dominum, reges, medicinam pluresque alios exercuisse, nec iniuria quidem: hominis nanque (cum eius gratia Peripatetici velint ac Stoici cuncta sub orbe lunae fuisse creata) res est huiuscemodi pertractare, quibus
20 id assequamur, sine quo nihil in vita iucundum. Quid nanque prodest cuiquam nivem sine sanitate? Insaniant, uti lubet, plaerique, parum distare incolumis ne quis vivat, an eget, garrientes; quid Orpheus[20] hymno decantaverit, de sanitate, repetito: vult is inutilia esse hominibus cuncta sine sanitate. Non abso-
25 num igitur in natura videtur, ut viri, tum sapientia, tum fortunis praecellentes, eam scire velint, eam exerceant artem, quae ut homines vivant incolumes efficiat. Nostros igitur nudos insulares regulos, ne mireris, mi Pomponi, medicinam artem velle cognoscere: potest et nudis natura dictare ut ingenium
30 ad bonas artes inducant, quandoquidem vestibus indutum neminem creaverit unquam. Quod mihi sit curae plaerunque ad te scribere, nescio quas agis gratias; verba simul et tempus incassum teris, Pomponi suavissime! Eo tibi emito precio quos nondum assequutus es; me autem, qui iure merito tuus sum,
35 ne istis ulterius ambagibus circuito. Et vale!

Madrito, quarto Idus Maii .M.CCCC.XCIX.

[19] Peter Martyr's reference is to (middle-Persian) Sapor I, the founder of a center for medical and philosophical studies, as well as to Mithridates VI Eupator, king of Pontus and a great erudite.

[20] Orph. *hymn.* 68, p. 48 Quandt.

about them. I do not think that you have forgotten what I wrote to you in the preceding days about the *boviti*, who are both doctors and priests; later on our people learned that it was a concern to those rulers that they be instructed by the *boviti* in the art of medicine just as, we read, the ancient rulers and sage men had once longed for: in fact you know (and it is unthinkable that you would not be aware of this) that many rulers and distinguished leaders, both Egyptian and Persian, were at the same time doctors and priests, such as Sapor, of the Medes, and Mithridates, who mastered twenty-two languages; and [you know] that many other rulers have practiced medicine, and not badly either: for it is characteristic of man (since both Peripatetic and Stoic philosophers claim that everything under the sphere of the moon has been created for man's sake) to study things of this kind and by so doing we secure that without which nothing in life would be pleasant. What good is it really to have white hair without health? Let most people rave unrestrained and try out that there is little difference between living in good or bad health; remember what Orpheus sang in his praise, about health: he views all things as irrelevant for men without health. It does not seem, then, to be out of tune with nature that men, excelling in wisdom and success, should wish to know and practice that art which makes men live healthily. Do not be surprised, then, Pomponius, that our chieftains, although naked, may want to learn the art of medicine: nature can induce even naked men to devote their ability to the good arts, since it has never created anyone dressed in clothes. I do not understand why you bother thanking me for my desire to write to you frequently; you use your words and time in vain, dearest Pomponius! With that currency, buy those whom you have not yet won over; but do not encircle me any more with those snares of yours since I am, and rightfully so, yours. Fare well!

Madrid, 12 May 1499

Pedro Fagiardo

Auspicato meas ex urbe Mediolano ad te literas discessisse credo; genealogice nunc cosmetriceque[21] tecum agere parum per est animus et, inflatis buccis, gloriari. Stirps haec ab Angleria nostra, ab avis atavisque, Mediolanensis est, ubi vates
5 ille noster Ausonius[22] mira esse omnia sapido cantat epigrammate. Quale genus hoc ab origine fuerit, ex libello trium quaternionum ad me cum Madriti tu caeterique optimates quotidie mihi domum implebatis, audituri, misso, potuistis colligere; legistis nanque circiter quadraginta ex hac familia reges recta
10 serie prodiisse, vastatamque, uti moris est rerum humanarum, quae vertunt fortunae vices, a Germanis Insubriam universam gentemque istam radicitus fere deletam, semilachrymans percurristi. Nonnulli tamen per varias tremuli latebras, donec furibundus ille Germanicus torrens ad alveum ripasque suas
15 rediret, evaserunt. Ab his domus Vicecomitum a qua se genitum iactat, ex Valentina avia, rex iste Ludovicus, Gallorum rex, emanavit. Germanorum igitur satiata rabie, in patriam e latibulis, qui supererant, rediere. Soli ubertas (est nanque fortunatissima tellus), ut ad priscum decorem cito rediret, effe-
20 cit. Hinc sanguis noster Anglerius, hinc mea progenies. Attamen, cum me utero mater gestaret, sic volente patre, Aronam, ubi plaeraque illis erant praedia domusque, concessit. Est autem Arona oppidum insigne, in Verbani lacus, quem iuniores *lacum Maiorem* appellant, ripa situm, munitissimum et bene fortuna-
25 tum, moenibus, in alae forma dispositis numerosis turribus, atque eminenti arce convexa moenibus, ab impetu hostium tutissimum, si qua hostes ingruant. Sunt nanque Aronenses Elvetiis Germanisque proximi, neque a Gallis et Hasta oppido maxime distant; ad ipsius etiam oppidi nundinas saepe concur-
30 runt, nundinarium nanque est et frequens mercatorum commercio. Equorum huc Elvetiorum Germanorumque multitudo ingens venum confluit. Lacus vero is Maior centum, ut aiunt, amplius milium passuum; duo ex Alpibus decurrentia flumina

---

[21] See *cosmeta* (= *ornator*), Iuv. VI 477.
[22] Auson. *ordo urb. nob.* XI 7, pp. 146-147 Peiper.

To Peter Fajardo

I trust my letters from the city of Milan have reached you in favorable circumstances; but now I wish to talk to you a bit about genealogies and blazons and boast, without restrain. Our stock of Anghiera, from my remote ancestors down, is from Milan, where our poet Ausonius sings in a delightful epigram that everything is admirable. You had the opportunity to judge the kind of stock our family was from its beginnings, from a booklet of three quaternions sent to me when you and other nobles used to fill my house in Madrid daily in order to listen to me; you have indeed read that some forty monarchs have come in direct line from this family; and, as is usual in human affairs subject to the vagaries of fortune change, you have realized, half in tears, how all of Lombardy and its people have been almost utterly destroyed by the Germans. Some, however, escaped frightened thanks to various hiding-places, until that raging German torrent went back into its channel and its proper banks. From the Anghieras the house of Visconti including Ludovico the king of the French, who boasts descent through his grandmother Valentina. When, then, the rage of the Germans had subsided, the survivors returned to their country from their hiding places. The fertil soil (it is indeed a very blessed land) contributed to its very quick return to ancient glory. From here comes our Anghiera blood, i.e. my stock. My mother, however, when she was carrying me in her womb, went away to Arona at the wish of my father, where they had most of their possessions and lands. Arona is indeed a notable city on the shores of Lake Verbano, younger people call it Lake *Maggiore*. It is quite prosperous and well protected by walls, numerous towers arranged in the shape of a wing, an elevated fortress equally surrounded by walls, and thus very safe overall from assaults, should an enemy attack. The inhabitants of Arona are actually very close to the Swiss and Germans and not too distant from either the French and the city of Asti; they often flock to the markets of this city teeming with merchants, for commerce there is very active. A large number of Swiss and German horses are brought here for sale. Lake Maggiore extends, as they say, for over 100

conficiunt lacum, fontesque innumeri a reliquis montibus de-
35 scendentes. Ticinus vero navigabilis fluvius, qui Padum ampli-
ficat, ipsius lacus aquas omnes ebibit, perque vastas eas planities
raptat; quibus et provincia multis montanis proventibus, trabibus utpote, lignis comburendis, et calce ac marmoribus fortunatur, instruiturque. Nec lacus opulentiam tacere intendo: di-
40 tissimus est accolis, turtures fluviales nutrit eximii saporis et
magnitudinis tantae ut sexaginta amplius librarum duo deuncialium fuerit aliquis repertus turtur. Vulgo librarum viginti
trigintaque aiunt captum saepe fuisse. Mirae inquiunt esse profunditatis lacum piscatores, tempestatibusque, veluti pelagus
45 ingens, agitari; pollet etiam piscibus aliis multiformibus, sed
raris alibi quibusdam, sub aurato quodam colore praecinctisque,
quos vocant *persacos*, luciis ingentibus, ipsorum appellatione
cavedinis, anguillis, bottistrysis, scationibus, piotis, agonibus,
tenchis, chepiis atque aliis, quorum nomina mihi deciderunt,
50 nec latina habere cognosco; est copia tanta ut vicina omnia,
tempore piscium, Mediolanumque ipsum saturent. Vis brevibus? Dulcium aquarum edulia sapidiora nullibi, nullibi plura.
Huc igitur ego ex itinere, quia ibi me mater dederat orbi, ad
veteres amicos affinesque diverti; quotquot in hoc iacent cor-
55 pusculo spiritus, quotquot animantes fibrae, miro intra sese
titillo garrientes prae laetitia, vires conduplicarunt. Ex natalis
ergo terrae complexu, ex veterum amicorum et affinium repetita
undecim dierum consuetudine, tam longae peregrinationis meae
fastidia excussi. Omnis lassitudo laboresque omnes cesserunt
60 illico. Caetera per exemplaria. Haec autem ex itinere ad Reginam, nuntio ad te mihi sese offerente, volui, ad animi mei
oblectamentum, describere. Grata ne tibi futura sint, an non,
parum curae est. Aequum fuit ut mihi semel, cum tibi aliisque
saepissime, satisfacerem. Vale!

Ex Caesareaugusta, quarto Idus Augusti .M.D.II.

miles, with two rivers flowing from the Alps to form the lake, and numerous other springs descending from its mountain ranges. In fact, the Ticino, a navigable river tributary of the Po, drains the lake's water distributed throughout the vast plains; with the water and many mountain products such as lumber, fire wood, lime and marble, the region prospers and is well supplied. And I do not intend to underestimate the lake's wealth: it is very rich for those who live near it; it feeds river turtles of exquisite taste and of such great size that one was found weighing more than 62 pounds, 12 ounces. 20 or 30 pounds catches are common. Fishermen say that the lake has exceptional depth and is stirred by storms like a great sea; it teems in fish of many shapes and varieties, rare elsewhere, such as those of a certain golden color with a streaking around which they call perches, big pikes called by them *cavedini*, eels, *bottistrisi* [i.e. *bottrisa, bottatrice*: burbots or freshwater eel-pouts], *scationi* [bull-head fish], *pioti* [mullets], *agoni* [*ago*, sea pike or gar fish] tenches, common shad [related to the herring], and others, whose names I have forgotten and am not sure they have Latin names; there is so great an abundance that the fishing season satisfies all the neighboring areas and even Milan itself. Do you want to know it in a few words? Nowhere else can you find more delicious fresh water fish or in greater quantity. Sorry for this interruption of my account related to my journey and visit of old friends and relatives, but I could not help it since my mother gave birth to me here: all the live spirits in my little body, and its living fibers that murmur inside me for joy through a wonderful tingling, doubled my strength. And so, thanks to the embrace with my native land and the prolonged intimacy of old friends and relatives for eleven days, I shook off the malaise of my long peregrination. All weariness and all toils immediately ceased. You will receive more news through other sources. The things above, however, I wanted to describe for my own pleasure right after the trip to the Queen, when a dispatcher headed for you became available to me. I am not primarily concerned whether or not they please you. It is only fair that this one time I satisfy myself, having very often before given satisfaction to you and to others. Fare well!

From Saragossa, 10 August 1502

Ludovico Furtato Mendocio, mei Tendillae Comitis filio

Petis quid habeatur ab orbe novo. Maiora in dies hactenus latentia deteguntur. De vasta quadam tellure quae sese offert nautis in laevam ab Herculeo freto[23] se vertentibus ad meridiem latam fecimus alias mentionem. In ea tellure provincias esse
5 vatias, *Pariam* puta, *Curianam, Cuchibacoam, Cauhietum, Saturniam, Caubanam, Urabaim, Zaraboroam, Beraguam* et multas praeterea diximus. Magnae illius terrae littora peragrantes Christophorus Colonus, primus tantae inventor magnitudinis, dehinc, illum aemulantes, Hispani, varia reperere flumina, tum ingentia,
10 tum parva et mediocria; praeter caetera in unum incidere latitudinis adeo immensae, ut incredibile sit posse id in natura fieri. Octoginta miliarium amplius aiunt et flumen esse asseverant, non maris sinum, quod dulcium sit aquarum, quod fluat in oceanum et insulis refertum sit neque fluxum patiatur aut
15 refluxum in internis. Quadraginta plaerique lequas cum caravelis, adverso eo flumine, adnavigarunt. Et diversos accolarum regulos salutavere mutuisque muneribus sese invicem amicitia devinxere, licet, ab initio, reicere hospites conarentur. Regulos *chiacones* appellant, flumini est nomen patrium *Maragnonus.* Sub
20 aequinoctiali locant linea plaerique nautae fluminis eius fauces, trans lineam ahi constituunt. Se ibi polum arcticum amittere fatentur omnes. Linguarum est in illis tractibus et nationum magna varietas. Animalium, volucrum pisciumque ac monstrorum diversitas est ingens; mores varii, ubique auro scatent,
25 unionibus abundant ubique regiones illae. Quarum sub eodem eius terrae discursu, aequinoctio plaeraeque subsunt, aliae citra, trans aliae. Elisias mille atque iterum mille provincias fovent illi tractus steriles etiam alias harenosasque ac horridas natura soli, Caribium sive Canibalium humanarum carnium helluonum
30 et venenatis sagittis advenientes hospites excipientium altrices alias, mitium et hospitalium incolarum alias. Frondescunt ibi arbores, maiori in parte, toto anno et prata virescunt. Vere tantum et autumno fruuntur incolae, hyemis horridae aut aestatis molestae expertes. Qui colles et decurrentium fluminum

---

[23] The reference here is to the narrow waterway near Hercules' columns or Strait of Gibraltar (see Sil. 1, 199).

To Louis Hurtado de Mendoza, Son of my Count of Tendilla

You ask what news we have from the new world. Day <
by day greater things, up to now hidden, are revealed. On
a previous occasion we mentioned a vast land, visible to sailors
who head South off the left side of Hercules Strait. In that
land we said that there are various provinces, that is, *Paria,
Curiana, Cuchibacoa, Cauhieto, Saturnia, Caubana, Urabá, Zaraboroa,
Veragua,* and many others besides. Traveling along the shores
of that great land, Christopher Columbus, first discoverer of
such vastness, and then the Spaniards, emulating him, discovered various large rivers as well as small and medium-size
ones, besides the largest one of such immense width that one
would not believe it could occur in nature. They say it is more
than 80 miles wide strongly declaring it to be a river, not
a bay of the sea, because of its fresh water: it flows into the
ocean, is full of islands and presents no tidal flows. Many have
sailed with caravels 40 leagues into it, going against its current.
They have also met a number of native chiefs and exchanged
gifts in reciprocal friendship, although at the beginning they
tried to fend off the foreigners. They call their chieftains *chiaconi*
and the river *Marañón.* Most of the sailors place the outlet of
that river at the line of the equator, others well below it. They
all admit that here they lose sight of the arctic pole. In those
regions there is a great variety of languages and nations. The
variety of animals, birds, fish, and monsters is great; diverse
are the customs; throughout those regions there is much gold
and an abundance of pearls. Most land if one sails this part of
the earth back and forth, is near the equator, with some on
either side. These areas encompass thousands of *Elisie* or provinces: from barren, sandy and horrible-by-nature grounds, to
some inhabited by Caribs or Cannibals, eaters of human flesh
who receive incoming foreigners with poisoned arrows, to
others yet full of gentle and hospitable natives. Most trees here
are green and the meadows flowering throughout the year.
The natives know only spring and fall, having no experience
of the rigors of winter or the vexations of summer. Those
who inhabit the hillsides and the banks of flowing streams live
happily. In few places, on high mountains, perennial snow is

35 ripas inhabitant, beate vivunt. In elatis montibus alicubi perpe-
tuae nives conspiciuntur, in profundis autem vallibus, ob ro-
rantes ad ima e montibus solares radios, calor ingens, quia vel
sub linea vel propinqui lineae sint aequinoctiali. Coloniae sunt
in ea terra duae destinatae, in Urabae magno sinu per Alfonsum
40 Hoiedam una, per Diecum Nicuessa in Beragua altera. Ad
Beraguam septingentorum hominum classe Nicuessa pervexit,
ad Urabam quadringentorum Hoieda; cui datus est comes Ioannis Cossa egregius et exercitus eorum littorum nauclerus. Sed
infoelici omnes fato et sinistris avibus periere tres ipsi primarii
45 et commilitonum pars maior variis adacti casibus. Particulares
aliquando de his inventis edemus libros, quae, meo iudicio,
maiora sunt et mirabiliora quam quae ab antiquis descripta
cosmographis. Iam vale!

Ex Valdoleto, .xviii. Decembris .M.D.XIII.

ep. 537 C = 540 A = 510 ms.   p. 541 G

Ludovico Furtato Mendocio

Ab orbe novo nuncios habemus. Vaschus Nuñez Balboa
manu promptorum favore, invitis magistratibus a Rege designatis, imperium sibi usurpavit in *Darienenses* Hispanos, eiecto
gubernatore Nicuessa et baccalario Anziso in carceres coniecto
5 (is erat iuris dicundi praetor). Balboa facinus adeo ingens aggressus est ac perfecit ut laesae maiestatis non modo veniam
fuerit assequutus, sed titulis onoratis insignitus. Fama didice-
rant, qui eas incolebant terras, esse trans montes altos, in ipsorum prospectu iacentes, mare aliud australe margaritis et auro
10 ditius; medios tamen reges sui iuris acres esse defensores, mille
propterea opus esse armatis hominibus ad illorum regum potentiam infringendam. Mittebatur ad eas vias ferro aperiendas
Petrus Arias, de quo supra, cum ea bellatorum manu. Interea,
dum sese apparant in Hispania, dum coguntur milites, dum
15 armantur, dum navigia construuntur, Vaschus Nuñez ille Balboa tantae rei fortunam tentare constituit. Centum nonaginta
viros ex Darienensibus coegit; in Kalendas Septembris anni

found whereas the low valleys under the all-embracing rays of the sun record intense heat all over, being either along or close to the line of the equator. Two colonies were founded in that land, one by Alfonso de Hojeda in the large gulf of Urabá, the other by Diego de Nicuesa in Veragua. Nicuesa reached Veragua with a fleet of 700 men and Hojeda Urabá with 400 men and Juan de La Cosa, a companion and most distinguished pilot expert of those shores. But all three, men of first rank, perished through ill fate and unfavorable omens, with most of their fellow soldiers experiencing various misfortunes. Someday we will publish special books about these discoveries, which, in my judgment, are more important and more extraordinary than those described by ancient cosmographers. For now, fare well!

From Valladolid, 18 December 1513

To Louis Hurtado de Mendoza

We have news from the new world. Vasco Núñez de < Balboa, with the support of some resolute men, against the opinion of the officials designated by the King, usurped command over the Spaniards in *Darién*, after driving out governor Nicuesa and imprisoning Enciso, who had the title of bachelor-at-arms being the magistrate in charge of administering justice. In so doing Balboa undertook and resolved such a great enterprise that not only was he given pardon for the charge of high treason, but was indeed covered with honors. Rumor reached our settlers living in these lands that across the high mountains in front of them there was another southern sea, richer in gold and pearls; however, the chiefs controlling the area in-between, were such fierce defenders of their right that it called for 1,000 armed men to break their power. Pedro Arias, of whom we spoke earlier, was dispatched in charge of soldiers to open those roads with weapons. But while preparations went on in Spain — gathering of soldiers, arms and

superioris .M.D.XIII iter capit: ferro partim, partim blanditiis
et nostratibus donis regulis pacatis, montes superat, mare salu-
20 tat. Petro Ariae ac sociis suis laborem illum atque una tantae
rei famam et gloriam surripuit. Mira scribuntur, quando certi
aliquid habebimus, scies. Ex Anglia scribitur regem illum esse
Caesari ac nostro Regi iratum, nuptiarum moram repudium
appellat. Regi Gallo despondisse sororem fertur nec placere
25 haec suis regnicolis. In Pannonia, *Ungaria* dico, (est et alia
Pannonia quae *Austria* dicitur) tumultus exortus est, ob cardinalem Strigonium. Qui, ex cruciata illis concessa in Turcas
a Pontifice, magnos dicitur coegisse cumulos pecuniarum, neque Ungaros ducat in Turcas, tali sese occasione oblata, Turco
30 implicito cum Sophio Persa ad quem traiecisse Taurum dicitur
in Armeniam, portis Caspiis aequatis, ita ut plaustris curribu-
sque commeatus et machinas trahentibus pateat iter. Ducentum
aiunt transmisisse bellatorum milia, certi adhuc nihil habemus:
scies quando sciemus. Ex Italia fertur Senenses a diversarum
35 partium factione pulsatos, extorres, tentasse reditum in patriam,
sed sua spe frustratos, moestos in exilium rediisse. Non desunt
qui credant quod favente Pontifice, eam sint provinciam aggressi. Sentiunt nanque alieno vivere Pontificem animo in Pan-
dulfos, urbis eius tyrannos. Vale!

Ex Valdoleto, .x. Kalendas Augusti .M.D.XIIII.

assembling the ships — Vasco Núñez de Balboa decided to test the fortune of so great an enterprise. He gathered 190 men from among the inhabitants of Darién; on the first of September of last year, 1513, he began the march and, having pacified the chieftains partly by the sword and partly by flatteries and gifts from our supplies, he crossed the mountains and reached the sea. He stole from Pedro Arias and his companions the toil as well as the glorious fame of so great an undertaking. Wonderful things are being written; when we have anything certain, you will know it. From England they write that that king, angry with the Emperor and with our King, views the delay of the wedding as a rejection. It is reported that he promised his sister in marriage to the King of France but that she was not liked by his subjects. In Pannonia, and I mean *Hungary* (there is another Pannonia which refers to *Austria*), an uproar broke out because of the Cardinal of Esztergom. He is said to have amassed huge riches from the crusade approved by the Pope against the Turks but did not lead the Hungarians against the Turks, although the occasion had presented itself being the Turks engaged with the Sophy of Persia, against whom it is reported that they had crossed the Taurus toward Armenia, having forced a passage in the direction of the Caspian Sea and thus opened the way for coaches and wagons carrying provisions and war equipment. It is claimed that they sent across two hundred thousand soldiers; presently nothing is sure; you will know it when we do. The report from Italy is that the exiled inhabitants of Siena, driven out by the various factions, did endeavor to return to their homes, but, disillusioned in their hopes, have gone back into exile with heavy hearts. There are some who believe they have done so with the support of the Pontiff, knowing for a fact that the Pontiff is hostile toward the Pandolfi, the lords of that city. Fare well!

From Valladolid, 23 July 1514

Ludovico Furtato Mendocio

E variis orbis partibus varia referuntur. Aperto Marte, Poloni Sarmathae censiti haeretici ab Ecclesia, in suum regem deducere illos ad Pontificis edicta nitentem arma sumpserunt et bis ad Borystenem fluvium, collatis signis, in eum certarunt. Conceptam
5 ab atavis superstitionem exuere cum vita volunt; utrinque iactura ingens oblata est, licet alterne se contriverint, suis tamen limitibus antiquis vivunt. Angliae regina peperit abortivum, ex concepta molestia ob discordiam viri et genitoris regum; prae nimio dolore, immaturum fertur eiecisse foetum. Exprobrabat innocenti reginae
10 vir patris eius desertionem et conquestus suos in eam expectorabat. Ab Urbe scribitur Iulianum, fratrem Pontificis, uxorem duxisse Sabaudiae ducis sororem. Distulerunt nostri, per Ioannem Vespucium, ad contrahendum nobiscum a Pontifice missum, rem concludere: sero sapimus aliquando. Ab orbe novo fertur habita-
15 tores Darienis aegrotos esse maiori ex parte, eo quod sedem in coenosi Darienis ripa primi elegerint atque circunsepti montibus sintque proximi aequinoctio: distant nanque gradus tantum septem, unde meridianis perpendicularibus fere, montanisque rotantibus ad ima radiis feriuntur. Si collium tamen culmina vel
20 montium latera elegissent, qua a ventis detur perflare aerem, in alicuius nitidi fontis aut fluminis vicinia, Elisiae sunt terrae illae, si praesertim oceanum spectent. Egestas primos coegit ibi figere pedem, quia illuc applicati, pagum reperere ditem et commeatibus patriis refertum. *Cemaco* loci regulo vi armorum eiecto, pagum
25 ipsi occupavere neque, de loco mutando, unquam iniere consilium. Elvetii se totis viribus tutaturos Maximilianum ducem Gallis, foedera petentibus, responderunt. Inter nostros milites et Venetos in agro Patavino quaedam feruntur post fugatum a Robigo proregem accidisse: sub lingua immurmuratur, parum igitur,
30 aut fere nihil esse debet, aut nostris damno cedere, quandoquidem non aperte loquuntur. Rex noster, putans locorum mutationem ad sui morbi levamen profuturam, ex Valdoleto Methymnam concessit, curia in Valdoleto relicta; sequor illum ego quocunque proficiscatur. Processit in hydropisim, neque motu, neque quiete,
35 serpens malum minuitur. Vale!

Ex Methymna Campi, pridie Kalendas Ianuarii .M.D.XIIII.

From different parts of the world various news is reported. The Polish Sarmatians, considered heretics by the Church, declared war and took up arms against their monarch who was striving to have them comply with the commands of the Pontiff, and twice they fought against him in open battles by the river Boristene. They will give up their ancestral fanaticism only with their life; a great loss was suffered on both sides and, although they wore each other out, they still live within their ancient borders. The Queen of England has had a miscarriage, brought on by her distress over the discord between the kings, i.e. her husband and her father, owing to her unbearable sorrow she is said to have delivered a premature fetus. The husband blamed the innocent queen for the desertion of her father and kept voicing to her his complaints. From Rome they write that Giuliano, brother of the Pontiff, married the sister of the Duke of Savoy. Our men delayed the conclusion of the agreement through Giovanni Vespucci, sent by the Pontiff to deal with us; sometimes we learn of things too late. From the new world we hear that the inhabitants of < Darién are for the most part sick, because they in the first place chose to live on the swampy area of the Darién and, although surrounded by the mountains, they are very close to the equator, being only seven degrees away and thus hit almost perpendicularly by the noon sun whose rays shine from mountain peaks to the deepest areas. Had they chosen hill tops or mountain sides, near some clear spring or river, where the winds are replaced by gentle breeze, their lands would be *elisie*, especially if facing the ocean. Need forced the first settlers there, for, upon landing they found a rich village with all kind of resources in place. After driving out *Cemaco*, the village chief, by force of arms, they took over the district themselves and never considered moving to a new location. The Swiss have replied to the French request for an alliance, that they would defend duke Maximilian with all their forces. Some episodes are reported to have occurred between our soldiers and the Venetians, in the territory around Padua, after the viceroy was driven out of Rovigo: it is muttered under the

Ludovico Furtato Mendocio

De antiquo more, sanctam acturus hebdomadam Ieronymorum coenobium, nomine *Melioratam*, se Rex contulit, a Met-
hymma distans miliaria quinque, ab Ulmeto municipio duo
tamen. Inde licet invalidus, Ulmetum ipsum petiit, dehinc Aran-
5 dam Dorianam, unde Reginam misit in Aragoniam, ad eos
conventus in Monzonum convocandos. Ventosillam, exiguam
paucarum domorum rusticanam villam, tenet, silvas frequentans
cervorum causa. Ab Urbe sentitur ancipiti animo esse Pontificem Gallo ne, si quid accidit, ob Gallicae foeminae, ductae
10 a Iuliano in uxorem, contractam affinitatem, sit adhaesurus an
nostro, qui contrahere, per propinquum, aliquando distulit.
Parmam petit Pontifex et Placentiam urbes, ducatus Mediolani
primaria membra, quae Iulius, eius praedecessor, fuisse quondam exarcatus Ravennae brachia dicebat. Elvetii in suis con-
15 ventibus, quos crebro celebrant, super hoc Pontificis petito
deliberant. Quae illi statuent facere oportebit; in Fortunae rotae
culmine nunc sedent, clavum figant ne rota labatur! Inter Gallum et Anglum reges fama est ridendum quoddam accidisse
stratagema: familiarem suum, quem ex imo loco rex Anglus
20 evexit et ducem effecit, nomine *Charolus Brandon* in Galliam
repetitum sororem viduam misit cum literis ad regem Gallum,
velle se nuptui dare sororem isti eidem familiari scribens. Creditur ista minime scripsisse quo fierent, sed rex Gallus verba,
non animum regis Angli librans, ne, si vidua haec ad potentio-
25 rem aliquando principem deveniret, formidolosum aliquid pa-
riat, sui regis literas ostendi iubet. His suspectis ut hinc et

112

breath, and therefore it must be of little or no consequence, or a bad loss to our men, since they do not talk about it openly. Our King, thinking a change of residence would bring relief to his illness, has moved from Valladolid to Medina, leaving the court at Valladolid; I follow him wherever he goes. His hydropsy got worse, such advancing disease is neither lessened by moving around nor by resting. Fare well!

From Medina del Campo, 31 December 1514

To Louis Hurtado de Mendoza

Following an ancient tradition, the King went to spend Holy Week at *Mejorada*, monastery of the Friars of Saint Jerome, five miles away from Medina and only two from the municipality of Olmedo. From there, although in poor health, he went to Olmedo itself, and then to Aranda de Duero, from where he dispatched the Queen to Aragon to convene the *Cortes* at Monzón. He is staying in Ventosilla, a small country residence made up of few houses, often going deer hunting in the woods. From Rome we hear that the Pontiff, were something to happen, is unsure whether to remain allied with the King of France, for the sake of the relationship by Giuliano's marriage to the French woman, or with our King, who once, through a relative, put off a union. The Pontiff wants the cities of Parma and Piacenza, important parts of the duchy of Milan, which his predecessor Julius claimed to have been at one time arms of the exarchate of Ravenna. The Swiss weigh carefully this request of the Pontiff in their assemblies, which they often convene. It will be opportune to do what they decide; they now sit at the top of the wheel of Fortune: let them hammer in a nail to prevent the wheel from spinning! Rumor has it that between the kings of France and England a ridiculous trick took place: the King of England sent to France a friend by the name of *Charles Brandon*, whom he had raised from very humble origins to the rank of duke, to request in marriage his widowed sister with letters for the King of France indicating he wanted this friend to marry her. It is believed that he did

fratris, inde domini mandata exequantur ambo, imperat; rex genialem parari torum iubet, despondet et una ut coeant datur opera ne dissolvi ulterius queat matrimonii vinculum, si forte
30 poenituerit ea scripsisse. Ita inter reges vivitur, artes artibus deludunt. Ab orbe novo scribitur Petrum Ariam ad australe pelagus misisse Gasparem Moralem, familiarem suum, quo ad insulam tenderet ex littore a Vasco Nuñez Balboa, primo illius pelagi repertore visam, sed non aditam ob tempestuosum anni
35 tempus. Quam unionibus abundaret proximi continentis reguli professi fuerant. Ivit, renitentem insulae regulum armis debellavit. Centum armatorum peditum habebat Gaspar manum contra inermem, licet ferocem. Non fuit opus magno labore. Mitis effectus regulus, nostros hospitaliter suscepit. Atria dicunt esse
40 domus eius rege digna; fortunatissima est arboribus et frugibus ac silvestribus animalibus et volucribus insula. Unum tulit unionem; nucem aequans mediocrem is, ad hastam positus inter Darienenses, precio mille ducentorum castellanorum fuit venditus. Vale!

Ex Aranda Doriana, .iii. Nonas Aprilis .M.D.XV.

ep. 548 *C* = 551 *A* = 521 *ms.*   *pp.* 546-547 *G*

Marchioni Mondeiaris

Audi quam varia siderum sint consilia. Quis hoc crederet? Regionis huius vineta .xv. Kalendas Augusti concreta gelu sunt omnia, uvae deperditatae. Vis ut quae ab exteris habeantur, uti

not at all write such a request with the intention for it to happen but the King of France, weighing the words, rather than any intention, of the King of England, so that, should this widow come to marry a more powerful prince, she would not cause some terrible consequence, ordered the letters by the king to be shown to him. After reading them, he commanded that they both follow the mandates of, on the one side, a brother, and on the other, of his lord; the King orders that the nuptial bed be prepared, celebrates the union and makes every effort that it be consummated, so that the marriage be valid and not subject to dissolution later, in case the english king regretted having so requested. Such is life among kings: plots beset by counter plost. From the new world they write Pedro Arias dispatched Gaspar de Morales, one of his followers, in the direction of the southern sea, so as to reach the island seen from shore by Vasco Núñez de Balboa, the first < discoverer of that sea, but never visited by him because of a stormy season. The chiefs of the neighboring continent had given assurance as to the island's abundance of pearls. He went with weapons and defeated the island's chief who was resisting. Gaspar had a formation of 100 equipped foot-soldiers against an unarmed, although ferocious chieftain. It was an effortless situation wherein the chief's attitude was changed and he received our men in a hospitable way. They report that his houses are palaces worthy of a king; the island is very rich in trees, harvests, wild animals, and birds. He brought a single pearl, of modest size resembling a nut: it was sold at auction among the inhabitants of Darién for the price of 1,200 *castelanos*. Fare well!

From Aranda de Duero, 3 April 1515

To the Marquis of Mondéjar
(Luis Hurtado de Mendoza)

Listen how varied is the influence of the stars. Who would believe it? The vineyards of this region were all frozen on July 18 and the grapes completely destroyed. You would like

patri tuo quondam, tibi significem. Non abnuo, quandoquidem
illius loco te sum habiturus suxerisque tu et meas literales
mamillas; hoc primum ad urbem Romam familiarem meum,
Orduñae capillati mei, qui tibi aliquando porrexit ientaculum
addiscenti apud me, fratrem, iuris peritum, qui me a Romanu-
sculis cavillationibus tueatur, misi. Litigiosae quaedam mihi
contentiones exortae sunt. Habebis egregium procuratorem, si
quid tibi negocii acciderit in Urbe. Dicitur licentiatus *Aguiñiga*.
Ad aliena pergamus. In Laurentino, Pontificis nepote, qui patrui copiis praeest, apertiora in dies apparent diversi animi
a nostris signa. Inde colligunt Pontificis animum alium esse
quam polliceatur. Per licentiatum illum meum, ad Pontificem
direxi de orbe novo pauca. Habebit aliquando plura. De particularibus hisce inventis libellos cudo; prodibunt si vixerimus.
Elvetii Lamparosam[24] vallem in Alpibus occupant, ea putant
Gallos tentaturos transitum. Aiunt perempta fuisse Vasconum
et reliquorum militum Gallorum milia decem, qui, subsequenti
exercitui ut viam aperirent tutaque redderent itinera praemissi,
fuerant. Forti animo tenent Elvetii angustias illas Alpium;
propterea quaesituros putant Gallos aliunde traiectum. Deter-
rent ab his inceptis Galli regem suum, difficultates et pericula,
maiorumque suorum exempla illi proponunt, argumentis eum
divertere ab hac provincia nituntur. Trivultius autem et reliqui,
extorres a patria, patriae ipsi calamitosi cives, iuvencm rcgem
stimulis adigunt, laudis et supinae illi gloriae munia enarrant,
retrocedere ostendunt esse ignominiosum, difficultates non esse
eas, quas meticulosi putant. Foederatos nunquam conventuros,
suspectos esse alterne omnes, Elvetios non esse uti solebant
unanimes, Galli regis exercitum potentem esse ad infringendas
totius orbis vires, iuveni regi persuadent. Ita trahunt iuvenis
animum in diversa. Processurum putamus, quia magnanimus
est et gloriae cupidus. Ita, prae intestinis odiis Guelforum et
Gibellinorum, sata semina Tartarea ex barbaris in barbaros,
Italiam ipsimet Itali dilacerandam coniiciunt. Rex noster, non
is qui solebat, est conversus ex Phoebeio, alacri et placido in
rabidum, ob infirmitatem, quae illum in dies magis ac magis

---

[24] This locality cannot be geographically identified: it could be the Lucerne valley
where a number of war-related events took place. It cannot be ruled but, however, that
Peter Martyr might have created such denomination on the basis of the Spanish adjective
lamparoso (from *lampara*) i.e. lamp.

me to share with you, as I did before with your father, the news from abroad. I do not refuse, since you are to replace him and because you too have been nourished by my teaching; for this reason, I first sent to Rome one of my followers, expert in law and brother of my young man from Orduña, who served you breakfast once when you were studying with me, so that he might defend me in captious questions at Rome. Some litigious disputes faultfinding me have arisen. You will have a most distinguished lawyer, were you to run into problems in Rome. His name is Doctor *Aguiñiga*. Let us proceed to other topics. Lorenzo, the Pontiff's nephew and in charge of his uncle's troops, shows daily more evident signs of a way of thinking opposite to ours. Therefore the implication is that the attitude of the Pontiff differs from his promises. Through my lawyer friend, I sent the Pontiff some news about the new world. Eventually he will have more of it about these discove- <
ries specifically I am compiling small books; they will be published, if I live. The Swiss occupy the Lamparosa valley in the Alps, where it is thought the French will try to cross. They say that 10,000 Gascons and other French soldiers, who had been sent ahead to open the way for the army marching behind them and to make it safe, have been slain. With great courage the Swiss occupy those narrow Alpine passes; still there is a belief that the French may seek to cross in another place. The French who try to dissuade their king from this undertaking, present him with difficulties, dangers and the examples of their forefathers argue to abandon this province. But then exiled people like Trivulzio and others, citizens pernicious to their own country, goad on the young king, underscoring the duties of fame and in the name of higher glory point out it is shameful to withdraw and that presumed difficulties are inexistent. They persuade the young king that the confederates will never agree, that they are all suspicious of each other, that the Swiss are not as unified as they used to be, that the army of the French king is able to annhilate all armies. Thus they draw the young man in opposite directions. We think that he will go forward, because he is ambitious and eager for glory. Similarly, because of internal hatreds between the Guelphs and the Ghibellines, the Italians themselves, like infernal seeds scattered everywhere cast Italy into the ruinous hands of greedy barbarians. Our King is not what he used to be: from hand-

40 gravat. Revocatum ex Aragonicis conventibus suum vicecancellarium, cum summa iussit ignominia capi ac duci ad oppidum Simancas, a Valdoleto lequas distans duas; quid causae
alias, nunc vale!

Ex Aranda, .xvii. Kalendas Septembris .M.D.XV.

ep. 557 C = 560 A = 530 ms.   p. 552 G

Marchioni Mondeiaris

Veh tibi, veh Hispania! Vita functus est Gonsalus ille
Fernandus Aquilaris a Corduba, *Magnus Imperator* antonomasice
ac iure merito appellatus, qui nomen tuum, primus, hac tempestate super astra locavit. Latuisti hactenus Hispania et tuorum
5 virtus militum sopita iacebat; eo alumno, tuo duce, o Hispania,
famam aeternam consecuta es. Is est a facie terrae ad Superos
revocatus, qui, more torrentis, obvia quaeque sternebat. Quae
gesserit, quando bellorum turbinibus implicabatur Neapoli, ex
meis ad te variosque tuae conditionis principes epistolis licet
10 colligere. Quartana illum rapuit in Kalendas Decembris; medicorum properata diligentia finem eius maturasse creditur. Regi
nuncium vehementer fuit molestum aut fuisse visum est: scru-
tator cordium Deus est solus. Fuit nanque viri eius magnani-
mitas aliquando Regi suspecta; vivere propterea illum in secessu
15 ociosum patiebatur. De hoc satis, licet nunquam satis. Ab Urbe,
gloriabundum nescio quid de me scripsit, procurator meus
licentiatus Martinus de Aguiñiga, Orduñae Cantabriae oriundus,
quem in Urbem impensamet mea sustineo ad litium tempe-
stuosas procellas. Pontifex, quo die sancti Michaelis solemne
20 agitur, sorori convivae cardinalibusque plaerisque ipse ipse
libellos quosdam, ex mea officina emissos, de orbe novo reci-
tavit cum summa laude de me, quod eam sumpserim provinciam, ne tam praeclara inventa in rapacis oblivionis fauces
collabantur. Ab orbe novo magna feruntur, maioraque in dies
25 expectantur. Appulso Petro Aria, missus est ad insulam Ditem,
ad australe pelagus, per Vascum Nuñez nuper repertum, Gaspar

118

some, cheerful and content Apollo he has become irritable daily because of an evermore weakening disease. He recalled his vice chancellor from the *Cortes* of Aragon and dishonorably ordered that he be taken and brought to the city of Simancas, two leagues from Valladolid; for what reason, I will tell you another time. For now, fare well!

From Aranda de Duero, 16 August 1515

To the Marquis of Mondéjar
(Luis Hurtado de Mendoza)

Woe to you, Spain! For the death of your famous Gonzalo Fernández de Aguilár of Córdoba, known by antonomasia and by right as the *Grand Captain* who first, in our time, placed your name above the stars. Up to his time, Spain, you had remained in obscurity and the valor of your soldiers lay dormant; under the leadership of this son of yours, Spain, you have obtained eternal fame. He, who, like a torrent used to sweep away everything in his way, has been called from earth to heaven. From my letters to you and several rulers of your rank, one can realize what he accomplished when he was drawn into the turmoil of war at Naples. In early December he was struck by quartan fever; we think the solicitous care of the doctors hastened his end. The news very much annoyed the King, or at least it seemed that way: God alone can fathom men's soul. The King was at times in fact suspicious of the magnanimity of this man; therefore he allowed him to live at leisure in a secluded place. Enough said on this topic, even if it is never so. From Rome my lawyer, Doctor Martín de Aguiñiga, originally from Orduña, Cantabria, whom I keep at my expense to defend me in the strong confrontations with Rome, has written something — I know not exactly what — about me, which fills me with pride. The Pontiff himself, on the day we celebrate the feast of Saint Michael, read to the sister who was a guest and to a large number of cardinals certain books that I wrote about the new world; he had great praise for me since I had taken on this task so that such

Morales, Petri Ariae familiaris: cum peditibus septuaginta ivit, cum regulo quater pugnavit; amicitiam, vicinis eam petentibus, inierunt. Dies egerunt ibi lautos quosdam, abundat nanque
30 leporibus et cuniculis caeterisque silvestribus quadrupedibus et volucribus insula, iure merito *Dives* appellata. Mutuis se muneribus colligarunt nostratibus calculis vitreis et tintinnabulis, aliqua etiam forte securi regulum donarunt. Compensat regulus muneribus munera, centum decem unionum libras octunciales
35 nostris impartitus est, fecitque se lubens Regi nostro tributarium annuarum centum librarum unionum. Res de unionibus famam superat. Diversi etiam centuriones, per diversas eius vastae telluris regiones tetenderunt indagatum. Quae afferent, habebis. Darienis aerem effectum esse aiunt salubriorem, quod
40 nemora silvasque adumbrantes oppidum disciderint; suffocatam nimium et opacam vallem arborum densitas detinebat, neque flatibus ventorum aerem purgantibus locus erat ullus. Vale!

Ex Madrito, quinto (Nonis) Decembris .M.D.XV.

ep. 558 C = 561 A = 531 *ms.*   *pp.* 552-553 G

Marchioni Bellecensi

Per illustrem oppidum Talaveram, dehinc Oropessam, Casataiatam et Valparaisum, post Torillum et Malpartitam, pervenimus Plasentiam, cum horrido ventorum et tonitruum procelloso nimbo, qui nos, ex insperato, repente, inter Torillum
5 et proximum flumen *de las Barcas* appellatum, adortus est. Alia via, venando, Rex paulatim advenit. Non citius venit quam cito discedere cogitavit, loca esse valitudinis suae causam imaginatus. Secessit ad Ducis Albae villam, quae dicitur *Abadia*; sub praetextu cervorum insectandorum, sub dio esse cupit
10 semper, abhorret a tecto. Ibi suscepit libens a nostro principe,

important discoveries would not slip into the rapacious jaws of oblivion. From the new world we receive great news, and even greater news is expected by the day. Once Pedro Arias landed, he dispatched Gaspar de Morales, one of his followers, < to the island of *Rica*, in the southern sea recently discovered by Vasco Nuñez: he went with 70 foot-soldiers and fought four times with a chieftain; they entered into friendship with the neighbors who asked for it. They spent some happy days there, because the island, rightly called *Rica* [rich], abounds in hares, rabbits, other wild creatures and birds. They sealed their friendship with an exchange of gifts; they gave the chief home-made glass marbles and bells, and even, by chance, some axes. Exchanging gifts with gifts, he distributed to our men 110 pounds of eight-ounce pearls and graciously paid a tribute to our King of 100 pounds of pearls a year. The reality concerning pearls actually exceeds all claims. Several other military commanders explored diverse areas of that vast land. You will have what they report back. They say that the climate in Darién is healthier, since they cut down tree groves and woodlands that shaded the city; the density of the trees kept the valley so stifled and dark and prevented the breeze flows which purify the air. Fare well!

From Madrid, 5 December 1515

To the Marquis of Los Vélez

After crossing the famous city of Talavera and then Oropesa, Casatejada and Valparaiso, and after that Torillo and Malpartida, we reached Plasencia in such a stormy blast of winds and thunder, which arose suddenly and unexpectedly between Torillo and the nearby river *Rio de la Barcas*. The King arrived with more ease by another route, having gone hunting. No sooner did he arrive than he quickly thought of leaving, blaming that place as the cause of his ill health. He retired to *Abadia*, the villa of the Duke of Alba, with the excuse of going deer hunting, he prefers always the outdoors

nepote suo Carolo, venientem oratorem. Is *Adrianus Traiectinus*
dicitur, vir gravis, prima senecta venerandus, Principis ipsius
praeceptor. Salutavi hominem, tractavi nondum. Bonum esse
ac literarum disciplina egregium audiveramus. Quantum licet
15 colligere, utriusque dotis et probitatis et doctrinae argumenta
prae se fert. Cuius et quanti sit ponderis tempus deteget. De
principe iam quindecenne quid sperandum sit, scrutabimur.
Lovaniae est hic orator academiae princeps, quem *decanum* dicunt. Ab exteris fertur Elvetios animo pervicaci, ut Galli pel-
20 lantur, vivere. Caesarem hortantur ut provinciam ducatus su-
mat. Triginta milia Elvetiorum, suamet impensa, conventura
offerunt, modo velit ipsorum postulatis annuere. Haud secus
ac si Caesareo stipendio essent merituri, se obtemperaturos
Caesari pollicentur. Galli regis oratores audiunt, auscultant
25 minime. Guilielmus, Bavariae dux, imperatorio nomine, cum
ignominia, Venetorum copias e Veronensi agro reppulit. Caesaris est is dux ex sorore nepos, egregius animo iuvenis. Rege
adhuc in ea villa moram trahente, miserunt ab orbe novo
Darienenses nuncium Henricum Colmenarem, de quo alias,
30 stemmata petitum, quibus noscat posteritas primos eius terrae
incolas honoratos titulos promeruisse: in scuto viridi castellum
auratum, cum depictis, in eo, a dextris leone, a sinistris autem
tigride, scutum sustinentibus, illos ornavit Rex. Circumeunt
autem scutum quattuor sagittarum totidemque arcuum mani-
35 puli. Rex autem, uti aiunt qui ad nos veniunt nuncii Palatini,
delectatus est, venatus fortuna secunda. Cervos nanque plures,
inquiunt, regia manu, sagitta tamen fuisse transfixos. Vale,
melius quam Rex valeat!

Plasentiae, pridie Idus Decembris .M.D.XV.

122

thus avoiding, staying inside. Here he willingly received an ambassador, coming on behalf of our prince, his nephew Charles. His name is *Adrian of Utrecht*, a serious man, worthy of respect for his upcoming old age, teacher of the Prince himself. I greeted the man, but I have not dealt with him yet. We have heard he is honest and renowned for his literary knowledge. As far as one can tell, he offers proof of both qualities, probity and learning. Time will disclose the degree and quality of his influence. We will try to find out what can be hoped from a prince by now fifteen years old. This ambassador, whom they call *dean*, is the highest member of the Louvain Academy. From abroad we hear that the Swiss persist in driving away the French while encouraging the Emperor to assume governance of the dukedom. They propose to assemble at their own expense 30,000 Swiss, provided he would consent to their demands. They promise to obey the Emperor no differently than if they had been hired with his money. The ambassadors of the French king hear them without paying any attention. William, Duke of Bavaria, in the name of the Emperor, has dishonorably driven back the Venetian troops from the territory of Verona. This duke, a young man of remarkable character, is the nephew of the Emperor by his sister. While the King still lingered at the < villa, the settlers of Darién sent a messenger from the new world, Enrique de Colmenares — of whom I spoke on another occasion — to ask for coat-of-arms by which their descendants would know that the first dwellers of that land were granted heraldic bearings. The King did award a coat of arms: a golden castle on a green blazon, with a lion to the right and a tiger to the left bearing a shield; four bundles of arrows and as many bows surround the shield. In the meantime the King is happy, as messengers who come to us from the palace tell us, because he has had good luck hunting. Indeed they claim that many deer have been downed by arrows from the royal hand. Be well, better than the King is!

Placencia, 12 December 1515

Leoni papae X

Quom incidissent in scripta quaedam mea, Galleatius Butrigarius, hic pro tua Sanctitate et Ioannes Cursius, pro sua Florentina republica, oratores, de orbe novo, placitura Tuae Sanctitati, si quando ad eius manus deveniet, mihi si-
5 gnificarunt. Eo suasu calamum resumpsi desidem effectum, persuasoribus ut ea colligerem deficientibus. Nostri agelli primiciae ad Te, Petri vicarium, in terris, deserebantur, cui rerum omnium decimae ac primiciae debentur; intercepit eas Gallus una cum viatoribus et latoribus ipsis. Successiva illis
10 habuit Tua Sanctitas, per meum familiarem licentiatum Aguiñigam, quem isthic mea impensa teneo contra Tuae Sanctitatis curiae litigiosos perturbatores. Ea relatum est Sanctitatem Tuam ipsam ipsam, Cardinalibus plaerisque et amata sorore astantibus, amota mensa, serena fronte, ad lassitudinem usque
15 legisse universa. Licet, angusta dextera, Tua Sanctitas mecum egerit, Catholici Regis postulata de me reiiciens, in *Reservarum supplicatione*, nuncio tamen eo delectatus, archetypis rerum earum e latebris scrinialibus extractis, transcribere illa feci et quo intercipientium iniurias vitarent, quo velate ista vagentur,
20 quae nova sunt et miranda, impressorum typis cudenda commendari permisi, id ita pertinaciter mihi persuadente Antonio Nebrissense Hispano, viro, erudito, qui Bononiae literalia suxit ubera. Si quid, in his quae ex nostra prodeunt officina, reperietur gustui doctorum sapidum, Tuae Beatitudini gratiae
25 debentur, cuius causa labor sumptus est, licet prima rerum frons, id est e tribus decadibus prima, diversos nacta sit autores, temporum curriculis id exigentibus. Vadit una *Babilonica Legatio* mea, ad Sanctitatem Tuam praefatione praeeunte, per quam intelliget an creditum mihi talentum in religione nostra
30 suffoderim, an duplicaverim.[25] Valeat Beatitudo Tua, ante cuius pedes sacros, animo, si nequeo corpore, stratus, me illi obnoxium perpetuo futurum polliceor. De Catholici Regis adversa valitudine nil scribo, quia sentio reverendum Archie-

---

[25] Peter Martyr's recalls the gospel's parable. See Vulg. Mt. 35, 14-30.

To Pope Leo X
(Giovanni de' Medici)

Since some reports about the new world were part of my writings, ambassadors Galeazzo Butrigario, representing Your Holiness, and Giovanni Corsi, representing the Florentine republic, indicated to me that those writings would please Your Holiness, if they ever heard of them. Persuaded by that advice I took up the pen again, which had become inactive when I lacked people urging me to compile the news. The first fruits of my small "labor" were given over to You, Vicar of Peter on earth, to whom tithing and first fruits of all things are due. The French king intercepted them, together with messengers and bearers themselves. Later reports Your Holiness has received through my dear friend Doctor Aguiñiga, whom I keep at my expense to confront the litigious agitators at the court of Your Holiness. It has been reported that Your Holiness himself read undisturbed, in the presence of most cardinals and of your beloved sister, and after the dinner table was cleared, all these news until weary. Although Your Holiness dealt with me with limited generosity, rejecting the demands of the Catholic King concerning me in the *Supplication of the Reserves*, nevertheless, delighted by that report, I took out the originals of those writings from my desk and had them transcribed, and in order to prevent that these new and wonderful things might avoid the indiscretion of interceptors or travel in secrecy, I authorized a publisher to print them on account of the fact that Anthony de Nebrija, a learned Spanish man who studied letters at Bologna, persistently urged me to do so. If there is anything coming out of my writings appealing to the taste of the learned, Your Beatitude is to be thanked because for your sake this task was undertaken, although the first part of this work, that is, the first of the three *Decades*, had found other supporters as time-related needs dictated. My *Legatio Babylonica* is appearing in the same volume, with a prefaced foreword dedicated to Your Holiness, thanks to which you shall understand whether I have buried or doubled the talent entrusted to me as per our religion. May Your Beatitude stay well, with my promise to be always obedient

piscopum Cusentinum, legatum tuae sedis apostolicae, late
40 cuncta significare.

Ex Guadalupe, septimo Kalendas Ianuarii .M.D.XV.

ep. 624 *C* = 623 *A* = 591 *ms.* pp. 581-582 *G*

Marchionibus

Iam res acta est de puella regina Leonora: vetulo regi,
Iulii die xiii, illam desponsavit. Regia corona ornata, prodivit
in publicum, honoratius esse regi, quam principi, nuptam per-
suasa. Unum et viginti milia ducatorum, precium sanguinis
5 virginei, per Galvanum Senensem mercatorem, trapezitam Valdoletanum, iam municipalem a multis annis, in Flandriam, ut
Galvanus ipse mihi rettulit, Guillelmus de Croi, dictus *Xebres*,
mavis latine *Caper*, misit. Hae fuerunt pecuniae ab oratore
Portugallico publice numeratae; quid de missis in archanis? De
10 Capro educatore satis. Ab Indis nova multa feruntur; civitates
repererunt Hispani, ab insula *Cuba*, quae *Fernandina* dicitur,
discedentes ad occidentem, meridionaliter tamen: in quibus
vivitur legibus mercimoniaque tractantur et induuntur. Libros
habent, interiectis lineatim regum et idolorum imaginibus, ut
15 apud nos videmus chalcographos historiales sive fabulosos or-
nare figuris codices, quo magis emptores alliciant. Vias stratas,
ex lapidibus et calce constratas domos et atria magnifica, templa
etiam egregia, ubi Zemibus, nocturnos lemures aemulantibus,
litant humanis victimis. Pueros puellasque, servos etiam precio
20 emptos, quotannis iugulant innumeros. Ad particulares de his
inventis narrationes, caetera remitto. Ex putato continenti feruntur unionum saepe numero cumuli; sunt iam edocti publi-
cani omnes quaestores neophitaeque de horum Gallorum et
Flamingorum familiarium studiis in rapiendo; uti sagaces odori
25 canes, quacunque quid emergat, olfacere invigilant. Cum quid
detegunt, ad Flamingos et Gallos hos certatim procurrunt, de
his quae cognoverunt faciunt certiores, partem de praeda illis

126

and prostrated in spirit at your holy feet, as I cannot do so physically. I do not write anything else about the ill health of the Catholic King, for I am aware that the Reverend Archbishop of Cosenza, legate of your apostolic see, relates extensively to this effect.

From Guadalupe, 26 December 1515

To the Marquises
(Pedro Fajardo – Luis Hurtado de Mendoza)

It is all over now for young Queen Eleanora: she was married to the old king on the thirteenth of July. She appeared in public wearing the royal crown, convinced that it is more honorable to be married to a king than to a prince. Guillaume de Croy, called *Chèvre*, *Caper* in Latin, if you prefer, sent 21,000 ducats — the price for virgin blood — to Flanders through the Sienese merchant Galvano, a banker and a citizen of Valladolid for many years, who told me this himself. The money was counted publicly by the ambassador of Portugal; what < happened to the money sent secretly? Enough about preceptor *Caper*. Many new things are reported from the Indies; the Spaniards have discovered some cities, setting out from the island of Cuba, called Fernandina, heading west and south: in these cities they live according to laws, conduct trade and wear clothes. They have books with images of kings and idols inserted between the lines, just as among us we see engravers decorating with figures, both historical and mythological, manuscripts, so as to attract more buyers. They have smooth roads, houses built with stone and lime, magnificent buildings and outstanding temples, where they offer human sacrifices to the *Zemi*, who resemble night ghosts. Every year they slaughter countless boys and girls, and even slaves who have been bought. For detailed accounts of these discoveries, I defer to other reports. Heaps of pearls are brought back from what is thought to be a continent; all the treasury's tax officials, even the neophytes, are now informed of the intentions of these friends of the French and of the Flemish to take things; like

127

pollicentur. Si a rege rem illam impetrarint, ad regem res defertur; facilius assentitur, quam ipsi postulent. Sunt arpiarum,
30 apud infoelicem iuvenem versantium, adeo rapaces ungues,
quod neque succum aut medullam illi relinquant. Cur haec tam
longa oratione protulerim, audite. Libras unionum, dicitis *perlas*,
centum sexaginta, uti fertur, attulerunt, ab Indis nostris occidentalibus, octunciales, de regis quinta collectas. Xebrica uxor,
per odoros neophitas monita, priusquam portarentur, impu-
35 denter illas poposcit; postulatas rapuit, neque regi videre tantum illas licuit, neque nubenti sorori vel unam ex illis unciolam
servavit. Sub hoc tenore cuncta procedunt. Valete!

Ex Augusta Caesarea, .xii. Kalendas Augusti .M.D.XVIII.

ep. 630 *C* = 629 *A* = 597 *ms.*   *p.* 584 *G*

Marchionibus

Christiani principes dormiunt, Selimsachus [26] vigilat solus
et vicina perturbat. Vafro est usus stratagemate. Rex Pannonus,
Ungarum dico, miserat eum salutatum congratulatamque victoriam, per oratores. Quod non tulerit in mandatis, de amicitia
5 ineunda, se moleste tulisse dissimulavit, suasitque oratori ut
hoc suo regi consulat, datque literas ad pacem et amicitiam
invitantes, quo securum reddat regem, ut imparatum queat
adoriri. Interea, per celeres tabellarios, praesidiariis confinium
praefectis imperat ut incursionibus Pannoniam infestent. Heri
10 mandatum executi sunt praefecti. Septem dierum itinere terram
vastarunt, in praedam, quidquid fuit obvium, dedere. Apud

[26] From *Selim šāh*: the Persian term used officially in chanceries to indicate the
Sovereign.

128

dogs with a fine sense of smell, they carefully sniff whereever a clue comes to the surface. The instant something is detected they competitively run to these French and Flemish, to inform them of what they have found, for a promised share of the booty. If they want to obtain something from the king, the matter is referred to him as he concedes more easily than they themselves may expect. The harpies' claws on the unhappy youth are so rapaciously greedy that no juice or marrow is spared. Listen to why I have brought these matters forth in a long discourse. They have brought from our West Indies, so it is told, 160 pounds of eight-ounce pearls as you refer to them, coming from the fifth of the king. The wife of Chèvre, advised by the keen-scented neophytes, impudently demanded them before they were brought; after her demand was satisfied she made them disappear, the king did not have a chance to see them or be able to save at least a twelfth part of them for his sister who is about to get married. Everything proceeds in this fashion. Fare well!

From Saragossa, 21 July 1518

To the Marquises
(Pedro Fajardo – Luis Hurtado de Mendoza)

The Christian princes sleep; the Sultan Selim alone keeps watch and disturbs his neighbors. He made use of a shrewd trick. The king of Pannonia, I mean Hungary, had sent ambassadors to greet and congratulate him upon his victory. The sultan did not led them on to his annoyance for the fact that in the messages there was no proposed friendship and persuaded, however, an ambassador to consult his king on this while giving him a letter promoting peace and friendship, so as to reassure the king that he would not attack him by surprise. At the same time, through speedy dispatchers, he ordered the governors in charge of the borders to attack Hungary with incursions. Yesterday the governors carried out his command. On a march of seven days they devastated the land and plundered everything in their way. Near Brescia there is a valley

Brixiam est valiis altis circunsepta montibus: ex crassis illius
vaporibus ob solis carentiam, est opinio generatum iri spiritus
varios; si de necromantia quid est credendum, daemonum opera
15 putantur eius vallis incolae uti ad veneficia. Magos magasque
deprehenderunt multos, octoginta combusserunt. Infantes peremisse innumeros, aerem terrasque, turbinibus et nimbis inso-
lentibus, saepe in regionum perniciem commovisse cum gran-
dinibus et horrendis typhonibus confessi sunt. Putant hac dira
20 contagione infectam esse provinciam universam. Ad nos. In
nostro senatu regio, de rebus Indicis conclusum est debere mitti
classem quae insulas, aromatum genitrices, perquirant. Duobus
transfugis Portugalensibus, a suo rege discedentibus, qui vicinas
earum terras longo tempore tractarunt, est provincia credita.
25 In Callecuto, Canenoro, Cochino et Mellaca, quam putant multi
Auream esse *Chersonesum*, horum alter septennio versatus est,
ad quarum urbium nundinas et fora venum ab illis insulis
aromata comportantur. Quattuor et viginti milia ducatorum
sunt, ad classem hanc instruendam, destinata. Si fauste res
30 successerit, Orientalibus et Portugalio regi commercia interci-
piemus aromatum et gemmarum, animos hominum effoeminantium. Fernandus Magallanes est primario nomen, Rodericus
Falerius alter: hic astronomiae peritiam profitetur. Ad alia.
Mortuo Magno Cancellario, suffectus est Mercurinus de Gatti-
35 nera, vir eruditus et iure consultus, longo tempore Burgundi
senatus princeps, et anno .M.D.X. ad Catholicum Regem Fer-
nandum, pro Maximiliano Caesare proque rege nostro Carolo,
dum puer esset, orator: iustus est et integer. Spero quae pro-
strata inter Scyllam iacent et Caribdim, huius consiliis resusci-
40 tatum iri, modo viam inveniat, qua de huius classis rectoribus
sciat evadere, ne ab eis suffocetur; tempus loquetur. Valete!

Ex Augusta Caesarea, .xv. Kalendas Octobris .M.D.XVIII.

surrounded by high mountains: from its dense vapors caused by lack of sunlight, various ghosts are believed to come alive; should anyone believe in black magic, the inhabitants of this valley are thought to use the devil's help for poisonings. They have captured many sorcerers and witches and have burned 80 of them, who confessed to have done away with countless children, often disturbing air and earth with whirlwinds and unusual storms, and to have brought ruin to those regions with hail and terrible hurricanes. The thinking is that the entire province was infected by this frightful contagion. Now, let us talk about us. Concerning matters of the Indies, it was decided in our Royal Council that a fleet should be sent to explore <
spice-producing islands. The enterprise has been entrusted to two Portuguese deserters, estranged from their king and who, for a long time, had been living in neighboring lands. One of them lived for seven years in Calicut, Cannanore, Cochin and Malacca, which some think to be the *Golden Chersonese*; the spices of those islands are brought to the markets and squares of those cities to be sold. 24,000 ducats have been allotted to prepare this fleet. If successful, this enterprise shall deprive the Orientals and the king of Portugal of effeminating products such as spices and gems and of their commerce. The name of one of the commanders is Ferdinand Magellan, the other is Ruy Faleiro: the latter displays knowledge of astronomy. About other topics. After the death of the Grand Chancellor, Mercurino da Gattinara took his place, a learned man and a jurisprudent, for a long time president of the senate of Burgundy and, in 1510, ambassador to the Catholic King Ferdinand for Emperor Maximilian and for our King Charles while he was a boy: he is a just and honest man. I hope that what lies listless between Scylla and Charybdis can be rejuvenated by his advice, provided it finds a way to escape the commanders of this "fleet," so as to not be suffocated by them; time will tell. Fare well!

From Saragossa, 17 September 1518

Marchionibus

Ab Indis et putato continenti proximis insulis, preciosi crebro afferuntur uniones. Sed quid Regi aut Hispanis tanti autoribus inventi prodest? Priusquam terram capiant in littoribus Hispanis, illos hi regii gurgites, ut caetera emergentia, olfaciunt; odoris canibus Hispanis plena sunt omnia regnorum loca, nil pullulat, a quo extorqueri possent opes quin mille accurrant satellites, arte iam intellecta, Gallis et Belgis rem significantes, quo ipsi partem assequantur: qui primus regem adit, is primus praedam rapit; facilius, quidquid petunt, rex condonat, quam ipsi petere audeant. Xebrensis vetula rapuit, primo certior effecta, unionum libras octunciales sexaginta, plures alii dicunt; sed auditu est rabiosum ut iam ementes ab eis et sacra et profana, in monetamque ipsam spuant, si duplicibus et quadruplicibus ducatis simplex aliquis vetus praecipue nitentibus et decoris immisceatur, ut ipsi iocose contumelioseque garriunt. De comitiis, mavis curiis Aragonicis, nil est ultra quod referam. Peracta sunt omnia, peracta est et spes Regis de donativo: gravamina illi de manibus partem rapuerunt maiorem. Si quid restitit, foeneratorum sitis id omne corrosit. Duodecies centena milia ducatorum, nos qui Regem secuti sumus, in hoc regno reliquimus. Sunt qui me stricte calculasse aiunt, quindecies amplius multi putant, ex misera Castella cuncta importata. Aragones ditavit, ditabit et Laletanos Rex, apud quos est rerum penuria dutior. In Ilerda aurato flumine Sicori, et Petrei atque Afranii fato Romanorum ducum, a Caesare in eius agro obsessorum, nobili urbe, sumus.[27] Hic, per incertam famam, relatum est Maximilianum Caesarem vita functum. A classe nostra, cuius est praefectus Ugus Moncada, fertur naufragii reliquias esse in insula Ebuso (dicit vulgus *Ibizam*), salinis egregiis notam. Tumultibus student milites, neque obolus illis praebetur; iam insulam universam depopulati sunt, fame adacti. Armenti aut gregis pecus iam Ebusanis restat nullum, nec quid comedant aut quid serant, uti ipsi conqueruntur.

---

[27] Peter Martyr's reference is to the long resistence encountered by Caesar at Ilerda, Spain by the hands of L. Afranius and M. Petreius, Pompeius's two trustworthy lieutenants, (see Caes. *bell. civ.* I 41 ff.; Lucan. IV 144, 261).

To the Marquises

(Pedro Fajardo – Luis Hurtado de Mendoza)

From the Indies and the islands near to what is thought to <
be a continent, precious pearls are often brought back. But with
what benefit to the King or the Spaniards, authors of so great
a discovery? Before these [pearls] touch the Spanish shores, these
royal sewers smell them out, as they do with anything emerging;
the entire kingdom is full of Spanish hounds with a keen sense
of smell; nothing potentially profitable can sprout without a thousand gangsters, who with remarkable cunning, run right to inform
the French and Belgians, so as to obtain a share for themselves;
he who first reaches the king, first seizes the booty; the king
gives permission for whatever they ask more easily than they
themselves would dare ask. Chèvre's old lady, having been
informed first, took 60 pounds of eight-ounce pearls, others say
more; it is indeed infuriating to hear that, as one buys from them
sacred and profane objects, they would spit on the very money if
any simple old ducat were to be mixed with the shiny and
beautiful ones worth two or four times as much, as they, jokingly
and injuriously claim. Concerning the assemblies, or Aragonese
Cortes if you prefer, there is nothing more to tell. Everything is
over; ended too is the hope of a King's donative: debts took
most of it from his hands. If anything remained, the greed of the
usurers has eaten it all away. We who have followed the King
have left in this kingdom 1,200,000 ducats. There are some who
say I computed the amount rigorously; others think it is fifteen
times more, all brought in from unfortunate Castile. The king,
who made the Aragonese rich, will do the same with Catalans
among whom poverty is harsher. We are at Lérida, a city famous
for its golden river Sicori and for the fate of Afranius and
Petreius, Roman commanders besieged by Caesar in his territory.
Here, an unreliable report, has it that Emperor Maximilian is
dead. We are told from our fleet leader, Hugo de Moncada, that
the survivors of the shipwreck are on the island of *Ébuso* (popu-
larly called Ibiza), known for its considerable salt mines. The
soldiers are eager to rebel; no compensation is given them; by
now, driven by hunger, they have ravaged the whole island. No
herd or flock remains for the residents of Ibiza, nothing left to

Ad Regem oratores miserunt; quos ego, lachrymis effusis, cum animi angore, audivi. Sic vivitur cum hac avara gente, sub Rege
35 clarissimo, tenebrosissima. Vos valete!

Ex urbe Ilerda, tertio Kalendas Februarii Millesimo Quingentesimo Decimo Nono.

ep. 650 *C* = 649 *A* = 617 *ms.*   *p.* 593 *G*

Marchionibus

Ex Afra urbe Thabarca, *Bugia* dico, venere nuncii ab obsessis nostris praesidiis; agrestibus herbis, neque illis ad saturitatem contentos quinque se aiunt menses egisse, arcibus inclusos: nequeunt sine vitae discrimine inde caput exerere. Ea se
5 pati extrema inquiunt, ne, si ab Afris deprehendantur, dedere arces cogantur; se tantum dedecus non admissuros, ut, spiritu anhelante, cedant hostibus remque a suo Rege creditam amitti patiantur. Quo animo id referant memoratu dignum est. Bis cocti tantum panis summulam ad esum et pulveris globulo-
10 rumque tormentariorum, quo accedentes hostes queant salutare, postulant sibi et sociis dari. Ita leviter super ea aerumna sermocinantur ac si de scaccorum ludo fieret mentio. Quanta sit in tuendis arcibus creditis vestrorum Hispanorum constantia, hinc colligite. Ab orbe novo scribitur Franciscum Garaium,
15 *Iamaicae* insulae gubernatorem (ea est Hispaniolae et Cubae australis), ad cultum redegisse tale Iamaicam, ut in ea colonias iam plures erexerit. Ubertate soli beata est ea insula, in qua, vix toto anno, diei ac noctis noscitur discrimen; ibi temperies gratissima, culturae magis quam auro legendo intendunt, licet
20 ibi aurum reperiatur. Armentis gregibusque referta est. Iam cogitat Garaius alias quaerere vicinas insulas, ad id naves instruxit sua impensa. Est aliud referendum. Moneor ut me apparem ad iter Valentiam versus; Hieronymo Cabanillae, praetoriae cohortis praefecto, futurus comes. Irrita puto fore quae
25 isti regio nomine petunt, ut scilicet Valentini iurent Regem absentem et donativum, praesenti dari solitum, post exactas curias, dent absenti. Neutrum arbitror assensuros. Audivimus

eat or to plant, as they themselves lament. They sent ambassadors to the king; I listened to them in tears with a grieving heart. Thus we live gloomily with these greedy and dismal people, under a most lustrious King. Fare well!

From the city of Lerida, 30 January 1519

To the Marquises
(Pedro Fajardo – Luis Hurtado de Mendoza)

From the African city of Thabarca, that is *Bugia*, came messengers from our besieged garrisons, saying they spent five months closed shut in fortresses, with wild herbs as their sole nourishment, at times even with insufficient quantity: they cannot stick their heads out without risking their life. They say they endure such an extreme condition, not to be faced with having to turn over the forts, should they be captured by the Africans; they could not conceive of so great a shame as to yield to the enemies for lack of strength or allow the abandonment of an enterprise entrusted by their King. The feeling with which they relate this is worthy of mention. They ask only that to them and to the allies be given a small quantity of bisquit bread to eat and powder and cannon balls with which to be able to "greet" the enemies when they arrive. Thus they discuss their hardships lightheartedly, as if talking about a game of chess. From this you may infer how great is the perseverance of your Spanish soldiers in defending the forts entrusted to them. From the new world they write that Francisco de Garay, governor of the island of Jamaica (South of Hispaniola and Cuba), has developed it to such a degree that already several colonies may be established. That island is blessed with a fertile soil; there is hardly a noticeable difference between night and day there throughout the year; the climate is very pleasant conducive to agriculture more than prospecting for gold, even though gold might be found; it is rich in herds and flocks. Garay is now thinking about looking for other islands nearby, and for this he has outfitted ships at his own expense. I need to report on something else. I have been

Valentinum populum de insurgendo in proceres et nobilitatem cogitare. Nos ibimus, quae successerint habebitis. Valete!

Barchinonae, Kalendis Decembris .M.D.XIX.

ep. 650 C = 650 A = 618 ms.   p. 593 G

Marchionibus

Scripsi alias ad repertas novas terras, *Olloam, Iucatanam,*
5 *Cozumellam* missos fuisse a Dieco Velazquez, Cubae progubernatore, milites, sub praetore Fernando Cortesio. Hi, videntes
eas quas prehenderunt terras, auro abundare atque argento
gemmisque variis, pedem figere et coloniam erigere constitue-
runt, nulla de Dieco Velazquez progubernatore, qui eos miserat,
10 facta mentione. Magistratus inter se diviserunt, ad loci populi-
que sedem aptantes regimen. Nuncios ad Regem destinarunt:
ecce illos cum donis ingentibus ex auro argentoque ac variarum
volucrum pennis, arte mira laboratis, a regulis, ex composito
et rerum nostratium permutatione habitis. Mira de terris illis
15 referuntur, de victimis humanis praecipue; de illarum regionum
rebus particulares cogito condere commentarios. Modum epistolae transcenderem, si de urbium illarum magnitudine, de
viarum platearumque ordine, deque legibus et libris caeterisque
vivendi modis, vellem impraesentiarum facere sermonem. Petasatus haec scribo. Valentiam tendo. Valete!

Quarto Nonas Decembris .M.D.XIX.

136

notified to prepare myself to set out for Valencia; I will be a companion to Jerónimo Cabanillas, chief magistrate. I think the petitions being presented in the name of the King shall go unheeded, namely, that the people of Valencia may swear allegiance to the absent King, and notwithstanding his absence go through with the donative customarily granted him in person at the dissolution of the *Cortes*. I do not think they will do either one. We heard that the people of Valencia are thinking about revolting against their leaders and the nobility. We will go there and you will know what happens. Fare well!

Barcelona, 1 December 1519

To the Marquises

(Pedro Fajardo – Luis Hurtado de Mendoza)

On other occasions I have written that to the lands newly < discovered, *Olloa, Yucatán* and *Cozumel,* have been dispatched soldiers by Diego Velasquez, vice governor of Cuba, under the command of Hernán Cortéz. Realizing that the conquered lands did have abundant gold, silver and different kinds of gems, they decided to stay and found a colony, without consideration for governor Diego Velázquez who sent them. They divided the responsibilitics among themselves, adapting the governing office to that place conditions and to the people. They have sent messengers to the King: here they are with great gifts of gold, silver and feathers of various birds — all exhibiting extraordinary skill — obtained from agreable native chiefs and in exchange for our products. Awesome things are reported about those lands, especially about human sacrifices; I am thinking about writing detailed descriptions of the situation of those lands. I would go beyond the scope of this letter, if I wanted to talk at this time about the greatness of those cities, the arrangement of their roads and squares, the laws, the books and different life styles. I write these things while I am ready to leave. I am off to Valencia. Fare well!

2 December, 1519

Magno Cancellario

Nec satis protenta est epistola, dormitant nimium iam nostrae literae. Dum haec morantur, ad manus habui a chalco-graphorum officina emissam, a facinorosis Toletanis huius Iun-cterae dementiae fotoribus, longam ac verbosam paginam, sub
5 spe concitandorum populorum contra vos, quae, quanto maior est, tanto minus efficax, quia facile potuit populo persuaderi falso fuisse confictam et a re valde alienam esse, neque vos unquam de huiusmodi tributis imponendis cogitasse. Ea est animus tibi significare, quo intelligas quam pestifera sit ista
10 contagio, quae tolli non poterit, nisi veneritis. Est carnium et piscium aliarumque rerum ponderibus subiectarum, pondus *arreldum* appellatum, id quadraginta constat unciis; pro singulo arreldo rerum, si vendantur in Regno, aiunt duos provinciales nummulos dictos *marapetinos* assignasse solvendos. Pro rebus
15 vero per designatos ministros ponderandis, pro singulo rubo (est rubus librarum sex deuncialium quinque ac viginti), quin-que nummos provinciales, ex cera aut abdomine, pro confi-ciendis candelis, e lana, e serico, e tabulis, tignis, trabibus, e pannis variis, e telis, e coriis, ex oleo, vino, aceto, metallis,
20 amygdalis, nucibus, acruminibus, sardellis et salitis piscibus ac recentibus, e pansis ficubus; ac mercibus quibuscunque aliis certam tributi portionem, si vendantur in Regno, sed si depor-tanda, in duplo. De gregibus etiam et armentis, caeterisque rebus aliis omnibus, quae vel permutando vel pecuniis solvendis
25 tractantur, per species quasque suas, precia nominant impo-nenda, quae praetermisi quia fastidio sunt apta gignendo. Fig-menta haec arbitror in frontes eorum fabam concussura, quo nanque latius fallax mendacium protendunt, eo se apertius de-cipi sentiunt populi qui, caeci, relictis artibus, lucri expertes,
30 impelluntur vagari, sibi familiaeque perniciem hac dementia construentes. Facinus infandum hoc clausula concludunt hor-renda, falsaque dicentes: exemplar hoc ab originali composito a Burgensibus traductum est, Segovianum vero nusquam ap-paruit, quia demersum est, quum neque Burgenses unquam aut
35 Segoviani tale facinus cogitaverint. Aio igitur sic, ne his nugis perturbemini; cito cadent omnia, si veneritis, uti pollicemini,

138

To the Grand Chancellor

(Arborio Mercurino da Gattinara)

This letter is not long enough; my writing is waning too much. During the delay a printed page came to my attention, a long sheet full of words, written by some rebelling people in Toledo, instigators of this insanity of the *Junteros*, who hoped to incite the people against you; although an increasing expectation it has little efficacy, because one could easily persuade the people that it was prepared with falsehood, that it is far from reality, and that you never thought of imposing taxes of this kind. I want to point out these things to you so that you may understand how harmful this contagion is: it cannot be eradicated unless you come. Meat, fish and other things that have weight are weighed and measured on the base of an *arrelde* which consists of 40 ounces; for each *arrelde* of merchandise, sold in the Kingdom, they say that the set tax is two provincial coins or *maravedis*. But for articles which need to be weighed by officials, they say that one has to pay five provincial coins for each *arroba* (an *arroba* equals six pounds of 25 ounces) of wax or fat for making candles, of wool, silk, boards, planks reams of cloths of different kinds, fabrics and leather, of oil, wine, vinegar, metals, almonds, nuts, sardines and fish, salty or fresh, and dried figs; they say that for any other kind of merchandise one has to pay a set amount of tax if sold within the Kingdom, and double that if exported. Also, concerning herds and flocks and all other things which are either exchanged or paid for, each-depending on its kind has a specific tax levied on it which I did not list because they are likely to cause disgust. I think they themselves will have to pay the price of these lies: indeed, the longer they stretch a deceitful lie, the more clearly the blinded people understand the deceit in having abandoned their crafts and lacking all income are forced to wander, bringing ruin to themselves and their families because of this madness. They complete this detestable action with a horrible clause, spreading lies: this sample was translated from an original composed by the people of Burgos, whereas the one from Segovia did not appear anywhere because it was stolen, although neither the people of Burgos nor those of

praecipue. Claudat ingentem tabellam de Indiis oceaneis nostris fama recens. Venisse naves Hispalim dicitur ab occidenti meridionali Cubae insulae, quae dicitur *Fernandina*. Reperisse aiunt
40 urbes munitas et vestitas ac ornatas gentes, quarum templa ingentia domusque calce ac lapidibus magnifice constructae sunt. Quando venerint, particulariter habebis. Vale!

Ex Valdoleto, cum superioribus ex defectu cursorum, pridie Nonas Martii .M.D.XXI.

ep. 717 *C* = 717 *A* = 685 *ms.*   *p.* 635 *G*

Marchionibus

Ab Indis vos quae habeantur, scitote. Scribit Cardinalis gubernator ad regem ista, ad vos ego, propterea devenient ilico ad Magni Cancellarii manus. Hispani ex insula Cuba, quae *Fernandina* dicitur, occidentem secuti meridionalius aliquantu-
5 lum, per Iucatana littora, prius tractata, in interna eius terrac salsum reperere pelagus, a mari distans lequas sexaginta amplius, more Caspii sive Hircani, sed maius multo: lequas enim aiunt continere in gyrum lacunam ipsam septuaginta circiter; fluit ac refluit ibi, ad oceani vices, nec qua egrediatur aqua
10 intelligitur; multa flumina in eam labuntur. Piscium aiunt lacunam esse volucribusque aquaticis refertam. Civitas est in eius lacunae medio fundata, nomine suo dicta *Tenustitam*, alias *Mexico*, a nostris novo nomine *Venetia "dives"* appellata, cuius rex potentissimus est nomine *Muteczuma*, ultima producta. Numero
15 domorum quinquaginta milium inquiunt constare civitatem illam, addunt multi dimidium ab hoc numero; sunt incredibilia quae de huius urbis et circumvicinarum aedificiis, commerciis et hominum frequentia referuntur. Domus sunt lapideae omnes; atria principum in ea sunt multa, quod huic Muteczumae regi
20 pareat procerum ingens multitudo, qui, certis anni temporibus, ex debito, regi assident, filiosque omnes a pueris mittunt eru-

140

Segovia ever conceived such a deed. I speak thus so that you may not be upset by these trifles; everything will quietly end, especially if you come as you promised. Let the latest report from our oceanic Indies close this long letter. They say that ships coming from the south-western part of the island of < Cuba, that is *Fernandina*, have reached Seville. They say that they have found fortified cities and populations with clothing and ornaments, whose great temples and houses are wonderfully built with lime and stones; you will know the details when they come. Fare well!

From Valladolid, together with previous letters for lack of couriers, 6 March, 1521

To the Marquises
(Pedro Fajardo – Luis Hurtado de Mendoza)

Here is the news we have from the Indies. The Cardinal < governor writes the King these things; I write them to you, and therefore soon they will reach the hands of the Grand Chancellor. The Spaniards, from the island of Cuba, called *Fernandina*, followed the route West, a little further South, along the earlier discovered shores of Yucatán; in the interior of that land they found a salt water mass, more than 60 leagues from the sea, similar to the Caspian or Ircanian Sea but much larger: in fact, they say that this lake's perimeter measures about 70 leagues all around; here the water ebbs and flows, like the ocean tides, but such phenomenon is not understood; many rivers flow into it. Reports describe it as a lake rich in fish and aquatic birds. In the middle of it there is a city named *Tenustitán*, otherwise known as *México*, referred to by our people as the *the rich Venice*, whose very powerful king is Montezuma, with the stress on the last syllable. They claim the city numbers 50,000 houses, with many adding half as much that number; incredible things are reported about the buildings of this city and of those nearby, about trades and population density. All the houses are built of stone; in it there are many palaces for the nobles, since a great multitude of leaders obey

141

diendos in eius regis palatio; terrarum est vasta intercapedo, quae huic regi paret. Circumeunt lacunam sex aliae civitates munitae lapideis et ipsae domibus constructae, in aqua partim,
25 in sicco partim, quinque aut sex milium domorum: a quibus circumcursitant, perpetuo tractu, naviculae uniligneae ad urbem ipsam primariam, suos ad eam vehentes proventus et ex urbe in patriam peregrinum aliquid revehentes, uti apud nos passim fieri videmus e villis et ruribus ad vicinas civitates et oppida.
30 Plateas habent ingentes, porticibus circunseptas, ubi mercatoriae sunt pulchrae constructae tabernae. Fora et nundinas exercent, ad quas aiunt sexaginta septuagintaque milia hominum concurrere, negociorum causa, ter in hebdomada. Quas tractent merces, longum esset narratu. Plaeraque tamen audite: vestes illo-
35 rum et supellectilia domorum, aulea ornatusque sunt ex gossampio, quod Italum vulgus *bombasum*, Hispanus *algodon* appellat; serico lanaque carent quod oves non assequantur neque boves aut capras habent; venatu et volucribus ac piscibus vescuntur. Miris fucant gossampium coloribus et pulchre telas
40 intexunt. Fructus provinciales sunt innumeri herbaeque hortenses variae, a nostris dissimiles. Moneta utuntur, non e metallo, sed ex quarundam arborum nuculis amygdalae similibus, quae paucis in locis aluntur, apricis puta aquosisque; est in his arboribus nutriendis summa opus diligentia, paucosque durant
45 annos. Plantatur haec arbor sub alterius altae arboris umbra, ne, dum tenera est, sole siccetur aestivo, aut atrocibus nimbis concutiatur; uti nutricis in gremio fovetur infans, ita sub alterius arboris tutela coalescit haec. Ubi vero iam induruit, nutrix arbor evellitur aut scinditur, quo illa frui iam queat aereo
50 spiritu ac solari, et radices eius in tellure vicina sese protendere possint. Preciosiores tamen merces vicissitudinaria tractantur permutatione. Sed huius nuculae nummalis audite quae sit utilitas: non est comestibilis, licet nucleosa sit, quia gustu est amariuscula et, quoniam tenera est, uri amygdala spoliata conteritur, et ex eo pulvere vinum efficitur nobile, principibus
55 tamen usuale solis; plebs autem populusque vino utitur ex maizii granis et fructibus confecto. Per caupones edulia venduntur assa elixaque; cervos, lepores, cuniculos, apros, aliorum etiam quadrupedum, nobis ignotorum, armenta pascit[28] illa

---

[28] See Ov. *met.* VI 395.

this king Montezuma, and, in specified periods of the year, assist him and dutifully send all their sons from childhood to be educated in the palace of that king; extensive lands are subject to this king. Six other fortified cities surround the lake, all with stone built houses, some 5,000 or 6,000 partly on the water and partly on shore: small boats made from single tree trunk sail continually all around to the most important city, carrying to it their own products and bringing back to their original site something foreign from the city, just as we see happening everywhere here between villages and countrysides and their neighboring cities and fortified towns. They have large plazas surrounded by arcades where beautiful shops for goods are found. They hold fairs and markets which, they say, attract 60 to 70 thousand people doing business three times < a week. What products they handle would be long to tell. Nevertheless here are the most important: clothes and house furnishings, blankets and ornaments made of cotton or *banbaso* as Italians call it, Spanish *algodón*; they are without silk and wool, because they do not have sheep nor oxen or goats; through hunting, they feed on birds and fish. They dye cotton with marvelous colors and weave cloths masterfully. The regional fruits are numberless, the vegetables and greens varied, different from ours. They have a currency, not of metal, but of small nuts, like almonds, from trees growing in few sunny and water rich places, the greatest care is needed in growing these trees which last only a few years. Saplings are planted in the shade of taller trees so as to withstand scorching summer heat and avoid being struck by heavy storms; just as an infant is suckled at the bosom of a nurse, so this young tree grows strong under the protection of another tree. Once this tree acquires vigor the nurse tree is uprooted or cut down, allowing for more air and sun and root expansion. The more precious goods, however, are exchanged with goods of like value. Yet, hear now the versatility of this little currency nut: although with kernel it is not edible, being rather bitter in taste; being tender as well it is crushed like a skinned almond, and from that paste good wine is made, although usually drunk only by the chiefs; the common people, however, drink a wine made from corn grains and fruits. Roasted and boiled foods are sold by wine makers; that land nourishes deer, hare, rabbits, boars and also herds of other four-footed animals unknown to us.

⁶⁰ tellus. De templorum magnitudine cultuque ac ornatu mira
referuntur. In his habent simulacra, quibus humana carne litant,
uri alias diximus, terras facere; variis deorum statuis vario
immolant effectu: huic pro frugibus, pro incolumitate illi, alii
pro victoria si ad manus veniendum sit cum hostibus in re
⁶⁵ bellica, sed cui pro frugibus, certis anni temporibus, immolant
sationis praecipue tempore, mox maturationis ob grandinum
formidinem, demum paulo ante sectionem. De his inventis
particulares cudo libellos decadibus, quas vidistis de orbe novo,
postligandos: tunc haec latius intelligetis. Nunc valete!

Ex Valdoleto, Nonis Martii Millesimo Quingentesimo Vigesimo
Primo.

ep. 758 *C* = 755 *A* = 725 *ms.*   *pp.* 662-663 *G*

Magno Cancellario

Haec ad vos attinent. Hispania, ut stetis iam tandem pro-
missis, de adventu desiderat. De rebus Italiae nihil ad vos ego,
quia propiores estis. De nostris: in Fortunae tabella Valentinum
excutitur regnum; facinorosos quosdam deprehensos prorex
⁵ punivit, qui sociorum exemplo, indicium timentes, aufugerunt.
Occupato Xativae municipio, ubi castellum est illud ingens,
afflictorum principum receptivum et impraesentiarum ducis
Fernandi Calabri domicilium non electum, conciliabula celebrat
praedonica fex illa, regem sibi elegit, audetque circumvicinia
¹⁰ omnia infestare. Pupus electus gregi male composito persuasit,
suis se carminibus effecturum ut proregis exercitui, solo suo
prospectu si veniret, arma de manibus caderent. Credit populus
oppidanus tributaque sibi ad milites alendos imponi passus est.
Haec sunt opprobria et ludibria quae crebrescunt deterentque,
¹⁵ nisi Caesarem adduxeritis. Integros profligarunt duos iam exer-
citus nobilium facinorosi. Dum haec in pluteo, apud me, adhuc
moraretur epistola, perlatum est don Diecum Mendocium proregem, ad miliare tertium ab Xativa, in alveo fluminis unius
apud oppidum, *Canales* nuncupatum, ripa latentem, ex insidiis

144

Impressive things are reported about the magnificence of the temples, about the cult and decorations. In these shrines they keep sacred images honored with human sacrifices, just as we said they do in other regions; sacrifices to different deities are for different purposes: one for crops, another for health, yet another for victory, if they have to engage in combat with enemies; to the one for crops, however, they make multiple offerings at specific times of the year, especially at sowing time, then at ripening for fear of hail, and finally a little before harvest. About these discoveries I am preparing detailed accounts to add to the *Decades* on the new world, which you have seen: then you will understand these things more completely. Now, fare well!

From Valladolid, 7 March 1521

To the Grand Chancellor
(Arborio Mercurino da Gattinara)

These reports concern you. Spain is awaiting your arrival so that you may finally make good on your promises. I say nothing about Italian matters for you are closer to them. Concerning ours: on the gaming board of Fortune the kingdom of Valencia is being shaken; the viceroy punished some criminals after they had been caught; and they, following the example of their companions, fled, fearing charges. After occupying the town of *Játiva* where there is a great castle which serves as refuge for persecuted nobles and now also as unwished residence for Duke Ferdinand of Calabria, those dregs of marauders hold assemblies, elect a king for themselves and dare to attack all the neighboring regions. The elected puppet persuaded his ill-assorted flock that with his spells he would cause the arms to drop from the hands of the army of the viceroy, right at first sighting. The city dwellers believe in him and allowed him to levy taxes to run his army. These are the disgraces and the mockeries which keep growing and will wear us down, if you do not send the Emperor. These criminals have already defeated two entire armies of nobles. While

20 cursores equites, levis armaturae, misisse, qui Xativanos vagos
ad certamen lacesserent. Decepti sicarii exeunt. Sequuntur pro-
vocatores, cadunt in insidiis; arma non decidunt nostris e manibus, uti pupus ille praestigiator dixerat. Primus ipse aufugit;
e sexcentum peditibus et equitibus quadringentis, circiter ter-
25 centum a tergo in nostrorum potestate mortuos et captos reliquerunt. Portis iam clausis se continent, cito labentur. Perempti
et ex proregianis plaerique, uti prorex ipse ad nos scripsit. Iam
se deceptos oppidani sentiunt, et pervicaciae poenitet. Erigere
tamen adhuc non audent caput, a profugis hospitibus pressi.
30 Est aliud dolendum, patientiae thoracem induito! Ex Hispaniola
unionibus et auro saccareisque massis et cassia fistula, navis
una nostris littoribus iam appropinquabat onusta. Pyrata Gallus,
nomine *Florinus*, in prospectu navium adortus, expugnavit,
accepit. Ea praeda sapidissima pellecti, nil tutum a nobis relin-
35 quent, quia praecipue don Petrum Bobadillam, qui, sua classe
credita, e Sancto Sebastiano evecta, terrore Gallica omnia littora
replebant, naufragio cum caeteris comitibus periisse intelligant.
Uti coclea sua cornua, vi aliqua succedente, contrahit, ita suos
animos suasque facultates a littoralibus locis ad interna cuncti,
40 Britanni praecipue remittebant. Proh, quantum incommodi ac
molestiae nobis est illius classis naufragium pariturum! Qui
hostes, ea favente, premebamus, prememur propediem ab hostibus, quando senserint se nullos obiices obviam habituros.
Neque enim nobis facultas est impraesentiarum classem alteram
45 parandi. Libentius dulcia, si dulcia emergerent, quam haec
fellita, tibi significarem. Quae tempus affert, ea capimus.

Ex Valdoleto, ut ad Pontificem proficiscar petasatus[29], decimo
quarto Februarii .M.D.XXII.

---

[29] See Cic. *ad fam*. XV 17, 1; Suet. *Aug*. 82, 2.

this letter was still waiting on my desk, it was reported that the viceroy, don Diego de Mendoza, hiding on the banks along the river channel three miles from Játiva near the fortified town of *Canales*, sent out from ambush speedy cavalrymen lightly armed to lure the scattered around people of Játiva in to fight. The cut-throats, deceived, came after these challengers falling into the ambush; the weapons did not fall from the hands of our men, as that puppet impostor had predicted. He himself fled first; of 600 foot-soldiers and 400 cavalrymen, they left behind in our hands about 300 dead and prisoners. Now barricated behind the gates, they shall soon fall. Most of the soldiers of the viceroy have also been killed, as he himself wrote to us. By now the town people realize they have been deceived and regret their obstinacy. However, they do not dare rebel, under the compelling influence of refugees still with them. There is another grief to bear; put on the breastplate of endurance! From Hispaniola, a ship loaded with pearls, gold, blocks of sugar and cinnamon was drawing near our coasts. The known French pirate *Florin* attacked the sighted ship, storming and capturing it. Enticed by that very tasty booty, they will leave nothing of ours safe, especially since they know that don Pedro de Bobadilla, who used to fill with fear all the French shores with the fleet entrusted to him, has died sailing out from San Sebastian in a shipwreck, together with the rest of his companions. Just as a snail pulls back its horns when something approaches, so they all, especially the Britons, resigned themselves and pulled back their forces from coastal areas farther inland. Oh how much trouble and affliction the shipwreck of that fleet will cause us! We, who used to chase enemies with it, will soon be destroyed by the enemy, when they realize that they will not have any obstacle in their path. Under present circumstances we do not figure on outfitting another fleet. I would more gladly pass on to you happy news if any should arise, rather than these bitter reports. We take what time brings.

From Valladolid, ready with my travel hat to go to see the Pontiff, 14 February 1522

Archiepiscopo Cusentino

    Uno halitu accipe multa. In horas Caesarem expectamus, uti ex Britannia suismet literis est pollicitus. A nobis interea de Fontis Rabiae captu iam nosti. Beovia est arx, in parvi cuiusdam fluminis ripa, qua vadosus est, sita. Ceperunt eam Galli,
5 quod itineris esset custos ad commeatus et suppetias Fontis Rabiae ferendas. En de Gallorum potestate erepta est. Sed, audi quali iactura hostium res acta sit et sustentata. Duce don Ludovico a Cueva, ducis Alburquerchi filio, parvo negocio primum est debellata, quum vero Galli, per eius capturam, fore
10 viderent ut, non sine magno discrimine et impensa, traducere quicquid ad auxilia ferenda Fontis Rabiae praesidiarii possent. Magna vi comparata, Beoviam adierunt; praeter finium et Baionae Gallicae copias, ex ipso Fontis Rabiae oppido Germanorum circiter mille a praesidiis exierunt pedites. Tribus tormentariis
15 vasis quatere arcem coeperunt, uno grandi cannono, praecipue sub divi Iacobi Hispaniarum patroni nomine conflato, simul cum Fonte Rabia perdito. Dum quaterent arcem hostes, super eminentem arci occupant collem Lipuzcani (quorum res agitur) duce uno e municipalibus Fontis Rabiae primario, eiecto a pa-
20 tria domo. Germani obsidentes, de colle redimendo cogitarunt, ascenderunt serptim. E margine ac labro collis ruit in Germanos Dux ille, cum sociis vix centum: saxis derotatis aut deiectis partim, vi telorum partim, Germanos omnes aut trucidarunt aut ceperunt; evasit nullus. Visa Germanorum strage, deserunt
25 obsidionem oppugnantes et fugiunt. A latere salit cum equitatu don Beltranus in fugientes. Fuit iactura ingens: in flumine obruti sunt multi, vadorum ignari. E Germanis superstitibus ad gubernatores duxere captos tercentum; ex illis centum ad Pontificem missi sunt, ut eorum opera utatur ad rem mariti-
30 mam, reliquis, bene depastis, data est libertas. Mites in victos Hispani nobiles sunt, uti nosti. De recuperato cannono veteri nostro, cum divi Iacobi simulacro, sitis laetitia summa. Inter primarios deosculati sunt et amplexi vas illud millies don Beltranus, praetor, et reliqui militum centuriones. Eodem, quo
35 anno superiore, fatali die profligati sunt in Navarra Galli, servata est Beovia. Sed quid? Ne laetum quicquam offeratur in

To the Archbishop of Cosenza
(Giovanni Ruffo)

In one breath, receive a lot of news. We are expecting the arrival of the Emperor any time now, just as he promised in his letters from Britain. In the meantime you received news from us about the conquest of Fuenterrabía. Beovia is a fortress located on the bank of a small river where it is fordable. The French conquered it being the check point of the supply and assistance route to Fuenterrabía. Now it has been taken back from the power of the French. But hear the kind of losses the enemy had to bear carrying out this sustained action. Under the leadership of don Ludovico de la Cueva, son of the duke of Albuquerque, at first it was overcome with little effort, with the French realizing its conquest not without great danger and cost would enable them with a garrison at Fuenterrabía, to provide all kinds of help. They prepared a great army and < attacked Beovia; besides the troops from nearby territories and from French Bayonne, some 1,000 German foot-soldiers left the Fuenterrabía garrison. With three artillery pieces they began to rock the Beovia fortress: a large cannon was lost, together with Fuenterrabía, precisely the one named after Saint James, patron of Spain, that was forged on it. While the enemies were destroying the fortress, the Lipuzcanes (the ones directly concerned) occupied the hill overlooking the fortress under the command of one of the elder citizens of Fuenterrabía, who had been driven out of his land. The Germans conducting the siege wanting to retake the hill started crawling upwards. From the sides and top of the hill the Duke broke through the Germans with scarcely 100 fellow soldiers: killing or capturing all of them, either with stones rolled or thrown from the top or with arrows; no one escaped. After witnessing the slaughter of the assailing Germans, the attacking forces abandoned the siege and fled. From one side don Beltrán brought on his cavalry against those fleeing. A great loss ensued: not knowing the fords, many drowned in the river. 300 prisoners from the surviving Germans were taken to the governors; 100 of these, were sent to the Pope, so that he could employ their skills for activities at sea while the rest was freed after being fed well.

ebria Fortunae taberna, quin moeroris tantumdem porrigat, eodem tempore raptata nobis fuerunt a pyratis Gallicis cadorum vini quod ad Sanctum Sebastianum vehebatur, milia duodecim.

40 Re Beoviae foelicibus auspiciis peracta, fines Gallicos, cum valida manu, don Beltranus adortus est; Sancti Ioannis Luci vicum vastavit ac naves multas, quae ibi erant in anchoris, aut combussit, aut disrupit submersitque. Mox ad Baionae Gallicae usque prospectum, obvia cuncta devastans, perrexit. Gregum 45 et armentorum ex vicinis locis copiam ingentem ad suos reportavit. Captae sunt a Lipuzcanis per idem tempus naves plures. Aemulatus aliorum praeclara facinora, tibi amicus Mirandae Comes, Navarrae prorex, debellandae arcis Maiae, in quodam Pyrenaeorum culmine sitae, provinciam cepit, quam 50 praesidio tenebat don Iacobus Velez Navarrus, Agramontesiae factionis eques, nobis aversus, cum decem aliis nobilibus exulibus; cum summis difficultatibus tormenta subvexit, obsedit. Primo impetu, sex e nostris, scopetarum iactu, peremerunt; directis in obsessos gravioribus nostris tormentis, murorum 55 pars ingens diruitur. Ascendere tentantes fortibus animis diu obstiterunt obsessi; plures nobilium iuvenes qui honoris et nominis adipiscendi gratia a gubernatorum curia ierant ad Comitem, saxorum ictibus deiecti percussique graviter fuerunt, nec evasit immunis Comes ipse, prorex. Instantem oppugnationi 60 fere peremerunt. Excussis tribus demibus vi saxorum, e murorum ruina deportatus fuit. Quum tandem se diutius non obstare posse intelligerent obsessi, Comiti sese dediderunt, nullo pacto alio a Comite concesso, praeterquam de vitae solius incolumitate. Diruta est arx illa, ne ultra posset esse praedonum aut 65 Gallorum receptaculum. A Maia, Atlantis filia, hanc et duas arces alias historiae quaedam Hispaniae veteres volunt esse nuncupatas. Ad Indos parumper navigemus! Classicula est advecta. Munera illa preciosa Caesari allata, miris modis laborata, in Valdoleto vidisti et hominum illorum acumen admiratus es. 70 Intellexisti etiam de magna illa civitate lacunari Tenustitana deque illius rege Muteczuma, potentissimo multorum regnorum et procerum domino, quem Fernandus Cortesius, illarum terrarum perlustrator invitum tenebat in suo contubernio, demum, uti fuerint nostri a barbaris male tractati et eiecti maiorique ex 75 parte trucidati (ea est provincia nuper vi armorum, cum auxilio tamen vicinorum populorum, Muteczumae regis inimicorum, recuperata). Particularem condo de his rebus decadem, quae

As you know, Spanish noblemen are lenient toward those conquered. Regarding our ancient cannon and its sacred image of Saint James, rejoice, because it has been recovered. Among the dignitaries, the commander don Beltrán and other centurions of the soldiers kissed and hugged that piece a thousand times. On the same ill-fated day on which the year before the French were defeated in Navarre, Beovia was liberated. But what else? So that no happiness be served in the wine-filled tavern of Fortune without an equal portion of grief being offered at the same time, 12,000 barrels of wine were stolen by French pirates while being transported to San Sebastián. Once carried to a good conclusion the matter of Beovia, don Beltrán, and a band of courageous men invaded the French territory, ravaged the village of Saint Jean de Luz, and either burned or destroyed and sank many ships anchored there. Then he reached French Bayonne, destroying everything in his way. From the nearby places he brought back to his people a great quantity of herds and flocks. In the meantime many ships were taken by the Lipuzcanes. Rivaling the renowned deeds of others, your friend, Count of Miranda and viceroy of Navarre, took possession of the Maia fortress, situated on one of the tops of the Pyrenees; don Jacobo Vélez, a knight of Navarre belonging to the faction of the Agramontese and our adversary, was holding that territory with a garrison, together with ten other exiled nobles; with the greatest difficulty he moved the mortars up from below and besieged it. At the first clash they killed six of our men with gun shots; after we pointed our heavier mortars toward the besieged, a great part of the walls was demolished. The besieged resisted those attempting to ascend for a long time with great courage; many young nobles, who had left the court of the governors to go with the Count seeking honor and fame, were driven back by rocks hurled at them and seriously hit; the Count and viceroy himself did not come out of it unharmed. They almost killed him as he pressed his attack. He lost three teeth by rock impact and fell over with the collapsing walls. When those who were besieged finally realized they could not hold out any longer, they turned themselves over to the Count at the sole negotiated condition of staying alive. The Maia fortress was destroyed so that it could not later be of refuge to robbers or the French. Some old Spanish tales say that the fortress and two others were

veteres meas subsequatur. De hoc satis! Hac hora, qua haec scribo, nuncius anhelans ad gubernatores cucurrit; Caesaris
80 classem e maritimis promontoriis esse visam inquit. Cito pariet haec praegnans fama. Pontifex vero sese apparat ut ad vos proficiscatur. Vale!

Victoriae, pridie Idus Iulii .M.D.XXII.

ep. 770 C = 767 A = 738 ms.   *p. 671 G*

Archiepiscopo Cusentino

Forte miraberis, cur a duodecima Kalendarum Augusti nullas ad te dederim; rara profecto sunt quae a me optantur, magis quam tibi satisfacere. Abiit, inscio me, cursor unus, ab eo tempore, uno igitur fasciculo plura ligabo. Turcarum prin-
5 cipem ais Rhodon cum exercitu, quali soletin hostes, petiisse. Ad medullam usque laesit tibi amicos omnes id nuncium. Optatos inde non expectamus successus, ob Christianorum principum dissidia et saevam ambitionis et avaritiae illos excitantium rabiem. Deus faxit ut aliter eveniat quam suspicemur. De Pon-
10 tificis vero motu ex Dertosia Tarraconem, nulla est mihi scribendi cura. Illum iam forte Romae habetis, quandoquidem ad nos iam pervenit, qui Genuae illum nuncius reliquerit. A nobis,

named after Maya, daughter of Atlas. Let us now sail a little while toward the people of the Indies! A small fleet has set out. You have seen in Valladolid those precious gifts, so beautifully made taken to the Emperor, and you admired the skillfulness of those people. You have even been informed of that great lagoon city of Tenustitán [Teotihuacan] and of its king, Montezuma, a most powerful lord of many kingdoms and eminent chiefs, whom Hernán Cortés, explorer of those lands, was keeping against his will in his military fort; and, finally, [you have been told] how our men were mistreated by the barbarians, driven off and to a large extent slain (that province was recently taken back by military force, with, however, the help of neighboring peoples, enemies of king Montezuma). About these topics I am composing another decade, which continues my previous ones. Enough of this subject! As I write to you, a dispatcher runs panting to the governors; he says that the Emperor's fleet has been spotted at sea from the promontories. Pregnant rumor will quickly deliver this news. The Pontiff, however, is getting ready to come to you. Fare well!

Vitoria, 14 July 1522

To the Archbishop of Cosenza
(Giovanni Ruffo)

Perhaps you wonder why I have not sent you any news since the twenty-first of July; few things surely do I wish more than to satisfy you. Without my knowing it the only dispatcher left, so starting with that time I will gather many news items in one packet. You state that the monarch of the Turks is heading for Rhodes with the sort of army with which he usually goes to war against enemies. This report has deeply affected all your friends. We do not expect here the successes we had hoped for because of the dissension among the Christian princes and the fiercely raging ambition and greed of those who instigate them. God saw to it that events turn out differently than we anticipated. I am not really concerned about

arbitror me alias scripsisse Gallicos fines fuisse graviter ab Hispanis infestatos direptosque fuisse vicos plurimos, cum ex
15 Baiona Gallica non audeant eorum praesidia caput exerere, ne illis accidat, quod saepe in re bellica solet evenire, ut victis admixti profligatores, patentes una portas, ingrediantur. Horrendum audi aliud exemplum: Iunctae popularis procuratores, in oppido Turdesillarum deprehensi, quando proceres oppidum
20 de Iuncterorum potestate vi armorum exceperunt, popularis levitatis fotae ab eis poenas luerunt. In municipio Methymnae Campi iugulati sunt numero septem; don Petrus vero Maldonatus a genitore, a matre Pigmentellus, Beneventani Comitis nepos ex sorore, in arce Simanchea detruncatus est: is ad Iun-
25 cteros Salamantina duxerat auxilia. Propius accedamus. Nudius quartus, qui fuit a Kalendis Septembris dies septimus, Caesar Valdoletum ingressus est. Post paucos inde dies ab Indis et orbe novo, immo et novissimo, literas habemus. Meminisse te oportet Barchinonae, in nostro senatu rerum Indicarum, fuisse
30 statutum, ut quinque naves ad insulas, aromatum altrices quaerendas, sub praetore Portugallico Fernando Magallanes, destinarentur, quod is Magallanes, quinquennio, versatus fuisset in Callecuteis, Cochineis et Canenoreis nundinis, ad quas ex illis insulis aequatori vicinis aromata per insularum commercia ve-
35 hebantur. Ierunt; Magallano ab insularibus quibusdam bello exagitatis interfecto quattuorque reliquis e classicula quinque navium deperditis, una tantum regressa est, dicta *Victoria*, cribro terebratior. Triennium in ea consumpsit navigatione. Particularem videbis de hac re ac diffusam et admirabilem
40 narrationem, quia universum ambivit orbem, solem semper secuta cadentem. Nunc vale!

Ex Valdoleto, tertio Kalendas Septembris .M.D.XXII.

154

writing on the Pontiff's transfer from Tortosa to Tarragon. You probably already have him in Rome, since already the messenger who left him in Genoa has arrived here. As far aswe are concerned: I think I have previously written, that the < French territory were gravely attacked by the Spaniards and that many villages were ravaged, since their garrisons did not dare stick their heads out from French Bayonne, so that what often happens during the course of war would not happen to them, i.e. that dissolute men, mixing with the defeated, might enter opening the gates wide. Hear another similarly horrible example: the officers of the people's junta, captured in the city of Tordesillas when the nobles took back the city by armed force from their power, have paid the penalty for the lies which they fed to the people. In the municipality of Medina del Campo seven men were executed; don Pedro, a Maldonado on his father's side and a Pimentel on his mother's, nephew of the Count of Benevento through his sister, was beheaded in the fortress of Simancas: he had brought Salamanca's reinforcements to the junta. Let us come to more recent events. Four days ago, that is, on the twenty-sixth of August, the Emperor reached Valladolid. A few days ago we received letters from the Indies and the new world, indeed the newest world. You should remember that in Barcelona during the meeting of our Council of the Indies it was decided that five ships be dispatched in search of the islands that produce spices, under the command of the Portuguese captain, Ferdinand Magellan, since he had frequented for five years the markets of Calicut, Cochin, and Cannanore, locations to which spices from islands near the equator were taken for local trading. They left; after Magellan was killed by natives exasperated by the war, four of the small fleet of five ships were lost, with only the *Victoria* returning with more holes than a sieve. It spent three years on that voyage. On this topic you will receive a detailed account, extensive and full of wonders, because it went around the globe always following the setting sun. For now, fare well!

From Valladolid, 30 August 1522

Marchionibus

Varias accipite, quibus labra confricetis, acridulas dapes!
Roma gravi peste urgetur, Pontifex, ob id in Vaticano palatio
inclusus. Papa Cardinalium efflagitationi non cedit, de loco
mutando ab ea contagione libero. A paucis visitur. Turcarum
5 princeps, qui Rhodon contundit obsidetque, ad terram ierat
in Graeciae continentem, quod bis suae acies oppugnatrices,
propugnatoribus Rhodianis, licet cum ingenti iactura, reiecti
fuerint. Vehementer excanduit, inflammatus ira, regressus est
in insulam et trans collem, ab ipsa urbe obsessa parum di-
10 stantem, tutus a tormentorum iactibus, sua locavit tentoria
castrensia, inde non discessurus, ut ait, re infecta, vel exercitu
Christianorum, qui eum inde propellat, accedente validiore.
Per leves biremes, dictos *bergantinos*, quae, per hostium classem, facile noctu dilabuntur, sollicite poscunt auxilia obsessi.
15 Satis de Rhodiis afflictis, Fons Rabia nos propius urget. Paucis
ante diebus Galli, frumentariae rei quaedam nobis, mari vecta,
rapuerunt, heminas, quae vehebantur ad nostros; e contra
nostri, quicquid Galli ad suos iam, prae rerum caritate lugen-
tes, multo maiora interceperunt. Sunt rei bellicae vices: ut
20 qui hodie psallit, cras uno scalpat digito caput. [30] Aliud habetote. Audivisse vos succincte arbitror, de repertis insulis aromatum altricibus a Castellanis. Res haec Portugallicum regem
remordet ad intima. Suburbana esse Malachae, quam plaerique
putant Auream esse Chersonesum, rura dicit Portugallicus,
25 quod vicinae sint, indeque per insularum commercia deferan-
tur ad Malacheas nundinas. Possessae rei manutentionem Caesar producet in medium intra suos limites assignatos ab Alexandro pontifice. Rex Portugaliae arguet, contentio exorietur:
uti graduum latitudo est facilis, ita longitudo difficilis discep-
30 tabitur; concludetur sero. Leguleiorum argutiis et contra po-
sitorum pelago, in re tanta non stabitur. Sunt eorum cavilla-
tiones aranearum telae. Quonam vero pacto, triennio consum-
pto, classicula, de qua puto vos non ignorare, paralellum

---

[30] See Iuv. IX 133.

To the Marquises

(Pedro Fajardo – Luis Hurtado de Mendoza)

Receive herein various astringent foods, with a tart taste that will make your lips shrivel! Rome is plagued by a grave pestilence which forces the Pontiff's confinement to the Vatican palace. The Pope does not give in to the demands of the Cardinals to move to a place free of the contagion. He is visited by few people. The sovereign of the Turks, who is crushing and besieging Rhodes, had reached Greece by land, because twice his attacking armies have been pushed back by those defending Rhodes, albeit with great losses. He felt enraged and, inflamed by anger, went back to the island. He set up his camp beyond a hill, a short distance from the besieged city itself, in a safe place away from the hurling of mortar, with the intention, as he says, of not leaving there until after completing his undertaking or forced out by a stronger Christian army. By means of light ships with two sets of oars, called *brigantines*, that easily slip through the enemy's fleet at night, the besieged are anxiously asking for reinforcements. Enough on the afflicted Rhodians; the matter of Fuenterrabía concerns < us more closely. A few days ago, the French stole certain quantities of food while being delivered by sea to our men; but then our men, on the other hand, intercepted in greater quantity whatever the French were taking to their men, who were complaining of lack of food. Such is the alternating fate of war: feast today, as tomorrow you may be bafflingly starving. Here is another report. I think you heard general talk about the spice-producing islands, discovered by the Castilians. This fact disturbs the king of Portugal deeply. He says that these territories sorround Malacca, which most people think of as Golden Chersonese, being near it where, through island trading, the spices are carried to the Malacca markets. The Emperor will claim his right of possession within the borders assigned by Pope Alexander. The king of Portugal will refute him, and a quarrel will arise: whereas is easily agreed on the longitudinal degrees it will be greatly argued about latitude; late will be a solution. In a matter of such importance, witty remarks by punsters and massive opposition shall be found

157

11

circuierit integrum, proras ad occidentem solem vertens sem-
35 per, donec ad orientem illarum una, gariophillis[31] onusta
redierit, et in eo discursu diem unum sibi defuisse repererit
(quae duo stomachis exilibus impossibilia videbuntur) per eius
rei ad unguem discussam narrationem, aliquando videbitis.
Decadem nanque formo quartam, tribus meis de orbe novo
40 iamdudum chalcographorum opera in vulgus emissis, succes-
sivam, de hisce rebus novis, ad Pontificem dirigendam. Nunc
satis! Valete!

Ex Valdoleto, pridie Nonas Novembris .M.D.XXII.

ep. 774 *C* = 771 *A* = 742 *ms.*   *pp.* 673-674 *G*

Archiepiscopo Cusentino

Haec tua sunt, quae in Hispania eveniunt. In Kalendis
Novembris e tabulato, in ingentis plateae centro erecto, Caesar
per praecones et scribas edictum super insanis motibus popularibus protulit huiusmodi: "Quoniam populi, suo contenti, vi-
5 tam agerent quietam, suis quique artibus, aut agriculturae,
seductoribus deficientibus, intenti, ex innata sua clementia rex
noster, electus Imperator, populis omnibus errores in eo casu
commissos remittit, seditionum vero autores, in laesae maiestatis crimen incidisse promulgat". Ad numerum usque ducentum
10 septuaginta, suis nominibus nuncupati, ei sententiae subiecti
sunt: Salvaterrae Comes et Zamorensis Episcopus ac don Petrus
Giron cum don Petro Lasso a Vega, Garci Lassi filio, et Ramiro Nunio Guzmano, cum universa eius domo ac filiis, uno
excepto, primos assequuti sunt tantae labis ictus. Caeteri ex
15 Salmantica, Abula, Toleto, cum doña Maria Pachieca, Ioannis
Padillae iugulati uxore, suisque sectatoribus, ac Valdoleto caeterisque huius dementiae receptoribus locis, quod humilioris
sint conditionis, tum procuratores, tum ductores copiarum, et,

---

[31] See Plin. *nat. hist.* XII 30: *est... in India piperis gravis simile quod vocatur caryo-phyllon...* The Medieval Latin form is *garyofolum* (see *ep.* 801, p. 170, 19).

wanting. Trivial quibblings are like spider webs. Thanks to a detailed narration you will someday understand how in the course of three years a small fleet, of which I think you were not unaware, completed an entire circuit, keeping its prows steadily on the setting sun, until one of its ships returned East loaded with cloves, in a journey that turned out to be one day short of a year (two facts that will seem incredible to weak stomachs). On these new matters I am indeed preparing a fourth *Decade* to be given to the Pontiff, now that my first three *Decades* on the new world have finally been done and published by the printers. Enough for now! Fare well!

From Valladolid, 4 November 1522

To the Archbishop of Cosenza
(Giovanni Ruffo)

These events happening in Spain concern you. On 1 November, from a platform erected in the large central square, the Emperor, through town-criers and scribes, issued a decree of this kind about the foolish popular movements: "*Because in the absence of rabble-rousers people lived a peaceful and satisfying life in a state of dedication to their respective crafts or agriculture, our King and Emperor elect, by his inborn compassion forgives all the people for the mistakes made during that circumstance; however, he orders the instigators of the rebellion to be brought to justice and charged* < *with lese majesty.*" About 270 people, listed by name, were then charged with treason: the Count of Salvatierra and the Bishop of Zamora, don Pedro Girón with Pedro Lasso de la Vega, son of Garcilasso, Ramiro Núñez de Guzmán with his entire household but for one son, received the first hit of so great a ruin. Because you do not know them at all and being they of humble origins, I leave out all the others from Salamanca, Avila, Toledo, including doña María de Pacheco, wife of Juan de Padilla who was beheaded with his followers, and those from Valladolid and all the other places which took in this madness, be they procurators, army commanders in charge, for these cities and towns, with overseeing that the people

in ipsis urbibus ac municipiis, ad populum in ea insania susti-
20 nendum, censusque ad alendum exercitum exigendos, praeter-
mittuntur, quodque tibi minime sint noti. Horum facultates
fisco, capita vero nobilium gladio, popularium ligno triplici
adiudicavit. Ad aliam iam: post regis Portugaliae obitum, ilico
Caesar Cabrensem Comitem et episcopum Cordubensem, don
25 Alfonsum Manrichum, ad sororem relictam viduam, doñam
Leonoram ad se reducendam destinavit. Addidit illis comitem
doctorem Cabrerum Aragonicum e senatoribus unum, quo si
opus fuerit agere quicquam iuridicum assit qui leges noverit.
Ad hunc usque diem in urbe Pacensi,[32] quae vulgo dicitur
30 *Baldaiozum*, Portugallicos fines tangente, morantur, ab rege
novo non admissi, ut praetereant in suos terminos; nescitur
adhuc quid causae insit. Doctorem tamen illum solum accersi-
vit. Quae concludentur, ab illius novi regis oratore, qui ad
Caesarem venit et proximus iam est, ad unius iter diei, sentie-
35 mus. Aiunt multi iuvenem regem amore intimo affici erga
novercam, cupereque uxorem: haec vulgo feruntur. Sapido iam
ferculo nares demulce. Ad Portugalensium insulas Cassiterides[33], vulgo *Azores*, tres appulsae sunt ab Fernando Cortesio
Iucatanarum et novissimorum aliorum orbium subactore naves.
40 De thesauris illarum, sed de ornatibus praecipue ac vestibus
diis eorum dicatis, quam variae sint ab illis, quas ab eodem
missas in Valdoleto vidisti, affectibus intimis referunt, et precio
et decore ab illis, in immensum differre aiunt. Qui una ex tribus
advecti sunt (duae nanque reliquae prae metu Gallorum pyra-
45 tarum in dictis insulis pedem fixerunt) octingentorum milium
ducatorum valorem in illis afferri audent dicere; sistunt ergo
donec ad eas advehendas alia classis ex Hispali mittatur, quae
iussa est parari, edocti nanque sumus exemplo molestissimo
quod nos vigilantiores efficiet, nisi nos fortuna obcaecaverit.
50 Anno quippe superiore, Florinus quidam, Gallus pyrata, navim
unam ab Hispaniola venientem, auro ad summam octoginta
millium dragmarum, unionum vero libris octuncialibus sexcen-
tis et ruborum saccari duobus millibus rapuit. Trium navium
harum princeps venit Ioannes Ribera, Fernandi Cortesii mit-

[32] See Plin. *nat. hist.* IV 117.

[33] Tin-producing islands (see Her. III 115; Strabo II 5, 15, 30) W of Gibraltar
(see Mela III 47; Plin. *nat. hist.* IV 119; VII 197), identified with the Azores by the
author.

160

living such folly paid taxes to keep the army. He confiscated their assets and actually ordered the noblemen to be decapitated whereas the commoners to the triple noose. And now let us go on to another topic: right after the death of the King of Portugal, the Emperor appointed the Count of Cabra and the Bishop of Córdoba, don Alonso Manrique, to bring back to him his sister, the widowed doña Eleonora. He sent along as well doctor Cabrera, a senator from Aragon so that, in case of needed compliance with the law, someone knowledgeable of it would be available. As of this day they are delayed in the city of *Pax*, usually called *Badajoz*, at the borders of Portugal, because the new king has not given them permission to pass into his territory; we do not know yet the reason for the refusal, but he summoned in the doctor alone. We will know what is stipulated through the messenger of that new king, who is coming from the Emperor and is now only a day's journey away. Many say that the young king has been affected by a very deep love for his stepmother and wants to marry her: people's gossip. For now, entice your nostrils with a tasty dish. Three ships of Hernán Cortés, conqueror of Yucatán and of other parts of the newest world, have made the Portuguese Cassiteridi Islands, commonly referred to as *Azores*. They report with deep emotion about the treasures of those islands, and especially the ornaments and garments dedicated to their deities, very different from those sent by Cortés earlier and which you have seen in Valladolid, claiming the difference is immense both for worth and beauty. Those who traveled on one of the three ships (the other two stopped in the above-mentioned islands for fear of French pirates) dare say their value reaches 800,000 ducats so they lay in wait until another fleet ordered outfitted, is sent from Seville to escort them, for we have learned from a most painful lesson, that has made us more watchful ever since, unless fate blinds us. Indeed, last year a certain Florin, a French pirate, seized a ship coming from Hispaniola carrying a total of 800,000 drachmas of gold, 600 pounds of 8-ounce pearls and 2,000 *robos* of sugar. Juan de Ribera, secretary of Hernán Cortés who sent him, came as commander of these three ships: in the name of his lord Hernán Cortés, he intends to give to the Emperor half of those riches; two other treasurers will give the remainder to the Emperor on behalf of the officers and the soldiers of those

55 tentis a secretis, qui, Fernandi Cortesii heri sui nomine, dimidiam illorum munerum partem est Caesari donaturus, reliquam
Caesari donabunt duo alii procuratores, magistratuum et militum terrarum illarum nomine. Hi duo cum navibus restant.
Ioannes Ribera tentare cum illarum trium una fortunam statuit
60 et evasit; quae hic afferat alias habebis: nondum exolvit quas
affert capsas suas tamen ad regem nihil ipse. In tribus illis
navibus tres afferebant a parvulis, in sua quanque cavea tigres
enutritas. Vi tempestatum in vasto oceano, una e caveis noctu
aperitur parumper. Summo conatu tigris tabulas discussit, exivit
65 in homines nil minus saeviens ac si nunquam hominem vidisset
quenquam, obvios affecit, uno ictu, vulneribus crudis; quinque
experrecti comites, quadrupedem feriunt hastis, persecutam in
mare deiiciunt. Ne idem accidat, in ipsa cavea secundam telis
transfixerunt; unam ergo tantum devehunt, quam faxit Deus
70 ut cum rebus aliis pyratarum evadat fauces; sunt nanque iam
nimium alia praeda pellecti, cum qua vires collegerunt validis-
simas, adeo ut iam nequeamus nostrum oceanum tuto pernavigare. De his aliquando latius, quandoquidem Romanae curiae
gratas esse meas de novis orbibus enatantibus, qui latuerunt
75 hactenus, oceano mersi, narrationibus. Iam vale!

Ex Valdoleto, decimo tertio Kalendas Decembris, Millesimo Quingentesimo Vigesimo Secundo.

ep. 782 *C* = 779 *A* = 750 *ms.*   *pp.* 678-679 *G*

Archiepiscopo Cusentino

Scribis Hieronymum Adornum Venetiis obiisse; fuit Caesari molestissimum id nuncium: bene de viro sentiebatur. Solator tamen animum! Eius loco suffectus est protonotarius
Caraciolus, quem nosti virum esse, longa rerum experientia,
5 prudentem. Speramus ut quae Adornus orsus fuerit, huius
industria rite perficiatur, quando praecipue Veneti videant nullas esse in Italia vires Gallicas, quibus queant inhaerere. A nobis
scito regionem hanc insolitis fulguribus et tonitruis infestatam
his diebus ita fuisse, ut multi in agro et in propriis laribus

lands. These two are staying with the ships. Juan de Ribera decided to try his luck with one of the three ships and successfully passed through; on another occasion you will learn what his cargo is: for he has not yet opened the cases which he carries as his own to the king. On those three ships they were transporting three tigers, reared since cubs, each in its own cage. Due to violent storms on high sea, one of the cages came open a bit one night. A tiger smashed the planks by brute force, hurled itself against the men, no less ferociously than if it had never seen people and with single strikes inflicted severe wounds on those it encountered; five fellow shipmates woke up, chased the animal wounding it with spears and threw it overboard. So as to prevent the same thing from happening, they darted the second tiger still in the cage; they only are transporting one which with God's protection may find secure passage with the load from the pirates' jaws who, having been greatly enticed by previous booty, which made them even more powerful, makes for an evermore treacherous ocean passage for our ships. One day I will report on these topics more extensively, since I understand the Roman Curia enjoys my < accounts on the new parts of the world now emerging and which up to this time lay hidden, as if completely submerged by the ocean. Fare well!

From Valladolid, 19 November 1522

To the Archbishop of Cosenza
(Giovanni Ruffo)

You write that Gerolamo Adorno died in Venice; this news greatly saddened the Emperor: that man was dearly esteemed. However, console your spirit! The protonotary Caracciolo, whom you have known to be a man of wisdom and long experience, took his place. Let us hope that what Adorno began may be brought to conclusion happily by the industry of this man, especially when the Venetians realize that there are no French forces in Italy which they can join. From us know that this region was affected these days by unusual light-

percussi fuerint; stupent homines, timentque ne coelorum hae minae mali aliquod portendant. Embrionem iam pepererunt. Veteranorum mille militum cuneus, Perpinianum iturus, ad fines Gallicos perturbandos, hac praeteribat. Cum praetorianis Belgis est orta seditio, curiam universam perturbarunt. Trucidarunt Hispani e praetorianis quinque; ex Hispanis unus fuit confossus. Non est ausus Caesar in observantiam ulcisci, ne deterius aliquid exoriretur. Quantocius fieri potuit, per suos centuriones educti sunt. Est veteranorum militum horum animi elatio tanta, ut se posse quorumcunque hostium copias triplicatas facile prosternere, sibi persuadeant. Hoc eodem die allatum est aliud infoelix nuncium. Scripsi alias e tribus navibus, quas ab extremis terris Fernandus Cortesius cum thesauris ingentibus mittebat, metu pyratarum, in Cassiteridibus, Azorum insulis, permansisse duas, donec classis nova ad eas perducendas mitteretur. Trium caravelarum fuit missa in earum tutelam classicula; nil profuit: ad Ioannis Florini praedonis Galli manus expugnata e duabus, praetoria ipsa, preciosis illis rebus onusta pervenit, evasit altera cum una tantum e duodecim magni capacibus capsis et una tigrium, de quibus supra memoravi. Pauca haec elapsa in immensum et precio et vestium elegantia superant ea quae vidisti dona, priusquam Caesar ad Galleciam ex Valdoleto, rediturus ad Belgas, discederet. Nec mirum quidem: a provincialibus populis illa, haec ab illius magni regis Muteczumae gazophylacio et reliquis proceribus atrii ac illorum egregiis templis asportata. Sexcentorum milium ducatorum amissa hoc saltu referunt valorem, qui res illas tractarunt, excedere: granati auri copia inerat ingens, vestes vero, diis eorum dicatae, multo erant auro comptae; ad quae visenda Venetum oratorem et nobiles plures duxi, ad eorum hospitia qui capsae illius curam habent, donec Caesari offerantur. Qualia fuerint caetera deperdita, praebent haec intelligendi materiam. Admirati sunt decorem et precium et arte mira laboratas imagines et contextas omnium florum, herbarum, animalium, laqueorum ac volucrum figuras; quod populi sint illi politici et ingenio acuti ac industrii, magno sunt argumento haec. Aliud accipe, quo epistola claudatur. Henricus, dominus Lebreti, regno Navarrae privatus, requisitus a Caesare, ut suis partibus inhaereat, traiiciendique per suas terras exercitus in Galliam assentiatur, dicitur respondisse se id, sine suarum rerum magno discrimine, annuere non posse, nisi per vim cogatur, quod intra fines Gallicos universum

ning and thunders in such a way that many have been struck in the fields or their homes; the people are stunned and fear that these threats from heaven portend some evil, indeed here is an embryonic sample. A squadron of 1,000 veteran soldiers, on its way to Perpignan to cause disturbances near the French borders, was passing by here. A revolt involving the Belgian pretorians ensued and it upset the whole court. The Spaniards killed five pretorians; one of the Spaniards was stabbed. The Emperor did not dare take revenge for fear that something worse might happen. With the help of his military commanders, the veterans were sent on as soon as possible. These veterans are so arrogant to be convinced they can easily defeat any troop of any enemy three times their size. The same day more sad news was reported. I wrote you earlier that of the three ships which Hernán Cortés was sending from very distant lands with huge treasures, two had remained in the Cassiteridi, the islands of the Azores, because of fear of pirates, until a new fleet could be sent to escort them. A small fleet of three caravels was sent as their escort; it did not do any good: of the two, the flagship, loaded with all that precious merchandise, fell into the hands of Jean Florin, the French plunderer; the other escaped, but with only one of the twelve large crates and with one of those tigers I spoke of earlier. These few things lost exceed greatly in worth and garment elegance those gifts which you saw before the Emperor left Valladolid for Galicia, with plans to return to the Belgians. And this is not strange since those things had been taken from the people of those regions, whereas these came from the treasury of the reknown king Montezuma, from other nobles of the palace, and from their extraordinary temples. The people who handled those objects say that the riches lost in this attack exceed 600,000 ducats: there was a great quantity of gold nuggets and the votive garments to their gods were as well trimmed in much gold; I took the ambassador of Venice and many other nobles to see the things of the remaining crate at the house of those who have custody of it until its presentation to the Emperor. They offer the opportunity to understand what sort of other things were lost. Admired were their beauty and worth, the inlaid images of remarkable skill, interwoven with all kinds of flowers, herbs, figures of animals, snares and birds; this is evidence those people have a political structure, sharp

habeat patrimonium. Quicquid delirant reges, miser plectetur[34]: si a Caribdi cavere studuerit, decidet in Scyllam. Sine magna eius iactura, nubila haec resolvi nequibunt.

Ex Valdoleto, tertio Idus Iunii .M.D.XXIII.

ep. 786 *C* = 782 *A* = 753 *ms.*   *p.* 682 *G*

Summo Pontifici Adriano VI

Uno halitu, post sacrorum oscula pedum, tres Charites, dico gratiarum actiones, accipiat Beatitudo Tua. Occaniae archipresbyteratum mihi est impertita et de pontificio more sub naviculae sigillo, breves accepi duas a Beatitudine Tua mem-
5 branas, ad Serenissimum Caesarem unam, qua suadens ut me summo prosequatur amore, fuisse me illius progenitoribus parentique Suae Maiestatis utrique gratissimum, significat, dehinc Suae Maiestati utilem, quo tempore suimet subdidi tumultuantes regna haec omnia perturbabant, dicitque mea fuisse obsequia,
10 non contemnenda, quando vos gubernatores, cum octodecim proceribus, insania popularis inclusos et fere obsessos premebat in oppido Turdesillarum, regnorum arce, quod ibi moretur aeternumque sit moratura Catholica Regina, Suae Maiestatis mater. Fuistis a me de rebus quae gerebantur moniti, nec parum
15 commodi, ad emergentia tunc negocia, significationes meas Caesareis rebus attulisse Vestra Beatitudo fatetur. Tale testimonium, Pater Beatissime, gratissimum mihi fuit, nec meae famae parum addidit incrementi apud bonos, quibus non invi-

---

[34] See Hor. *epist.* I 2, 14: *quicquid delirant reges, plectuntur Achivi.*

166

intellect and are industrious. And now hear one more news item, which closes this letter. Henry, lord of Albret, who lost the kingdom of Navarre, was summoned back by the Emperor so that he might join his cause and allow his army headed for France through his territory but, hearsay has it that Henry replied he could not go along without great danger for his possessions, unless compelled by force, because all his wealth was in French territory. The weakest bears whatever toll a king demands: his care to avoid Charybdis, will not free him from Scylla. These clouds cannot be dispelled without great loss on his part.

From Valladolid, 11 June 1523

To the High Pontiff Adrian VI
(Adrian of Utrecht)

Your Holiness, please accept in one breath with the kissing of your holy feet, three distinct "thanks," expressing gratitude. You have granted me the deanery of Ocaña and, following papal protocol, I have received from your Holiness two briefs with the navicella seal. The first, for his most Serene Majesty the Emperor, recommending that I be received by him with great benevolence stating that I was in the good graces of his ancestors and both parents of his Majesty, and therefore useful to his Majesty at a time when his own rebellious subjects were disturbing all these realms pointing out as well that mine were true services, not to be underestimated at a time when people's madness kept you governors and 18 other nobles shut in and virtually besieged in the city of Tordesillas, a stronghold of the kingdoms, being the present and future residence of the Catholic Queen, mother of his Majesty. You were advised by me on what was really happening and Your Holiness acknowledges that my information brought no small advantage to the cause of the Emperor with the events unfolding at the time. Such testimony, most Holy Father, has been highly pleasing to me and has increased greatly my reputation among the judicious men to whom, not with restrain, but rather with

tus immo et gloriabundus membranam ipsam legendam porrigo
20 additumque amorem Caesaris sentio erga me. Membranarum
altera imperat, ut prosequar de orbe novo quicquid, post Tuae
Beatitudinis discessum ab his regnis, oceanus ab utero suo
praegnanti detegere Hispanos permittit. Non invitus laborem
sumam: tres aliae, ab impressis, meae decades propediem ex
25 mea prodibunt officina, quae Beatitudinis Tuae nomen in fronte
gestabunt. Circuierunt nanque integrum Hispani paralellum et
insulas aromatum altrices repererunt. Immensamque illam civitatem lacunarem Tenustitanam, cum amplissimis novis regionibus, nostro Caesari restituimus. Caetera Cusentinus Archie-
30 piscopus, tui pontificatus dexter oculus. Valeat Tua Beatitudo,
ante cuius sacros pedes prostratus, dico humilem commenda-
tionem!

Valdoleto, Idibus Augusti .M.D.XXIII.

ep. 791 *C* = 787 *A* = 758 *ms.*   *pp.* 685-686 *G*

Archiepiscopo Cusentino

Haec ad te caeterosque rerum apud nos emergentium cu-
pidos. Ex insulis Hispaniola, Cuba, Iamaica et putato continenti, cassiae fistulae (cuius proventus in Hispaniola sunt ar-
borei fructus iam immensi) ac saccari, auri etiam, non conte-
5 mnenda pervecta est copia. Particularius aliquando haec; ad
propiora nunc. Magnus noster Comestabilis, astu suo, quosdam
e Fontis Rabiae portarum custodibus seduxit. Uno tantum
e tribus filiis Ioanne Tovaro secundogenito, iuvene magnanimo
comitatus, sine lecto, sine iumentis ac famulis obsequiariis,
10 blanditiarum omnium oblitus, per Lipuscae Biscaiaeque Canta-
brorum anfractuum regiones, plebeio habitu montano contec-
tus, pererravit ignotus. Exploratores, qui Fontem Rabiam, noctu, clam ingrediebantur, ubinam Comestabilis esset pernoctatu-
rus, locum nanque quotidie mutabat, soli sciebant. Quando iam
15 ad optatum finem rem perduxisse arbitrabatur, fortuna solitis
est artibus usa; qua nocte conventum erat de porta nostris per
vigiles aperienda quingenti et quater mille Germani bellatores,

pride, I present your parchment so they may read it and have noticed that the benevolence of the Emperor toward me has increased. The other brief orders that I continue to write about the new world after your Holiness's departure from these kingdoms, to report on whatever the ocean allows the Spaniards < to discover in its pregnant womb. I will face such task with pleasure: very soon three more *Decades* of mine after the published volumes will leave my office bearing the name of your Holiness on the title page. The Spaniards have indeed travelled a whole parallel and have found the spice-producing islands. We have restored to our Emperor that immense lagoon city of Tenustitán and its largest new territories. The Archbishop of Cosenza, the right hand of your pontificate, will relate the rest. May your Holiness be well! Prostrated at your holy feet, I humbly entrust myself to you.

Valladolid, 13 August 1523

To the Archbishop of Cosenza
(Giovanni Ruffo)

These reports are intended for you and others eager to earn of our ongoing novelties. From the islands of Hispaniola, < Cuba, Jamaica and from what is believed to be a continent, a considerable quantity of cinnamon (whose abundant production in Hispaniola is harvested from trees), sugar and also gold have been taken out. More details on this later; for now let us turn to events closer to us. Our Grand Constable with his cunning has corrupted some sentries at the gates of Fuenterrabía. Accompanied only by one of his three sons, his second-born Juan Tovar, a generous young man, he wandered incognito through the territory of Guipúzcoa, Vizcaya, and rugged Cantabria without carriage, horses or servants and conveniences, merely dressed in mountaineer's ordinary clothes. The scouts who used to enter Fuenterrabía secretly at night, were the only ones who knew where the Constable would spend the night, as he moved on every day. When he thought he was close to bringing this undertaking to its

acciti a Caesare praecedente vespera, Sancti Sebastiani portum
captarunt. Re intellecta, Gallorum duces obsessi, de repentino
20 congressu aliquo suspecti, prioribus mutatis custodibus, recentes
ac numero plures successerunt. Ita boni Comestabilis vigilias
et labores, novercali suo more, fortuna frustravit, neque his
contenta, similem casum astruxit ilico. Moniti nostri per tran-
sfugas a Baiona, urbeculam eam, Gallorum finium propugna-
25 culum validissimum, ex inertia praesidiorum, saepe protento
crure secure dormientium, imparatam posse reperiri, de impetenda mari ac terris uno crepusculo, cogitarunt. Tentatum est,
sed quo tempore copiae terrestres ad muros oppugnaturae sese
applicarunt, maritimae classi cum instrumentis et ferris, prora-
30 libus carinis, ad oppositas cathenas disrumpendas paratae, venti
defecerunt. Ita, desperatis animis, nec sine iactura, oblata occasione amissa, vulneratis e turritis moenibus multis et plaerisque
peremptis, re infecta, redierunt. Classiarii vero, ne frustra penitus laborasse viderentur et prae dolore tanti facinoris evasi,
35 despumantes, in Gallica littora descenderunt. Bene munitum
oppidum Cabretonum cum vicis et locis aliis circumvicinis
pluribus debere in praedam. Inter caetera opima spolia, resinae
ad stipandarum rimas navium, qua indigebant, aptae copiam
ingentem se reperisse iactant. Sed vereor rerum vices: non
40 dormitabunt in quaerenda vindicta hostes, qui nunc praeda
onusti psallunt; forte aliquando spolia lugebunt, aut, eorum
causa, innocentes vicini. Iam vale!

Lucronii, unde propediem discedemus, Nonis Octobris .M.D.XXIII.

desired outcome, fate spun her web: the night which the <
sentries had agreed to open the gate to our men, 4500 German
soldiers, summoned by the Emperor the previous night, took
possession of the port of San Sebastián. Realizing what happened, the commanders of the besieged French suspecting
a sudden attack changed their sentries, replacing them with
many more new ones. And so fate, in its stepmotherly role,
denied all watches and efforts by the good Constable, and
not to be overdone, plotted a reverse calamitous action right
afterwards. Our men, advised by the deserters from Bayonne
that that city, a very strong French border bulwark, could be
caught unprepared given the negligence of their garrisons
who often slept worry-free with their legs stretched out,
decided to take it by sea and by land one evening at sunset.
As the attempt was underway and the land forces approached
to attack the walls, the wind fell the fleet, stilling the readied
war equipment and armed ships on the verge of breaking
anchor. And so, with all hope gone, with damages and a lost
opportunity, many suffered wounds from the turreted walls
or were killed: the remainder pulled back from an unsucces-
sfull undertaking. The soldiers of the fleet, however, so as
not to seem to have toiled uselessly and feeling sorry to have
lost such a unique chance, landed full of anger on French
shores and plundered the well-fortified city of Capbreton with
many surrounding villages and localities. They brag to have
found among other rich spoils a huge quantity of resin, which
they needed, suitable for sealing the leaks of the ships. But
I fear the ever changing fortune of events: the enemies, who
now rejoice full of booty, will not remain passive in searching
for revenge; perhaps, someday, either they or innocent neighbors will weep because of these spoils. For now, fare well!

Logroño, from where we will leave shortly, 7 October 1523

Archiepiscopo Cusentino

Ab Indis naves habemus. Ab oppido *Panama* et insula, re
ac nomine *Dite*, quod sit foecunda unionum, australe putati
continentis latus ad occidentem, lequas scribit Egidius, vulgo
Gil Gonsalus, vir claro genere natus, sexcentas percurrisse. Par-
5 ticularia de huius navigationis inventis quae tu summo Pontifici
poteris ostendere, quandoquidem (post visa, quae ad Adrianum,
eius praedecessorem, scripseram, sero allata, quod mortuum
repererint), id optare Suam ais Beatitudinem, magna quidem et
narrata ac Summis digna sunt Pontificibus. Nunc ad septen-
10 trionale huius putati continentis latus redeamus. *Panucus* est
amnis ingens navigabilis, nuper inventus a nostris, ab ingenti
Tenustitana civitate lacunari lequas distat sexaginta circiter.
Franciscus Garaius, Iamaicae gubernator, velle in eius ripa
deducere coloniam instat. Eius erigendae veniam a Caesare
15 impetravit et, quod maius est, ut aeterno appelletur nomine
Garaiana Panuci regio illa permissum. Fernando Cortesio Te-
nustitani stratori magni imperii id esse molestum intelligimus.
Ne detrimenti aliquid hinc exoriatur, timemus. Tempus dicet.
Parte alia scito, post accessum Victoriae navis gariofolis onustae
20 quae orbem circuivit (de qua re particularem vidisti, viditque
Pontifex narrationem ad Adrianum directam), statutum fuisse
ut nova classis instruatur ad idem iter, quo coepta possessio
manu teneatur ac frequentetur. Regi Portugallico id est perniciosum, inde male sapidum; ut effectus eius rei differatur effla-
25 gitat, sui esse iuris arguit. Caesar ut audiatur imperavit. Classis
impensa ingens est, differre damnosum; suspenditur tamen. In
civitate Pacensi, vulgo *Badaioz*, quae fines Portugaliae claudit
cum Castellae regnis, Castellanorum et Portugalensium utrinque
quattuor et viginti scientiarum omnium et rei maritimae peri-
30 torum fuit conventus. Diu discussum est et sillogismatum utrinque. Ultimus dies Maii elapsi, is est terminus a Caesare datus
suis iudicibus, illi concioni. Sic finis fuit. Re infecta, redierunt
nostri. Rem Caesaream satis aperte probasse inquiunt, quod
extra lineam ab Alexandro sexto Pontifice Maximo concessam
35 iaceant illae insulae. E contra, Portugalenses intra suos limites
esse arguebant. Protrahere rem illis expediebat, nobis proscin-

To the Archbishop of Cosenza
(Giovanni Ruffo)

Now the ships have returned from the Indies. Egidius, <
commonly called *Gil Gonzáles*, a renowned man by birth, writes
that he travelled from the city of *Panama* and from *Rica* island,
rich by name as it abounds in pearls, along the southern side
of what is thought to be a continent for 600 leagues in the
westerly direction. The details discovered through this exploration you can reveal to the supreme Pontiff since (after your
review of the news I had written to his predecessor Adrian
but delivered only after he had died) You say that his Holiness
wants them; the accounts are indeed important and worthy of
the Supreme Pontiffs. Now let us return to the northern coast
of this territory which is thought to be a continent. The *Panuco*
is a large and navigable river, discovered recently by our men,
about 60 leagues from the great lagoon city of *Tenustitán*.
Francisco de Garay, governor of Jamaica, presses on with his
desire to found a colony on its banks. He obtained from the
Emperor, upon requesting it, permission to build it and, what
is more, that the *Panuco* territory be called forever *Garayana*.
We understand that this annoys Hernán Cortés, who has destroyed the vast empire of *Tenustitán*. We fear some trouble
will come from this. Time will tell. On the other hand, know
that after the arrival of *Victoria*, a ship loaded with cloves,
which had sailed around the earth (on this topic you saw the
detailed account sent to Adrian, and the Pope has also seen it),
it was decided that a new fleet be equipped for a second
journey, so that this newly conquered possession, be maintained
and inhabited. This is ruinous for the king of Portugal and,
consequently, not at all appealing; he insists and argues that it
is his right that completion of this project be delayed. The
Emperor ordered that he be heard. The cost of a fleet is
enormous, to delay is damaging; nevertheless, everything is
on hold. In the city of *Pax*, commonly called *Badajoz*, which is
at the border of Portugal and the kingdom of Castile, there
was an assembly of Castilians and Portuguese with 24 representatives from each side, experts about every discipline and
about life on the sea. There was much discussion, and argu-

dere. Demisso capite ac moesti Portugalenses regressi sunt; semiminabundi ferro tutaturos, ni argumenta proderint, fere insinuarunt. De hoc nunc satis, in particularibus latius. Comiti
40 Nasauti, qui Xebri loco apud Caesarem suffectus, data est in uxorem Ceneti marchionissa. An primogenitus sit a paterno sumpturus nomen, an a Mendociis materno, controversatum est aliquantulum, de redditibus etiam non nihil. Impensa tandem Caesaris conclusum est. Quid aut quantum, ipsi viderint
45 quorum interest. Est aliud ridiculum, non praetereundum, quod de pluviis anni quarti ac vigesimi blateratum est: re ipsa super nos evenit. Fluvius hic toto fere anno vadosus, alveum adeo, per alluviem, superavit, ut Caesarem in palatio velle obsidere videretur. Ad equorum uteros intra regiam crevit inundatio,
50 suburbium obrutum. Via tibi nota, quae dicitur *Hortus Regius*, summersa, plateae duae illae ingentes, tenus hominum pectoribus, aqua plenae. Currus et plaustra innumera, quae commeatus ad fora vexerant raptavit furor torrentis traxitque ad fluminis alveum non pauca horrea triticea ordeaceaque in planis illis
55 domibus clausa, multa putrefecit; domus plaeraeque collapsae. Si ab hac rabie indemnes evasistis, prosit! En aliud diu vaticinatum: Galleca infestant Galli nostra littora. Exerere caput e portubus nemo audet. Villas straverunt plaerasque. Mercatorias et piscatorias naves rapuerunt plures; littora cuncta labe-
60 factant. Sunt rerum vices. Sic vivitur. Vale!

Burgis, duodecimo Kalendas Iulii Millesimo Quingentesimo Vigesimo Quarto.

ments were presented from both sides. The last day of this past May was set by the Emperor for his judges as the last day of that assembly. So it has ended. Our representatives came back with matters unresolved. They say the rights of the Emperor were recognized quite openly, because those islands are located beyond the borderline set by the supreme Pontiff, Alexander VI. On the other hand, the Portuguese maintained they were within their side. It was to their advantage to prolong the discussions; to ours to cut them short. The Portuguese left heads low in discontent and hinted menacingly, that they would engage in war unless evidence was produced. Enough for now on this topic; I will give more details later. To the Count of Nassau, who took the place of the Count of Chièvres in the Imperial court, was given in marriage the Marquise of Cenet. There was considerable discussion about whether the firstborn should take his father's name or be a Mendoza like his mother, and to a certain degree also about his revenues. Finally, the matter was closed by intervention of the Emperor. What or how much will be decided by those concerned. I cannot ignore another piece of ridiculous news since much talk accompanied the rains of '24: it really happened to us. This river, fordable most of the year, with the rains overflowed so much that it seemed to want to besiege the Emperor in his palace. The water level inside the palace rose up to the abdomen of the horses; the suburbs were flooded with water. A street you know, *Huerto Real*, was submerged and its two large squares filled with water up to men's chest. The rage of the torrent swept away countless carriages and wagons that brought goods to the markets and carried toward the river-bed a considerable amount of corn, wheat, and barley which was kept in those low houses besides a lot that rotted; most of the houses tumbled down. If you escaped this rage without loss, good for you! Here is another calamity long foretold: the French are attacking our Galician coasts. No one dares venture out of the ports. They have razed most of the villages to the ground, siezed several merchant and fishing vessels and keep spreading ruin along the entire shore. Such are fate's circumstances through which one lives. Fare well!

Burgos, 20 June 1524

Archiepiscopo Cusentino

Quartana pressum habemus Caesarem, tristis est curia. Parum negociatur. Ad alia. Misimus artis maritimae peritum virum quendam, nomine *Stephanus Gomez*, cum una tantum navi, *caravela* vulgo. Ex Clunio discessit, fretum quaesiturus
5 inter *Floridam* tellurem et *Baccallaos*. Cataium inde se reperturum inquit; eat bonis avibus! Maluchea classis paratur. Augusto mense credunt aliqui vela facturam, neque Ianuario arbitror ego, quod non intelligam ita paratas esse naves, aut coacta tanto viatico necessaria. Ibit tandem, Deo favente, nulla de Portuga-
10 lensium habita ratione, in hoc tanti momenti negocio. De casu tui meique amici licentiati Vargas audisti forte, quanti valoris vir esset in magnis et arduis tractandis negociis nosti. Cupidineis in senecta vexatus stimulis monialis cuiusdam, genere clarae (ministram quam *freilam* vocant, cui nomen non est dandum),
15 exarsit. Noctu, per scalas coenobii muris appositas, ad eam proficiscebatur. Nocte intempesta una dierum, re peracta forte praeter vires aetatis, invasit horror hominem, sive ex conscientia sceleris admissi vel ex hebetudine cerebri et medullarum, ita ut semilanguidus redeunti per scalas, ensis e manu primo deciderit;
20 sequutus ensem ipse gravi rotatu, uti pulliculus animam exhalavit. Id prodigium divino iudicio ab omnibus asctiptum est et apertum est argumentum nil simile admissum relinqui a Superis impunitum. Germani, Caesareo conducti stipendio, Rosilionem versus mittuntur. Ad me ipsum parumper. Quam liber a fortu-
25 nae bonorum cupiditate tuo tempore vixerim, quamque opulentis ambitiosi fumi foetore sese pascentibus magis miserear, quam invideam, tute ipse testis es; unde, quandoquidem aliquid ultra propheticum illud optatum, neque divitias, neque paupertatem, ex Catholicorum vitam functorum benignitate, sum
30 assequutus, animum iusseram meum a postulatis quiescere, sed una me ratio movit, ut praeter statutum expergiscerer. Caesarem ego nuper his verbis adortus sum: "Inclite ac invictissime Caesar, quod me Tua Maiestas diligat, praebitus honor senatorius et oratorii muneris aliqua designatio testantur. Quod satis
35 est in fortunae blandimentis habeo mihi sumque Tua Caesarea Maiestate ditior, quia parvo contentus vivo. Perturbant nanque

176

To the Archbishop of Cosenza
(Giovanni Ruffo)

We know that the Emperor is ill with quartan fever. The court is sad. Few important matters are being dealt with. Let us turn our attention to other topics. We have sent a certain < man, an expert in seafaring art named *Estevão Gomes*, with a single ship, commonly called caravel. He left from La Coruña in search of straits between *Florida* and the land of *Bacallaos*. From there he claims he will find Cathay; may he go with good omens! A fleet is being prepared for the Moluccas. Some believe it will set sail next August but I do not think it will happen before January, because there does not exist a properly outfitted ship, nor have needed supplies for so great a journey been gathered. It will leave finally, with the help of God, without consideration for the Portuguese in this venture of such great importance. You perhaps heard of the misfortune of your friend and mine, doctor Vargas, a man reknowned for his ability in dealing with vast and difficult issues. Tormented in his old age by desires for a certain nun from a noble family, (they refer to this religious woman, whose name need not be given, as *freila*) he fell in love. At night he used to go to her climbing the walls of the convent with ladders. One time, in the middle of the night, having performed an act perhaps beyond the strength of his age, he was overtaken by fear, either from his realization of having committed a crime or from deep brain torpor, first he dropped the sword from his hands almost passing out while descending the ladder; chasing after the sword, he lost his balance and, like a young cock, breathed his last. This incident was regarded by all as a sign of God's judgement and clear evidence that no such action is left unpunished by heaven. The Germans hired with money from the Emperor are being sent around Rossiglione. And now let us talk a little of what concerns me. You yourself are a witness of how free from desire for the goods of fortune I have lived in your time, and how much more pity than envy I have felt for men striving after the allure of senseless ambition; consequently, since I have received from the goodness of the deceased Catholic Sovereigns something more than longing de-

libertatem amantis ingenium equorum et mularum agmina, familiarium molestiae multo gravius, quibus nunquam satis praebetur et longi temporis fastidia. De minutis et his paucis
40 obsequiis, grandia dicunt et appellant servitia et conquestibus perpetuis aethera complent. Exteriore tamen amoris aliquo erga me signo indigeo, ad honorem, cuius ferculum nemo unquam abiecit, propter oratores mihi conterraneos Mediolanensem, Venetum, Florentinum, Genuensem, Ferrariensem, Mantuanum
45 (qui omnes me nobilibus ortum parentibus Mediolani ac aetatis meae, quicquid boni fuit, in hac tuae Maiestatis domo consumpsisse sciunt), aliter Tuae Maiestati me gratum esse nequeo illis persuadere". Placuit sermo Caesari. Iamaicae, novo nomine *Sancti Iacobi*, foelicissimae insillae abbatialem mihi designavit
50 antisteam. Appello foelicissimam, quod ibi sit toto anno fere par nocti dies, quod non horrida vigeat aestas, non hyems rigida, quod perpetuis fruatur vere ac autumno; ab aequinoctio gradus tantum sexdecim et alicubi pauciores distat. Literas habetote Caesareas ad Pontificem supplicativas! Bullas expedite!
55 Sed alterum in casu hoc habeto. Regressus ad Caesarem cum gratiarum actione repetii: "Quo Tua Maiestas intelligat vera esse quae postulatis miscui, de solius amoris erga me signo, non avara cupiditate, in ipsius Abbatiae templo erigendo primi anni redditus integros, nullis impensis deductis, me praebiturum
60 polliceor. Pius est Caesar, pium est opus, utere tua pietate in hoc, uti soles in caeteris, aperiat et Tua Maiestas manum". Subrisit. Tantumdem imperatum est ut e regio fisco tribuatur. Expilabo in dies magis, quando iam sit opus incoeptum. E meis familiaribus mittam ad id opus aliquem; quae sequentur intel-
65 liges. Monitus ab Mapheo, postarum magistro, quod iam esset cursor petasatus, haec celeriter scripsi. Mentitus est: quattuor ultra dierum spacium intercessit. Hinc habeto paucula forte nulla, post haec, per dies aliquot. Comes Potentiae, Neapolitanus, ad curiam veniebat. Captus est et in arcem ductus Siman-
70 cheam, quod, Caesare inconsulto, ausus fuerit Pescariae Marchionem ad singulare certamen provocare, quo tempore Sua Maiestas, Marchionis opera contra Gallos lacessentes indigebat. De Gallis nescio quid summurmuratur, quod Rosilionis comitatum incursionibus infestarint. Est aliud maius. Indicum sena-
75 tum Caesar renovavit, a caeteris negociis explicitos delegit. Principem senatus, quem Hispanus *praesidentem* appellat, Oxomensem Episcopum, confessorem suum effecit, addidit collegas

sires, beyond riches or poverty, I refrained from requests; but one reason stirred me to overcome my self-imposed limit. Recently, I addressed the Emperor in these words: "O glorious and invincible Emperor: the office of Senator offered to me and the appointments as ambassador give evidence that Your Majesty loves me. I consider these sufficient delights of fortune, and I am richer than Your Imperial Majesty, for I live content with little. Indeed, numerous horses and mules disturb the freedom of the person who prefers talent, even more so the bothers of courtiers, to whom never enough is given, which seem endless. Their services of little significance, are, in their view, great feats of servitude, thus fill the air with incessant complaints. Nevertheless, in my honor I need an outward sign of your love for me, whose hospitality no one has ever turned down, on account of the ambassadors my countrymen of Milan, Venice, Florence, Genoa, Ferrara, Mantua (they all know I was born from noble parents in Milan and that during my time I have spent whatever good I have in the service of Your Majesty), whom otherwise I cannot convince that I am in Your Majesty's grace." The Emperor liked my reasoning and appointed me prelate of the newly named Saint James abbey in the so felicitous island of Jamaica. I label it so because there, <
throughout the year, day equals night, full summer is not unpleasant and winter is unrigorous, thus one perpetually enjoys springs and autumns; it is only 16° from the equator and at some point even less. Here are the supplication letters from the Emperor to the Pontiff. Prepare the bulls! But here is a later development in this case. When I went back to the Emperor to thank him, I repeated: "So that Your Majesty may understand that the words I mixed with the requests are true, a concerned expression of love alone toward me, not out of greedy desire, I promise to offer the entire income of my first year, without subtracting any expense, incurred while building the church of the named Abbey. The Emperor is a devout man and his works are godly; use your piety in this as you usually do in other instances, and may your Majesty open his hand." He smiled. It was ordered that just as much be contributed from the royal treasury. The "profit" will grow more each day as the work gets underway. For this task I will send one of my close friends; later you will know what happen. Advised by the postmaster Mafeo that the courier was now

Canariensem Episcopum, iurisperitos duos, tibi notos, ambos
doctores iurisdicundi, Beltranum et Maldonatum. Suo Caesareo
80 chirographo me imperat adesse. Ad aliud. Hac iter fecit regis
Portugaliae cursor, quod Florinus pyrata Gallus navim regi suo
raptaverit ab Indis venientem, qua merces vehebantur gemmarum et aromatum ad ducatorum centum octoginta milium summam conqueritur. Ubi primum huc appulsi sumus conclusum
85 est, ut Catherina, nubilis Caesaris soror, tibi nota, detur regi
Portugallico, eius consobrino, in uxorem. Vale, fastiditus, ut
arbitror, tam longa filateria!.

Ex Valdoleto, quo .iii. Nonas Augusti accessimus .M.D.XXIII.

ep. 806 *C* = 802 *A* = 765 *ms.*   *pp.* 698-699 *G*

Archiepiscopo Cusentino

Catherinam sororem Caesaris in Portugaliam ad virum
consobrinum misimus; pridie quam discederet, matrem adivit.
Se nuptam esse recensuit, ad virum ire oportere obortis lachrymis ait. Acies paratas esse Castellanas et Portugalenses ad
5 conflictum ni properaverit, dixisse fertur. Ad haec mater:
"Puellula es (hoc semper suo idiomate appellavit symbolo,
quod est *nigna*), nondum nubilis, ne cures". "Hem quam magna

ready to leave, I quickly added this. He lied. Four days more have gone by. After this you will, perhaps, have little or no news, for some days. The Count of Potenza, a Neapolitan, was coming to the court. He was arrested and taken to the fortress of Simancas, because, without consulting the Emperor, he dared challenge the Marquis of Pescara to a duel, at a time when His Majesty needed the help of the Marquis against the relentless French. Whispers, of one sort or another, about the French are going around since they have made incursions into the county of Rossiglione. There is other more important news. The Emperor has restored the Council of the Indies and chosen men free from other tasks. He appointed as head of the Coun- < cil, the *president* for the Spaniards, the Bishop of Osma, his own confessor, and has added as colleagues to the Bishop of the Canaries two law experts known to you, both doctors in law, Beltrán and Maldonado. With an imperial document he orders me to be present. On to something else. The courier of the king of Portugal came by and complains that the French pirate Florin has taken from his king a ship coming from the Indies with its cargo of pearls and spices worth about 180,000 ducats. As soon as we arrived here, we concluded that Catherine, the unmarried sister of the Emperor, well-known to you, would be given in marriage to the king of Portugal, his cousin. Fare well, even if you are by now annoyed, as I suppose, by such a long rambling!

From Valladolid, where we arrived, 3 August 1524

To the Archbishop of Cosenza
(Giovanni Ruffo)

We have sent to Portugal Catherine, sister of the Emperor, to her husband, a cousin. The day before leaving, she went to her mother. She reflected on the fact that she had been married and, with tears in her eyes, said it was proper to go to her husband. She is reported to have said that the armies of the Castilians and Portuguese were ready to fight, unless she hurried. To this her mother replied: "You are a child (she has

sunt in promptu scandala, ni ego iero". Mater ad haec: "Ne timeas nigna, ne timeas, non accidet mali quicquam". Eluce-
10 scente altero mane, matre nil ultra salutata, discessit. Ad Indos ab Hispanis inquietis spiritibus. Multa emergunt in dies, quae natura illis infixit nascentibus. Quattuor appulsa sunt navigia. Ab Senatu partibus illis praebente leges, ex Hispaniola literas habemus. Quae ad iusticiae administrationem attinent praeter-
15 missis, ad Cubam, alias Fernandinam insulam, ab *Nova Hispania* et Fernando Cortesio illarum terrarum domitore, appulsum esse quendam centurionem ab Cortesio missum, nomine *Christopho-rum Olitum* scribunt. Afferre illum in mandatis aiunt ab Corte-sio, ut inde in latus putati continentis, dictum *Figueras*, alias
20 notum, traiiciat ibique coloniam erigat. Quadringentorum pe-ditum et equitum triginta numerum habet secum. Ad locum eundem vadit Gil Gonsalus, praefectus regius. Ferunt et Pe-trurn Ariam, putati continentis et Aureae Castellae gubernato-rem, mittere copias ad locum eundem. Sperant omnes se illic
25 fretum optatum reperturos, terras a terris dirimens; veremur ne, si occurrerint, se invicem de suo more, quod sint sodalitatis impatientes, mutuo conficiant. Hispaniolae Senatui datur sum-ma potestas, ut ferventibus eorum animis eant obviam. Ab hoc Olito nuncium quoddam infoelix emanavit. Franciscum Ga-
30 raium, Iamaicae, meae sponsae, gubernatorem, dixi, alias, de colonia in Panuci magni amnis ripa deducenda, semper cogi-tasse. Septingentorum peditum, quattuor et quadraginta supra centum equitum coegerat manum. Ambagibus longis in tempus aliud relictis, ecce: ivit cum eo comitatu Garaius. Olitus hic,
35 in Cuba insula sistens, dixit Garaium fuisse profligatum, mox in Cortesii potestate obiisse. Per incertam hanc famam se ha-buisse Hispaniolae senatores, ad nostrum regium, dico Senatum Indicum, scripserunt. Quando apertius habebimus, habebitis. Hic annus rebus Indicis, episcopis praesertim, acrem se ostendit,
40 praeter seditiones ducum, quas timemus. Vita functi sunt plures episcopi: Alexander Geraldinus Italus noster, in antistea sua Sancti Dominici et Conceptionis Hispaniolae, raptatus est; obiit et putati continentis alius. Prior vero Melioratae, ad utranque antisteam Sancti Dominici et Conceptionis Hispaniolae desi-
45 gnatus, expectare nolit vestra pontificia plumbata diplomata: dum illic expeditio tractaretur, exhalavit fluxu ventris animam, quippe mitem et providam. Evenit et aliud adversum. Ex ostio Baethis duodecim navium classis, ad Indos itura, vela fecerat;

always called her with the Spanish diminutive *niña*), not yet of an age to be married, do not worry about it!" "New scandals are at hand, if I do not go." And her mother replied: "Do not be afraid, *niña*, do not fear; no evil will befall you." At sunrise the following day, with no further good-bye to her mother, she left. From the restless Spanish spirits, let us move on to the Indies. Day after day new aspects of the character nature im- <
pressed on them from birth come to light. Four ships have landed. We have letters from Hispaniola sent by the legislative Council of those regions. Leaving aside matters pertaining to the administration of justice, they write that a certain centurion by the name of *Cristóbal de Olid*, sent by Cortés, has landed in Cuba, otherwise known as *Fernandina* island; he is coming from New Spain on behalf of Hernán Cortés, conqueror of those lands. They say he is charged by Cortés with sailing along the coast called *Figueras*, another known name, of what is thought to be a continent, and of founding a colony there. He has with him 400 foot-soldiers and 30 cavalrymen. Gil González, the royal governor, is going to the same place. They say that Pedro Arias, governor of the presumed continent and of *Castilla del Oro*, also is sending troops to the same place. They all hope to find there the desired strait, or land divider; we fear that, if they meet, they will destroy each other, in their usual manner, as they do not consider being friendly. The Council of Hispaniola enjoys full power to keep in check their inflamed spirits. Some sad news came from this Olid. I said elsewhere that Francisco de Garay, governor of Jamaica, now linked to me, always had in mind to found a colony on the banks of the great Panuco river. He had gathered a group of 700 soldiers and 144 cavalrymen. Leaving for another time lengthy descriptions, here it is: Garay went with that group. Olid, as he stopped at Cuba, reported that Garay had been defeated and soon after died in the hands of Cortés. Members of the Council of Hispaniola inform our Royal Council, that is, the Council of the Indies, that they consider it an uncertain fact. When we find out anything more precise you will know it. This year is showing itself harsh for affairs of the Indies, especially for the bishops, in addition to the chiefs' rebellions, which we fear. Several bishops have died; our Italian Alessandro Geraldini has been snatched by death in his see of Santo Domingo and Concepción in Hispaniola. Another died on the presumed continent. The prior of Mejorada,

vi tempestatum quassata, magnam opum partem in mare, quo
50 se exoneraret, coacta est proiicere ad portumque redire unde
prodierat. Regressa tandem est et, foelicibus in puppim flanti-
bus ventis, coeptum iter peragit. Ad nos ab Indis redeamus!
Caesar, suae quartanae profuturam credens aeris mutationem,
Turdesillas, ubi mater eius pessundata Saturno sedet et sedebit
55 aeternum, se contulit. Neapolitanus quidam, cum unguento sibi
noto, quo renes uncturus sit, quartanam abrasurum sese obtulit.
Admissus est, neque obstitit medicorum argutia. Inungit. Prima
facie visum est profuisse. Regressa mox est. Conqueritur un-
guentarius quod nimis propere medelam abiecerint medici:
60 longiore parumper tempore opus fuisse ait; dimissus est un-
guentarius. Forti animo langorem patitur Caesar. Mare quoque
nobis infensum est. De carrachis pluribus obrutis et disturbatis
vi tempestatum, vos apertius scitis, quia Italae omnes erant.
Iacobus de Vera insignem in Hispania tuo tempore unam con-
70 struxerat: ad manus pyratarum Gallorum ea venit, cum mille
quingentis saccis lana Hispana sarcitis, rebusque aliis ad valorem septuaginta ducatorum milium; ad Belgas et Antuerpienses
nundinas proficiscebatur. Sed aliud accidit magis mirandum,
quia inauditum hactenus. De statione Bilbaii et fluminis eius in
75 oceanum fluentis commodo audivisti saepe. Intra fluminis fauces valde superne stabant in anchoris multae naves, plenae
mercibus, coactae ut, uno facto agmine, ob pyratarum metum,
exirent, ad Belgas iturae. Nactum ausi sunt Galli pyratae fluvium pernavigare. Putarunt Cantabri, navium domini, amicas
80 esse. Duae e navibus, ab anchoris erutas, abduxerunt; expergi-
scentur posthac vigilantius ignavi navium domini. Vale!

Ex Valdoleto, unde nullas a me ulterius habebis: cras naque ut
Madritum (Mantuam Carpentanam) proficiscamur, discedemus. Decimo
quarto Kalendas Decembris .M.D.XXIIII.

however, appointed for both the sees of Santo Domingo and Concepción, in Hispaniola, did not want to wait for your pontifical documents with leaden seals: while the expedition was being organized, afflicted by dysentery, he breathed forth his kind and wise soul. Another adversity also occurred. From the mouth of the Guadalquivir, a twelve ships fleet had set sail to go to the Indies; badly shaken by violent storms, it was forced to throw out at sea a great part of its goods in order to lighten the ships, and sail back to the port of departure. Finally it returned and with favorable winds completed the journey it had begun. From the Indies let us come back to ourselves. The Emperor, believing that a change of air would be beneficial to his quartan fever, moved to Tordesillas, where his mother is and will always be, under the negative influence of Saturn. A Neapolitan offered to rid him of the quartan fever using an ointment known to him, which he will smear on his sides. He was admitted, and the physicians' "cleverness" was not an obstacle. He spread it on him. At first it seemed to help; the fever soon came back. The anointer complains because the physicians have rejected the medication too soon claiming more time was needed; he was dismissed. The Emperor bears his illness with courage. Even the sea is hostile to us. You are more than aware of the many carracks destroyed and smashed by violent storms, being all Italian. During your time, in Spain Jacobo de Vera had built a remarkable one: that carrack fell into the hands of French pirates, with 1500 bales of Spanish wool and other goods worth 70,000 ducats; it was headed for the Belgian markets, especially Antwerp. An even more unusual incident happened, one never heard before. You have often heard of the port of Bilbao and the advantages of its river, that flows into the ocean. In its delta, quite a way up, were anchored many ships full of goods, about to go to the Belgians and forced to proceed in one convoy for fear of pirates. The French pirates dared to sail the river to catch them. The Cantabrians, owners of the ships, thought they were friendly ships. They led away two of the ships removing their anchors; from now on, the careless owners of the ships will be more vigilant and on alert. Fare well!

From Valladolid, from where you will not receive any more letters from me: tomorrow we will leave to go to Madrid (*Mantua Carpetana*), 18 November 1524

Archiepiscopo Cusentino

Ab argumentis quibusdam non fauste Gallos in hac insania Martiali procedere arbitramur. Leutrecus, dux confinium Angiae, a suo Christiano rege revocatur; ut, confinibus relictis, properet ad se cum praesidiariis omnibus suis imperare
5 dicitur. Huius urinae spectatores medici aegrotum vel aegroto proximum esse iudicant stimulatorem, dum interea quid rabida sors allatura sit apertis fàucibus operiuntur. Ad Indos transeamus. Tres habemus ab Hispaniola naves, saccareis panibus et coriis boum, quorum est iam tanta in insulis copia,
10 ut ignorent, qua mittere illos queant, mercibusque aliis onustas. Iacobus Velazquez Fernandinae, quae Cuba est, gubernator, qui ditem Crassum opibus superabat, Codro miserior et paupere paupetior[35] obiit: in construendis novis classibus ad novas terras quaerendas et Fernandi Cortesii fortunam
15 infringendam, ingentes consumpsit thesauros. Frustra omnia, Cortesii nanque genius supereminet. Vita et functus est in ipsius Cortesii potestate Franciscus Garaius Iamaicae, meae sponsae, diu gubernator. Is et ipse novarum terrarum cupiditate se ipsum expilavit ac, tandem in calamitate redactus,
20 calamitose abscessit e vita. Haec latius in particularibus rebus Indicis, de quibus propediem duas decades habebitis, ad Mediolani ducem directam unam, ad Pontificem alteram. Sed audi quid inter nos versetur de Indorum libertate, super qua variae sunt opiniones diu discussae. Nihil adhuc repertum
25 conducibile. Iura naturalia pontificiaque iubent ut genus humanum omne sit liberum, imperiale distinguit, usus adversum aliquid sentit; longa experientia hoc censet, ut servi sint, ne liberi sint hi: quod a natura sint in abominabilia vitia proclives ad obscoenos errores, ducibus et tutoribus deficientibus,
30 ilico revertuntur. Accitos in Senatum nostrum Indicum bicolores Dominicos fratres et pede nudos Franciscos, illarum partium longo tempore colonos, quid fore putent satius consuluimus. Nihil a re magis alienum sanxerunt quam quod

[35] See A. GERBI, *La natura delle Indie Nove* Milano: 1975, 265-268.

To the Archbishop of Cosenza
(Giovanni Ruffo)

From certain indications we think that the French in this crazy war do not have any luck. Lautrec, frontier commander at Anjou, was recalled by his "Christian" king; he is said to have ordered him to hasten to him with all his garrisons after leaving the borders. The physicians who examine the urine, think that its owner is sick or very close to being sick, and they wait with open jaws to see what angry fate will bring. Let us go on to the Indians. Three ships have arrived from Hispaniola, loaded with loaves of sugar, ox pelts so abundant in the islands that they do not know where to ship them, and with other goods. Jacobo Velázquez, governor of Fernandina, that is Cuba, who surpasses rich Crassus in wealth, died more wretched than Codro and poorer than a pauper: he consumed great treasures in building new fleets to search for new lands and weaken the fortune of Hernán Cortés. All in vain, for the genius of Cortés surpassed him. Francisco de Garay, governor for a long time of Jamaica, linked to me, also died in the < hands of the same Cortés. He too ruined himself because of his desire for new lands, and in the end, reduced to calamity, died wretchedly. I will report more extensively the details of these matters in the Indies: in a short while, you will have two *Decades* about them, one addressed to the Duke of Milan, the other to the Pontiff. But listen to what we say among ourselves concerning the freedom of the Indians, about which various opinions have been discussed at length. No expedient has been found up to now. Natural and canon law dictate that the whole human race be free, but Roman law has made a distinction, and consuetude proved the opposite at times; experience, however, has long established, that they are slaves, not free men: since by nature they are inclined to loathsome vices, having no guidelines and tutors, they quickly repeat shameful mistakes. Having summoned to our Council of the Indies the two kinds of Dominican friars and bare-footed Franciscans, who lived a long time in those areas, we have consulted them on what they think might be better. They declared nothing would be farther from the truth than leaving them free. I will

liberi relinquantur. Latius haec et quae referent in particula-
35 ribus. Nunc satis. Vale!

Ex Mantua Carpentana *(Madrito)*, octavo Kalendas Martii Millesimo Quingentesimo Vigesimo Quinto.

ep. 812 *C* = 809 *A* = 770 *ms.*   *p.* 703 *G*

Archiepiscopo Cusentino

De rebus placidis, gratis, honorificis, humano generi
utilibus ad te, de petulantis fortunae scloppis ad alios. In
portu Clunio classis est, ad Maluchas insulas aromatum al-
5 trices destinata; quando discedet, intelliges. Ab Hispania
Nova, domita nuper a Cortesio, thesauris onustae duae naves appulsae sunt ad Cassiterides. Earum una, thesauris in
terram expositis, tentare fortunam decrevit; pyratarum praedonum evasit rabiem. In hac vectus est Lupicus alumnus
10 meus, a teneris [36], quem dilexisti a puero, iam barbatus, qui
paulo post tuum discessum, cum bona mea venia, duce Roderico Albornocio, a rege ad partes illas misso, cum magi-
stratu computatoris, rerum novarum auditu pellectus profectus fuerat. Thesauros afferunt et tigrim a catella in cavea
15 nutritam, colubrinam [37] et unam, quam esse auream fama
ferebat, apportant. Eam non tanti esse scribit Lupicus; exiguo auri gradu fulctam dicit. Nondum est appulsus; ab Hispali ad nos veniet et multa intelligemus. Caesar magna
multaque impartitus est suis. Ioannem Fonsecam Burgensem
20 et Rosanum antistitem obiisse nosti. Palentinum in Burgensem transmutavit, Palentiam Pacensi designavit; doctorem
Mansum Pacensem effecit; licentiatum Suarez, senatorem
haereseos inquisitionis, nominavit Tudetensem, in Granaten-
sem elegit Civitatensem. Hanc dedit antisteam doctori Mal-

---

[36] See Quint. I 2, 18.

[37] A long and thin artillery piece used from the XV to the XVII century. So
named after its snake-like shape. From classical Latin *colubrinus, a, um*. See also Provençal
colovrina.

report more extensively on these matters and on what they will entail. Enough for now. Fare well!

From Madrid (Mantua Carpetana), 22 February 1525

To the Archbishop of Cosenza
(Giovanni Ruffo)

I report to you about matters which are pleasing, peaceful, bring honor or useful to the human race, but to others about the blows of insolent fortune. The fleet is in the port of La Coruña headed for the Moluccas, spice-producing islands; you will know when it leaves. From New Spain, recently subdued by Cortés, two ships loaded with treasures made the Cassiteridi Islands. One of them, having unloaded its treasures on land, decided to try its luck; it avoided the rage of the pirate robbers. On that ship, sent off by the king as an accountant, travelled Lopique, my pupil since he was little and now grown, whom you held dear from a tender < age; he set out with my benevolent permission under the guidance of Rodrigo de Albórnoz a little after your departure, attracted by what he had heard of the new discoveries. They are carrying treasures, a cub tiger that was nourished by a dog in a cage, and also a culverin, the only one believed to be made of gold. Lopique writes that it is not solid gold, only plated with a thin layer of it. He has not made land yet; he will come to us from Seville and we will have much news. The Emperor has imparted to his own many great gifts. You are aware that Juan de Fonseca, bishop of Burgos and Rozas, died. He transferred the bishop of Palencia to Burgos and has assigned Palencia to the bishop of Badajoz with the see of Badajoz going to doctor Manso; he nominated the licentiate Suarez, member of the College of the Inquisition on heresy, for the see of Tuy and chose the bishop of Ciudad for the see of Granada. He has given this prelature to doctor Maldonado, my colleague on the Council

donato, mihi collegae in senatu Indico, evexit et multos ad commendarias. Vale!

Madriti, .iii. Nonas Martii (quo die putamus iactam esse aleam[38] in agro Papiensi, multoque sanguine foelicem alias tellurem esse irroratam) .M.D.XXV.

ep. 814 *C* = 811 *A* = 772 *ms.*   *p.* 704 *G*

Archiepiscopo Cusentino

A nobis ad Indos, ab Indis ad nos frequentior est classium concursus, quam sarcinariorum iumentorum a nundinis ad nundinas. Sexto Kalendas Maii vela fecit una classis navium viginti quattuor. In ea Ioannes Mendigurrenus Cantaber, familiaris
5 meus tibi notus, vehitur. Mitto salutatum sponsam meam, Iamaicam insulam, foelix regnum, septuaginta leucarum longitudine ab oriente, in occidentem latitudine triginta, ubi non hyems rigida, non aestas torrida, ubi fere nullum est diei et noctis discrimen, quod proxima sit aequatori ad gradus octo-
10 decin et paulo plus, pauloque minus pro latitudine. Ibi toto anno frondescunt et una fructibus onustae acerbis et maturis arbores, ubi semper prata florescunt. In particularibus latius. Sunt in ea insula erectae duae coloniae quas, licet paucis habitatas civibus, vult Caesar civitatum nomine ac praerogativis
15 frui. *Sibillam* appellant unam, *Oristanam* alteram; in utraque, quod ex trabibus et paleis essent erecta, combusta sunt templa. Statui ut e redditibus meis primariae, quae Sibilla est, lapideum inchoetur templum et lapideum saltem fiat sacrarium, in quo tuta sit cum ornamentis Eucharistia, ne tanto ulterius discrimine
20 subiiciantur. Tantundem, meo supplicatu, mandat Caesar expendi. Is meus, ut oeconomi et in redditibus colligendis quaestoris officio fungatur, missus est a me. Optandum est ut foelicibus sulcent oceanum auspiciis. En dum ista versarem, Lupicus meus ab Cortesio quaedam et magna Caesari ad aurem dicenda

---

[38] See Suet. *Caes.* 32,3.

of the Indies; he has also raised many to positions of trust. Fare well!

Madrid, 4 March 1525 (the day I think the die was cast in the territory of Pavia marking the blood-shed time for that land — formerly lucky).

To the Archbishop of Cosenza
(Giovanni Ruffo)

The coming and going of fleets from us to the Indies < and from there to here is more frequent than that of beasts of burden from one market to another. On the 26th of April a fleet of 24 ships set sail. On it travels, Juan de Mendigorría from Cantabria, one of my retinue whom you know. I send greetings to the island of Jamaica, now linked to me, a happy kingdom at 70° longitude from the East and 30° latitude to the West, where there is no icy winter or scorching summer and where there is almost no difference between day and night because it is very near the equator, just over 18°, a little less in latitude. There, where the meadows are always in bloom, trees are green the whole year and loaded with both unripe and ripe fruits at the same time. You will have the details later. Two colonies have been founded on that island and, although inhabited by few people, the Emperor wants them to enjoy the fame and privileges of cities. They call one *Seville*, the other *Oristán*; in both, the church burned down because they were built with lumber and straw. With the revenues I receive from the more important of them, which is Seville, I decided to begin building a stone church with at least a sacrarium in stone as well, so that the Eucharist and its vessels might be safe and no jonger subject to such a great danger. Upon my request, the Emperor also ordered that such expense be matched. I sent my man to be the steward and treasurer in the office collecting the revenues. We must wish that they sail the ocean with favorable auspices. As I was reflecting on these matters, my dear Lopique brings some

25 portat. Ea praetermittamus impraesentiarum, detegentur aliquando. Publica sunt haec. Contra magistratuum regionum assensum, Fernandus Cortesius it cum exercitu valido ad delendum Christophorum Olitum, ab eius imperio alienum. Hinc strages expectatur Hispanorum, hinc labefactatis eorum viribus,
30 timetur Indorum defectio; sunt impatientes Hispani: non priores modo, sed neque pares aequo animo ferunt. Ad eundum tendunt locum Gil Gonsalus et a Petro Aria putati continentis gubernatore, praefectus alter, nomine *Franciscus Fernandez*. Misit et mari Cortesius in Olitum e suis ducibus unum, nomine
35 *Franciscus de Las Casas*. Sub spe freti reperiendi, tendunt omnes. De Indis satis nunc, alias plura. Distulit discessum cursor, inde longam habes epistolam. Addo parumper. Galli oratores veniunt. Ab rege Anglo tertium habemus: bellum, quam pacem hi mallent et matrimonii vinculum. Obstat puellae non aptae
40 viro aetas. Marchio Brandalburchensis obiit. Per equos dispositos, ad uxorem, quondam reginam, Valentiae morantem, proficiscebatur. Ubi primum appulsus est, lassus ex equorum et curruum quassatu quod esset procerus valde, non abstinuisse a coitu dicitur. Ad solandam reginam misit Caesar Episcopum
45 Conchensem, tibi amicum. Coactus Castellae conventus stricte supplicant ut Caesar uxorem capiat gignendae proli aptam; Catherinam Portugallicam viro maturam, sapientem, decoram, venustam et bene Caesare dignam capiat uxorem, instant. Donec rex cum Gallo, miro fatorum ordine, in Caesarea clauso
50 cavea, componatur, meo iudicio, conclusio differetur. Promissam vobis ducalem decadem et a vobis efflagitatam, secum attulit Camillus Gillinus ad herum illustrissimum ducem, Mediolano regrediens, inde se missurum exemplar ad vos pollicitus est; pontificia subsequentur propediem. Si de magni cancellarii

important news from Cortés to whisper in the ear of the Emperor. Let us leave them aside for the moment; they will be revealed one day. The following matters are of public knowledge. Hernán Cortés, against the opinion of court officials, is off with a strong army to destroy Cristóbal de Olid, who opposes his rule. Thus, we anticipate a slaughtering of Spaniards and once these are out, we fear the Indians' rebellion; the Spaniards are impatient: not only the leaders, but those in the ranks as well, do not bear it with good spirit. Gil Gonzáles heads to the same place with another admiral by the name of *Francisco Fernández*, who is sent by Pedro Arias, governor of the presumed continent. Against Olid by sea Arias dispatched commander Francisco de Las Casas as well. They all proced with the hope of finding a strait. Enough for now about the Indians; another time we will say more. The courier postponed his departure, therefore you have a long letter. I add some more news. The French ambassadors are coming. From the English king we have a third item: they would prefer to have war rather than peace and a marriage. The problem is the age of the young girl, not suited for a husband. The Marquis of Brandeburg died. With horses arrayed for travel, he was going to his wife who, since becoming queen lived in Valencia. They say that, as soon as he arrived, although weary — being rather tall — from the jolting of the horse-drawn wagons, he did not abstain from sexual pleasures. The Emperor sent your friend the Bishop of Cuenca, to console the queen. The *Cortes*, convened at Castile, pressure the Emperor to take a wife suited for child bearing; they insist he marries Catherine of Portugal, who is of age for a husband, wise, beautiful, amiable and well worthy of the Emperor. As long as the king, by fate's strange dictates, is in league with the "*Gallo*" [rooster-the Frenchman] shut up in the imperial cage, it is my opinion that a settlement will be put off. Camillo Gillino brought with him for the very illustrious Duke the decade dedicated to the Duke, promised to you upon your request, and he has assured me that upon his return from Milan he would send you a copy; those dedicated to the Pontiff will follow shortly. If you hear something concerning the resentment of the grand chancellor Mercurino da Gattinara, your friend, toward the Emperor for receiving many people privately, against the authority of his

55 Mercurini a Gattinera, tibi amici, turbato in Caesarem animo, quod plaerosque a secretis admittat contra sui magistratus autoritatem, aliquid audiveris, ne putes in stationes male fidas navem hanc collisum ituram. Caesar indiget eius obsequio, neque alteri locus in promptu aequus. Ipsi convenient. Tu vale!

Toletum venimus, octvo Kalendas Maii, ergo data Toleti, Idibus Iunii Millesimo Quingentesimo Vigesimo Quinto.

office, do not think that this ship is going to come into unsafe ports. The Emperor needs his regard and it is not a position easily accessible by someone else. They themselves will agree. Fare well!

We reached Toledo the 24th of April and this, therefore, was consigned at Toledo the 13th of June 1525.

INDEX OF CROSSREFERENCED PASSAGES

Listed below are the crossreferences between the chosen letters and the passages of the De Orbe Novo Decades. *In the latters the topics barely dealt with in the* Epistolary *are discussed at length.*

(The number references are from the Graz photooffset reprint)

Opus epistolarum	Decades de Orbe Novo
131, p. 360	I 1, p. 39
134, p. 361	I 1, pp. 39-42
135, pp. 361-362	I 1
136, p. 362	I 2, p. 44
139, p. 363	I 2, p. 47
141, p. 364	I 1, p. 42
143, p. 365	I 1-2, pp. 40, 43-47
145, p. 366	I 2, p. 47
147, pp. 367-368	I 2, pp. 43-44
153, pp. 370-371	I 2, p. 45-47; I 3, p. 48
157, p. 373	I 2, p. 43, 47; I 3, p. 48
159, p. 374	I 1, p. 39
165, p. 377	I 3, p. 50
169, p. 379	I 6, pp. 62-64
177, p. 383	I 9, pp. 72-73
180, p. 384	I 9, p. 73
181, pp. 384-385	I 9, p. 73
189, p. 388	I 9, pp. 72-74
190, p. 389	I 9, pp. 73-75
201, p. 394	I 8, p. 68
205, p. 396	I 9, pp. 73-74
529, p. 537	I 9, p. 70; II 1, pp. 78-79; II 6; II 10
537, p. 541	II 2, pp. 83-84
542, p. 543	II 1, p. 81; II 4, p. 89; II 5, p. 92
544, pp. 544-545	III 10, pp. 139-140
548, pp. 546-547	I-III

Opus epistolarum	*Decades de Orbe Novo*
557, p. 552	III 9, p. 139; III 10, pp. 139-140
558, pp. 552-553	II 7, p. 95
559, p. 553	III 9, p. 139
624, pp. 581-582	III 10, p. 141 ss.
630, p. 584	V 7, p. 187
635, p. 587	III 10, p. 140
650, p. 593	V I, p. 160
650 bis, p. 593	IV 3, p. 148
715, p. 633	IV 1, p. 146
717, p. 635	V 3, pp. 169-175
758, pp. 662-663	V 8, p. 196
766, pp. 668-669	IV
770, p. 671	V 7, pp. 187-192
773, pp. 672-673	V 7, pp. 192-194
774, pp. 673-674	V 8, p. 196; V 10, pp. 200-201
782, pp. 678-679	V 10, pp. 200-202
786, p. 682	V 3
791, pp. 685-686	VII 4, pp. 224
801, pp. 693-694	VI 1-2, pp. 205-206; VI 9, p. 213; VII 5, pp. 224-225; VIII 3, p. 245
804, pp. 696-697	VI 10, p. 214; VII 4, p. 223; VII 6, pp. 226-227; VII 7, p. 228; VII 9, p. 233; VIII 1, pp. 240-241; VIII 9, pp. 260-261
806, pp. 698-699	VII 5, p. 225; VIII 2, pp. 243-244; VIII 9, p. 262
809, p. 702	VII 4, pp. 222-223; VIII 2, pp. 243-244
812, p. 703	VIII 9, pp. 260-261
814, p. 704	VII 1, pp. 214-215; VII 2, p. 217; VIII 9, p. 260; VIII 10, pp. 263-266

From the *Decades of the New World*

As for the epistolary, we prepared a detailed summary of the topics dealt with by the author in the Decades of the New World *I 1-7 and III 4; for the other books, narrating events that took place in the New World or those related to it, but not strictly connected with Columbus, we simply mention the contents for a more general orientation.*

DECADE I

Book 1: Preface with dedication to Cardinal Ascanio Sforza (p. 206); Christopher Columbus unfolds his project to the Sovereigns (p. 206); departure of Columbus with the caravels given him (p. 206); stop of the fleet at the Canaries, brief digression on these islands (p. 206); discontent of the sailors and intervention of Columbus to restore order (p. 208); land sighted, discovery of six islands, two of which particularly large, Juana [Cuba] and Hispaniola; landing at Hispaniola and first contacts with the natives (p. 208); customs of the natives, description of the canoe (p. 212); the Cannibals or Caribs and their cruel customs (p. 212); the food of the natives, maize, *ages, yuca* (p. 214); the gold of the islands (p. 214); flora and fauna (p. 216); friendship pact with the cacique Guacanagarí and decision to leave thirty-eight men to explore Hispaniola (p. 218); the language of the natives (p. 218); return to Spain (p. 218); honors accorded to Columbus by the Sovereigns (p. 218); Columbus appointed Admiral and his brother Bartholomew named *Adelantado*; preparations for a second expedition entrusted to Juan de Fonseca and subsequent departure of the fleet from Cádiz on 25 September 1493 (p. 220).

Book 2: The Sovereigns at Medina del Campo are informed of the return of the ships from the expedition (p. 222); in the absence of Columbus, who remained at Hispaniola to explore, the commander of the fleet, Antonio Torres, presents the report (p. 222); discovery of the islands named by the Spaniards *Dominica* and *Galana* (p. 222); description of the dwellings of the Cannibals in another island (p. 224); the islands of *Guadeloupe* and *Carucueria*, description of parrots (p. 226); upon returning to Hispaniola, they discover many islands including *Madanino*, inhabited only by women; description of their customs (p. 228); discovery of other islands: Montserrat, Santa María la Redonda, San Martín, Beata Virgen de la Antigua, Santa Cruz (p. 228); clash with the Cannibals (p. 230); discovery of a group of islands or archipelago and of *Burichena* island, named by the Spaniards San Juan (p. 232); arrival at Hispaniola, where native interpreters flee during the night (p. 234); Columbus learns of the slaughter of the thirty-eight men he had left with the brother of Guacanagarí (p. 234); digression on the natives, happy with their natural state but tormented by the desire for power (p. 236); escape of native women from the Spanish ships, under the leadership of Catalina, reminiscent of the Roman Clelia (p. 238); Melchor is sent by Columbus to find Guacanagarí, accused of the slaughter of the thirty-eight men, and discovers a bay he names Puerto Real (p. 240); meeting with another cacique (p. 240); expedition of Hojeda and Gorvalán, who find rivers laden with gold (p. 242); the cacique Caonabó (p. 242); digression on astronomy: height of the pole on the horizon (p. 242); choice of a place for the founding of a city (p. 244); description of hot spices (p. 244).

Book 3: Dedication to cardinal Ludovico of Aragon (p. 246); description of Hispaniola: nature of the island, fertility of the soil (p. 246); exploration of the territory of the Cibao province (p. 248); construction of the fortress of Santo Tomás (p. 250); the gold of Cibao (p. 250); exploration of Luján (p. 252); mention of the bull of Alexander VI concerning the *raya*, the line dividing the ocean between Spaniards and Portuguese (p. 254); exploration of Cuba (p. 254); the island of Jamaica (p. 256); exploration of the places along Cuban shores, cape Alpha-Omega (p. 256); friendly exchange with the natives: the Spaniards taste iguana meat for the first time (p. 258); description of the fishing method of the natives, who use the *guaicano*, sea-lamprey (p. 260); meeting with other natives (p. 262); discovery of narrow canals with water that is milky and thick (p. 262); meeting with a man dressed in white followed by other men who suddenly vanish (p. 264); description of the flora and fauna of Cuba; the varied dialects of the natives of Cuba (p. 266); the bad condition of ships and supplies force Columbus to turn back (p. 266); good reception by the natives (p. 266); meeting with an elderly native who passes on to Columbus some wisdom (p. 268); description of the happy life of the natives, reminiscent of the mythical golden age (p. 270); return of Columbus, now sick, to Isabela (p. 270).

Book 4: Upon his return to Spain, Columbus, learns of slanders against him and goes to the Sovereigns to justify his actions (p. 272);

behavior of the Spaniards toward the natives (p. 272); cacique Guarionex, the rebellion of cacique Caonabó and his capture (p. 272); the mission of Alfonso de Hojeda to Caonabó (p. 274); upset of the natives over the building of new fortresses (p. 276); gold mines and electrum alloy on the mountains of Cibao, forests of scarlet trees near the fortress of Concepción (p. 276); Columbus defends himself from charges of low profits from the new lands (p. 278); tribute of the natives of Cibao in exchange for assurances for their lives (p. 280); armed clash between the brother of Caonabó and the Spaniards (p. 282); capture of the brother of Caonabó (p. 282); description of a violent hurricane (p. 282); death of Caonabó and of his brother during the return voyage to Spain (p. 284); while new caravels are built to replace those destroyed by the hurricane, Bartholomew Columbus is sent to explore the gold mines 60 miles from Isabela (p. 284); on 11 March 1495 Columbus returns to report to the Sovereigns, leaving his brother in the New World with full powers (p. 284).

Book 5: Bartholomew Columbus builds the fortress of Fortaleza del Oro (p. 286); return to Concepción to collect the tributes brought by caciques Guarionex and Manicautex (p. 286); arrival of three caravels with food supplies from Spain (p. 286); dispatch of three hundred native prisoners to Spain (p. 286); building of the fortress of Santo Domingo (p. 286); meeting with king Bechio Anacauchea, not far from the river Naiba, where there is no gold (p. 288); festive reception by the natives, games and performances (p. 290); return to Isabela where Bartholomew finds many sick men whom he distributes among the fortresses that have been built (p. 292); departure for Santo Domingo (p. 292); uprising of Guarionex, his capture and subsequent release (p. 294); hospitality of Anacaona, sister of Beechio Anacauchea: the *Adelantado* tastes and enjoys iguana meat (p. 296); reports on the cuisine of the natives (p. 296); the treasure of Anacaona (p. 298); gifts and tributes to the *Adelantado* (p. 298); uprising of Roldán (p. 300); cacique Maiobanex helps Guarionex against the Spaniards (p. 302); return of Columbus to the New World (p. 304).

Book 6: Beginning of the third journey of Columbus (p. 306); description of route and climate (p. 306); sighting of land: the stop at a port near Punta del Arenal (p. 308); meeting with a canoe on which travel twenty-four "white" men: Columbus's hypothesis on the different look of these men (p. 308); the frightened natives take off (p. 310); the strait Boca del Dragón and Margarita island (p. 312); disembarking on the land of Paria (p. 312); happy welcome by the natives and description of their dress (p. 314); exploration of the province of Paria: Cumaná, Manacapana and Curiana (p. 314); digression on astronomy: the pole star and some incredible natural phenomena (p. 316); Columbus sails toward Hispaniola (p. 318); hypothesis of Columbus about the land of Paria (p. 320).

Book 7: Uprising of Roldán and his followers at Hispaniola (p. 322); the *Adelantado* fights against the people of Cibao, who are defeated (p. 324); negotiations between the *Adelantado* and Maiobanex for the handing over of Guarionex (p. 326); after some ups and downs the territory is peaceful again and the caciques captured (p. 328); plots against Columbus and appointment of governor Francisco de Bobadilla to investigate Hispaniola (p.332); the Columbus brothers are taken to prison in Cádiz and then freed by order of the Sovereigns (p. 332).

Books 8-10: Accurate narration of the journey made by Pedro Alfonso Niño along the coasts of Paria in 1499-1500, taken from his account; journey to Brasil by Vincent Yáñez Pinzón, who left from Palos in December 1499, and his return in 1500, from information given by the survivors; the superstitions of the islanders in Hispaniola and their legends; mention of Columbus.

DECADE II

Attempt at colonization made by Alfonso de Hojeda, appointed governor of the Urabá province, and by Diego de Nicuesa, governor of the province of Veragua; conflicts and sad living conditions among the Spaniards of Darién; power struggles between Vasco Núñez de Balboa and Enciso; return of Enciso to Spain to obtain a ruling of condemnation against Balboa; expedition of Balboa against the caciques of the bordering territories; the cacique Comogro informs Balboa of the existence of an immense sea and islands rich in pearls; Balboa conceives a bold plan of action to be pardoned from the King for usurping power; appointment of Pedro Arias as governor and his departure for Darién.

DECADE III

Books 1-3: Detailed account of the expedition of Balboa and the abundance of treasures found: gold and pearls; feelings of those adventurers at the sight of the new South sea.

Book 4: Departure of Columbus from Cádiz for the fourth voyage to Hispaniola (p. 336); the island of Guanassa (p. 336); the land of Quiriquetana called Ciamba by Columbus: exchange of gifts with the natives (p. 338); the region of Taya and Maya (p. 338); digression on the look of those lands and on the language (p. 340); discovery of the islands Cuatro Estaciones and the Limonares islands (p. 342); the Río de los Perdidos (p. 342); the port of Cariai (p. 342); fight between a monkey and an archer (p. 344); capture of a wild boar which fights with a monkey and gets the worst of it (p. 344); the regions of Cerabaró and Aburema (p. 346); the rivers of these regions (p. 346); the region of Xaguaguará and its inhabitants (p. 348); Spanish ships attacked by the *broma* (p. 348); the *Adelantado* is sent by Columbus to explore the region of Veragua (p. 350); conflicts with the natives who refuse to accept the Spaniards as permanent inhabitants (p. 352); return to the island of Jamaica because of the ships ruined by the *broma* (p. 352); mission of Diego Méndez to the extreme edge of Hispaniola (p. 352); other reports on the nature of Veragua and the natives of Cerabaró (p. 354); the rivers Marañón and Dabaiba: the beliefs about Dabaiba (p. 358); gold and precious stones of those regions: Andrés de Morales buys a huge diamond from a native of Paria (p. 360).

Books 5-10: Crossing of the new governor, Pedro Arias, to Darién; valuable information on Sebastian Cabot, explorer of the glacial sea; description of the island of Hispaniola; references to other islands of the Antilles; news about the expedition of the deputies of Pedro Arias sent to conquer the areas east and west of Darién.

DECADE IV

Discovery of the Yucatán by Francisco Hernández de Córdoba in 1517; exploration of the Atlantic coast of Mexico by Juan de Grijalva in 1518; beginning of the undertaking by Hernán Cortés in 1519.

DECADE V

Bold enterprise of Hernán Cortés; march through the country of Cempoal; alliance between the cacique and the Spaniards; ascent to the Mexican Cordillera up to the plateau of Anahuac; hard fight against the people of Tlaxcala who, never defeated by the generals of Montezuma, after the death of their leader Sinotencatl surrender to Cortés; march with the inhabitants of Tlaxcala through very rich territories; Montezuma's attempts, with gifts, to stop the march of the victorious army;

description of the colossus of Popocatepetl and Mexico City valley; end of the fortune of Montezuma; struggle between Cortés and Pánfilo de Narváez, sent by Velázquez to strip him of his authority and capture him; overcoming of the danger; general insurrection of the people against Cortés; slaughter of the Mexicans; sacrifice in the temple of many men of Cortés and the people of Tlaxcala; major strategic retreat of the Spaniards with serious losses.

DECADE VI

Gil Gonzáles is charged with exploring the coasts of the South sea in search of a passage toward the Atlantic; exploration of the western coast of Yucatán, of inland areas of Central America, especially of Nicaragua; gathering of supplies and gold in huge quantity; reports concerning the structure and the geography of the region and the conditions of its inhabitants; return to Hispaniola; reference to the disagreement between Spain and Portugal over the possession of the Moluccas, rich in spices, during the assembly at Badajoz convened to solve that issue; decision of the Royal Council to submit for approval by the King the sending of a fleet of six ships, under the command of Estevão Gomes, Magellan's traitor pilot, to search for a passage to Asia north of Florida.

DECADE VII

Precious contributions to the knowledge of the coasts north of Florida from the talks with Cabot and Lucas Vázques de Ayllón, member of the Royal Audience of Santo Domingo; founding of a colony in a favorable area; reports on the conditions imposed by law on the slaves, as opposed to the arbitrariness of the conquistadors; Bartholomew de Las Casas, while waiting for a new law, pleads the natives' cause; charges by the exploiters against the natives; ill-fated undertaking by Francisco de Garay, governor of Jamaica; treason of Cristóbal de Olid; plan of an expedition by Sebastian Cabot to the Moluccas, through the Strait of Magellan.

DECADE VIII

Details on the undertaking and death of Francisco de Garay; his probable death by poison given him by Cortés; description of Jamaica, of which Garay was governor; treason of Cristóbal de Olid and unsuccessful expedition organized against him by Cortés, despite the boldness of commander Francisco de Las Casas, who, imprisoned, has himself killed by his companions; conquest of Guatemala by Pedro de Alvarado; greater borders of the New Spain; description of the native customs of the people of Chiribichi, which contrast those of Mexican civilization; march of Cortés, unaware of the outcome of the expedition headed by Las Casas in Honduras; dissention in Mexico City, while Cortés is away; accusations against Cortés and secret investigation into the charges against him; arrival of coded dispatches and appointment of an impartial lawyer, Luis Ponce de León, with full powers.

TEXT AND TRANSLATION

I 1: *ad Ascanium Sfortiam Vicecomitem, cardinalem, vicecancellarium*

Solebat grata vetustas pro diis habere viros, quorum industria et animi magnitudine ignotae maioribus eorum terrae
panderentur. Nobis autem, qui Deum habemus unicum sub
triplici Persona, quem colamus, restat ut huiuscemodi genus
5 hominum, si non coluerimus, admiremur tamen. Reges vero
observemus, quorum ductu et auspiciis, datum est illis cogitata
perficere, utrosque etiam extollamus et, pro viribus, illustremus
iure merito! Quare, de insulis maris occidui nuper repertis et
rei autoribus, quid referatur habeto. Hoc siquidem tuis litteris
10 vehementer cupere videris, ab ipsius ergo initio rei, ne sim
cuiquam iniurius, exordiri est animus. Christophorus Colonus,
quidam Ligur vir, Fernando et Helisabethae, Regibus Catholicis, proposuit et suasit se ab occidente nostro finitimas Indiae
insulas inventurum, si navigiis et rebus ad navigationem atti-
15 nentibus instruerent, a quibus augeri Christiana religio et margaritarum, aromatum atque auri inopinata copia haberi facile
posset. Instanti, ex regio fisco, destinata sunt tria navigia: unum
onerarium, caveatum, alia duo mercatoria, levia, sine caveis,
quae ab Hispanis *caravelae* vocantur. His habitis, ab Hispanis
20 littoribus, circiter Kalendas Septembris anni secundi et nonagesimi supra quadringentesimum et millesimum a nostra salute,
iter institutum cum viris Hispanis circiter ducentis viginti Colonus coepit. A Gadibus, in alto oceano Fortunatae, ut multi
putant, insulae, quae ab Hispanis *Canariae* nuncupantur, iam-
25 pridem repertae, distant millia passuum mille et ducenta, secundum eorum rationem. Dicunt enim distare ter centum lequas, singulas autem lequas, navigationis periti, quattuor millia
passuum continere, suis computationibus, aiunt. *Fortunatas* insulas, ob coeli temperiem, appellavit antiquitas: neque enim
30 gravis urget incolas hyems neque atrox aestas. Sunt tamen qui
eas velint esse Fortunatas quas *Capitis Viridis* insulas Portugalenses appellant. Canarias ad haec usque tempora hominibus
nudis, eo quod extra omne clima Europae ad meridiem et sine
ulla religione degentibus, habitatas, Colonus, aquandi et refi-
35 ciendarum navium gratia, priusquam se tam duro labori crederet, adivit. Non insuave futurum arbitror, quandoquidem in
Canarias incidimus, si ex ignotis quomodo notae, si ex incultis

I 1: To Cardinal Ascanio Sforza, Vice-Chancellor

As a sign of gratitude, ancient people used to consider as gods, men who, by their genius and greatness of spirit, discovered lands unknown to their forefathers, whereas we, who have one God in three Persons to adore, rather than worship such men, do at least admire them. Therefore, let us show our respect to the Sovereigns, under whose inspiration and auspices those men were allowed to bring to completion their plans: let us also praise and exalt both of them rightfully to the best of our abilities. Hear then what is told about the recently discovered islands of the western sea and about those who carried it out. Since in your letters you have expressed a strong desire for pertinent news, in order to avoid doing injustice to anyone I will then start from the beginning of said venture. A certain Ligurian, Christopher Columbus, presented his plans to Ferdinand and Isabella, the Catholic Sovereigns, convincing them he could discover the islands near the Indies by sailing West, if they would provide him with ships and whatever else was necessary for navigation, and that thus the Christian religion could be spread further and a quantity beyond expectation of pearls, spices and gold could be easily obtained. Because of his insistence, they provided him three ships with funds from the royal treasury: a [square-rigged] cargo ship with topsail, and two light merchant ships with lateen sails known as *caravels* to the Spaniards. After he obtained the ships, at the beginning of September 1492 A.D., Columbus began his planned voyage, sailing away from the Spanish shore with about 220 men of Spanish nationality. The Fortunate Isles, which the Spaniards call Canaries, had already been discovered long ago way out in the ocean: indeed, many reckon, at a distance of 1,200 miles from Cádiz; experts of the art of navigation say, on the other hand, that they are 300 leagues off Cádiz, in their calculations each league equals 4,000 paces (four miles). The ancients called these islands *Fortunate* because of their mild climate: indeed, the inhabitants suffer neither severe winters nor torrid summers. However, there are some who think that the Fortunate Isles are none other than the Portuguese Islands of *Cape Verde*. Columbus stopped at the Canaries, still inhabited by naked men

quomodo cultae sint effectae, narraverimus. Longa namque annorum curricula, incognitas iam oblivioni tradiderant. Hae insulae septem Canariae dictae, anno circiter millesimo quadringentesimo quinto, a Gallo, nomine *Betanchor*, ex concessione reginae Catherinae, regis Ioannis, filii sui dum infans esset tutricis, repertae forte fortuna fuerunt. Pedem ibi fixit per aliquot annos Betanchor; duasque ex illis occupavit ac redegit in cultum: Lancelotum et Fortem Venturam. Eo mortuo, heres eius Hispanis viris precio insulam utranque praebuit. Fernandus dehinc Peraria et uxor eius Ferream et Gomeram invaserunt; nostris temporibus tres reliquas, Canariam Magnam scilicet, Petrus de Vera, nobilis Xericii civis, et Michael de Moxica, Palmam autem ac Tenerifen Alphonsus Lugo, sed impensa regia. Gomeria deinde ac Ferrea non, cum magno labore, subditae sunt, sed Alphonsus Lugo duriuscule rem perfecit: gens enim illa nuda, silvestris, saxis et fustibus bella gerens, semel eius exercitum fugavit trucidavitque circiter quadringentos, tandem eos devicit. Ita Canariae omnes ad Castellanam additae sunt potentiam. Ab his igitur insulis Colonus, occidentem solem semper secutus, licet in laevam paulisper, tres et triginta continuos dies coelo tantum et aqua contentus, navigavit. Hispani comites murmurare primum secreto coeperunt, apertis mox conviciis urgere, de perimendo cogitare; demum vel in mare proiiciendo consulebatur: se deceptos fuisse ab homine Ligure, in praeceps trahi qua nunquam redire licebit. Post trigesimum iam diem, furore perciti proclamabant ut reducerentur, ne ulterius procederet stimulabant hominem, ipse vero, blandis modo verbis, ampla spe modo, diem ex die protrahens, iratos mulcebat, depascebat. Proditione quoque taxandos esse a Regibus, si adversi quicquam in eum molirentur, si parere recusarent praedicabat. Optatum tandem terrae prospectum laeti suscipiunt. Patefecit navigatione hac prima sex tantum insulas atque ex iis duas inauditae magnitudinis: quarum alteram *Hispaniolam*, *Ioannam* alteram vocitavit, sed Ioannam esse insulam non pro certo habuit. Illarum quarundam littora cum abraderent, cantantem inter condensa nemora philomenam[1], mense novembre,

---

[1] Medieval graphic variant for *Philomela* (Verg. *georg.* IV 511), the protagonist turned nightingale in mythological tales. A metamorphosis perhaps inspired by the bird's groaning shrills (Ovid. *met.* VI, 428 ff.).

living to the South in a climate altogether different from European climates and without religion, to replenish his supply of water and repair the ships, before setting out on such a difficult venture. Speaking of the Canaries, I do not think it will be gratuitous to recall here how those islands became known and civilized, from unknown and barbarous. Actually the passing of time put them almost into oblivion. These seven islands, i.e. Canaries, were discovered by chance around 1405 by the Frenchman *Béthencourt* by consent of queen Catherine, guardian of her son, King John, who at that time was a child. Béthencourt lived there for several years; he occupied and colonized two islands: Lanzarote and Fuerteventura. Upon his death, his heir sold both those islands for money to some Spaniards. Later, Fernando Peraria (Peraza) and his wife occupied Hierro and Gomera islands. In our times the Spaniards conquered the other three as follows. Pedro de Vera, a nobleman from Xeres, and Miguel de Moxica conquered Grand Canary, whereas with subsidies from the royal treasury. Alfonso de Lugo got Palma and Tenerife, Gomera and Hierro were then subdued without great resistance, but Alfonso de Lugo brought violence with his conquest. In fact, the wild natives, although naked and unarmed but for sticks and stones, put his soldiers to flight one time killing 400 of them but were, finally, subdued. And so, all the Canaries were added to the possessions of Castile. From these islands, then, Columbus, who had always headed West, although slightly deviating to the left, sailed for 33 consecutive days, surrounded only by water and sky. His Spanish companions at first began to murmur in secret, then followed up with open protests and thoughts about getting rid of him, to the point of even considering to throw him overboard: they felt deceived by the Ligurian and dragged to a precipice with no hope of returning. After thirty days and by then enraged, they demanded to be taken back appealing to him not to go any farther. Yet Columbus, now with sympathetic words, then with soft promises, sought to postpone the return every day and did soothe and calm their angry hearts. He kept saying that if they attempted anything against him refusing to obey him, they would also be accused of treason against their Sovereigns. Finally, with great joy, they come within sight of the desired land. During this first crossing, he discovered only six islands and among them two of extraordi-

audierunt. Dulcium aquarum ingentia flumina, nativos portus, magnarum classium capaces, adinvenit. Ioannae littora lambens, ad occidentem a septentrione, recto latere, non multo minus octingentis millibus passuum percurrit, aiunt enim cen-
5 tum et octoginta lequas. Continentem arbitratus, quod neque terminus neque termini ullius signum in insula, quantum oculis prospectus inserviebat, appareret, retrocedere instituit. Redire etiam illum pelagi tumores coegerunt: nam Ioannae littora, per varios inflexus, tantum iam ad septentrionem se
10 vertebant et curvabantur, quod boreales flatus naves acrius infestarent, quoniam hyems vigebat. Ad orientem igitur proras vertens, Ophiram insulam sese reperisse refert, sed, cosmographorum tractu diligenter considerato, Antiliae insulae sunt illae et adiacentes aliae. Hanc *Hispaniolam* appellavit, in cuius
15 septentrionali latere, tentare locorum naturam cupiens, terrae appropinquabat, cum in planam quandam et caecam rupem aquis coopertam carina grandioris navis incidens aperitur et perstat. Saxi latentis planities fuit illis ne submergerentur adiumento; cum reliquis igitur duabus properantes, viros
20 omnes incolumes educunt. Ibi, primum ad terram egressi, homines indigenas viderunt qui, venientem inauditam gentem conspicati, facto agmine, in condensa nemora omnes, veluti a canibus gallicis timidi lepores, sese fugientes recipiunt. Nostri, multitudinem insecuti, mulierem tantum capiunt; hanc
25 cum ad naves perduxissent nostris cibis et vino bene saturatam atque ornatam vestibus (nam ea gens omnis utriusque sexus nuda penitus vitam ducit, natura contenta), solutam reliquerunt. Quom primum ad suos mulier concessit (sciebat enim illa quom fugientes diverterent) ostendissetque mirum esse
30 nostrorum ornatum et liberalitatem, omnes ad littora certatim concurrunt: gentem esse missam e coelo autumant. Aurum, cuius erat apud illos aliqua copia, ad naves natando portant, pro frusto aut paropsidis fictilis aut vitrei crateris aurum commutabant. Si ligulam, si tintinnabulum, si speculi frag-
35 mentum, si quicquam aliud simile nostri impartiebantur, tantum auri quantum petere libebat aut unusquisque eorum assequebatur exhibebant. Cum iam res ipsa ad familiare commercium devenisset et gentium mores nostri perquirerent, reges habere gentem illam per signa et coniecturas cognove-
40 runt. E navibus descendentes nostri a rege et reliquis indigenis honorifice recipiuntur: nostris omnibus, quibus poterant et

nary vastness: he named the first *Hispaniola* and the other *Juana*, without being positive the latter was an island. While sailing along some of the islands during the month of November, they heard Philomela [nightingales] singing in the thick forests. He found large rivers of fresh water and natural harbors, capable of holding big fleets. Sailing North-West off Juana's shores in a straight line he traveled no less than 800 miles, that is 180 leagues. Thinking this was a continent, since he could not see either an end or signs that the island's land ended, as far as the eye could reach, he decided to turn back. He was forced to return also by the fury of the sea and the fact that Juana's shoreline had many inlets facing North i.e. exposed to the north winds that, during the winter season, hit the ships more fiercely. So, turning the prow eastward, he claims to have found the island of Ophir, but, considering carefully the cosmographers' reckoning, it must have been the Antilles and nearby islands. He named this island *Hispaniola*. Wanting to examine the nature of places on its northern coastline, he came too close to land and the keel of the largest ship hitting unexpectedly against a flat, and hidden rock, broke and was grounded. The flat, hidden rock below prevented anyone from drowning; the other two ships quickly rushed to the rescue and all men were brought to safety. It was here that, on landing, they saw for the first time the natives, who, upon seeing all those strangers, fled in flocks to take refuge in the thick forests, like timid hares fleeing the hounds. Our men in pursuit of the crowd, captured only a woman whom they took on board their ships, fed her well with our food and drink and dressed her nicely (for those people of both sexes live absolutely naked, quite happy in their natural state) and let her go. As soon as the woman returned to her people (she knew where the fugitives were hiding) and proved to them our wonderful welcome and generosity, they all raced each other to the beach: they thought these newcomers to be people sent from heaven. Swimming toward the ships, they brought gold, in some quantity, which they exchanged for objects of little value, a pottery dish or a glass. If our sailors gave them a little spoon, a hawk-bell, a mirror fragment or anything of the kind, they gave in exchange as much gold as they were asked or as much as each of them carried. As these trades increased the familiarity, our men observed better their customs

sciebant, modis assurgebant. Sole ad occasum vergente nostris, dato salutationis angelicae signo, genua Christiano ritu fiectentibus, itidem illi faciebant, crucem, quocunque modo Christianos colere conspicerent, adorabant. Ex navi, quam saxo illisam diximus, nostros homines et quicquid in ea vehebatur, ita celeriter atque animo laeto gens illa in terram, suis lintribus[2], quas *canoas* vocant, eduxerunt, quod affines affinibus apud nos, nulli maiore misericordia tacti, succurrant. Canoas autem illas, ex solo cavato acutissimis lapidibus ligno, longas, sed angustas construunt; *monoxyla*[3] propterea esse dicemus. Octoginta remigum capaces plerasque se vidisse multi affirmant; usus ferri apud eos nullus invenitur. Propterea quomodo sive domos, quas mira arte laboratas videbant, sive alia quaecunque, ad eorum usum pertinentia, fabricarent maxima nostros detinuit admiratio; sed ex fluvialibus quibusdam durissimis lapidibus, praeacutis, omnia apud illos diduci certum est. Esse non longe ab illis insulis quorundam ferorum hominum insulas, qui carnibus humanis vescantur, fama didicere. Id esse causae quod ita trepidi adventantes nostros confugerent, postea rettulerunt, *Canibales* arbitrati (sic truculentos illos sive *Caribes* vocant). Horum obscoenorum insulas, itinere fere in medio ad has insulas, ad meridiem reliquere. Suas insulas ii mites a Canibalibus non aliter incursionibus crebris vexari perpetuo ad praedam conqueruntur atque, per nemora, venatores, per vim et per insidias, feras insectantur. Quos pueros capiunt, ut nos pullos gallinaceos aut porcos, quos ad obsonia volumus pinguiores et teneriores educare, castrant; grandiores et pingues effectos, comedunt. Aetate autem iam matura cum ad eorum manus perveniunt, peremptos partiuntur; intestina et extremas membrorum partes recentes epulantur, membra sale condita, ut nos pernas suillas, in tempora servant. Mulieres comedere apud eos nefas est et obscoenum, si vero, quas assequuntur iuvenes, ad sobolem procreandam non aliter atque nos gallinas, oves, iuvencas et caetera animalia curant et custodiunt. Vetulas ad obsequia praestanda pro servis habent. Insularum, quas nostras iam possumus appellare, tam viri quam foeminae, cum Canibales adventare praesentiunt, aliam

[2] See Verga. *georg.* I 262; Liv. XXI 26, 8; Plin. *nat. hist.* VI 104, 105.

[3] It is a one-oar vessel carved out of a single tree trunk, see Plin. *nat. hist.* VI 105; Verg. *mil.* III 7: *monoxylos, hoc est paulo latiores scafulas ex singulis trabibus excavatas.*

and understood from signs and conjectures that those people had chiefs. When our sailors got off the ships, they were welcomed with honor by a king and other natives: the natives bowed to our men the best they could and knew how. At sunset, at the sign of the *Angelus*, when our peole knelt according to our Christian custom, the natives did the same venerating the cross and parroting whatever the Christians did in veneration of the cross. From the shipwreck reported earlier and caused by a rock, those people very quickly and spontaneously brought to safety our sailors and its cargo, using their boats which they call canoes; they did so driven by an even stronger sense of compassion than we would among ourselves to help our relatives. They build ther canoes long and narrow, making them out of single tree trunks hollowed with very sharp stones, so we call them *monoxyla* [single-oar canoes]. Many report that they have seen most canoes with 80 rowers; yet among the natives we have not seen any use of iron. For this reason, the highest admiration was generated in our men, as well as for the way they build their houses, admittedly constructed with great ingenuity, and any other object of need; we are sure that they make their tools from very sharp and very hard river stones. The Spaniards learned by hearsay that not far away from those islands there were other ones inhabited by fierce people, who ate human flesh. Later they found out that this was the reason why the natives fled so fearfully at the arrival of our sailors, for they thought they were *Cannibals* (so they call those cruel men, or also *Caribs*). They left the islands of these monsters to the South, almost half-way on their sailing to these islands. These peaceful islanders complained that their islands were constantly upset by frequent attacks by the Cannibals, in much the same way that wild beasts are chased by hunters in the forest, violently and insidiously, to catch them. They also castrated the children that they captured, just as we do with chickens and pigs raised for delicacy to be fatter and juicier and once fattened they eat them. But if captured by the cannibals at a mature age, they are killed and cut into pieces; they eat the intestines and the end of fresh parts, preserving the limbs for the future by salting them, just as we do ham. The cannibals consider it a shameful crime to eat women; but if they capture any of them young, they take care of them and keep them for procreation, not unlike our taking care of hens,

quam fuga salutem nullam inveniunt. Sagittis arundineis,
praeacutis licet utantur, ad Canibalium tamen vim et furores
reprimendos parum prodesse comperere; decem enim Canibales centum ex aliis facile, si concurrant, superaturos omnes
5 indigenae fatentur. Quid utraque gens, praeter coelum atque
eius lumina adoret non satis exploratum habuerunt. De reliquis insularium moribus brevitas temporis atque interpretum
inopia plura noscere non permiserunt. Radicibus, ii mites,
nostris napis et magnitudine et forma, sed, gustu dulci, casta-
10 neae tenerae adhuc similibus, ad cibum utuntur. Has *ages*
vocant ipsi. Est et aliud radicis genus quam *iuccam* appellant:
ex hac et panem conficiunt. Agibus vero magis assis aut elixis
utuntur, quam ad usum conficiendi panis. Iuccam vero sectam
et compressam (succosa namque est) pinsunt et in placentas
15 coquunt. Sed mirum hoc: aconito lethaliorem esse aiunt iuccae
succum; qui epotus illico perimit. Panem autem ex eius massa
sapidum et salubrem esse omnes experti sunt. Panem et ex
frumento quodam, panico, cuius est apud Insubres et Granatenses Hispanos maxima copia, non magno discrimine, confi-
20 ciunt. Est huius panicula longior spitama, in acutum tendens,
lacerti fere crassitudine; grana miro ordine a natura confixa,
forma et corpore, pisum legumen aemulantur: albent acerba,
ubi maturuerunt, nigerrima efficiuntur, fracta, candore nivem
exuperant, *maizium* id frumenti genus appellant. Et est apud
25 eos aurum alicuius aestimationis: nam auricularum torulis et
naribus perforatis insertum in tenuissimas diductum laminas
ferunt. Cum tamen neque ad eos commeare mercatores, nec
ipsos alia littora noscere praeter sua nostri didicissent, quaerere ab eis per signa coeperunt unde sibi id aurum compara-
30 rent. Quantum signis colligere licuit, ex fluviorum arenis, ab
altis montibus collabentibus, id neque magno labore, lectum:
in pillulas, priusquam diduceretur in laminas, astringebant,
non tamen in ea insulae parte, quam rex ille tenebat (quod
postea patuit experimento). Nam, cum inde iam discessissent,
35 forte in flumen inciderunt cuius arenam multo auro mixtam
esse, cum in terram aquandi et piscandi gratia exilissent, perpenderunt. Nullum animal quadrupes se vidisse dicunt, praeterquam tria genera cuniculorum. Serpentes insulae nutriunt,
sed minime noxios; anseres silvestres, turtures, anates nostris
40 grandiores et cigneo candore, capite purpureo repererunt.
Psittacos, quorum alii virides erant, alii flavi toto corpore,

218

sheep, heifers and other animals. Old women, however, are kept as slaves to do chores. Men and women of there islands, that we may view as ours, as soon as they hear the Cannibals coming, have no other way of saving themselves but fleeing. Although armed with pointed arrows made of reeds, they are quite aware of their irrelevance to prevent the violent fury of the Cannibals; indeed all the natives agree that ten Cannibals could easily overpower one hundred of them, if pushed to fight. The Spaniards could not fully comprehend what both peoples worshipped, other than the heaven and its stars. Short time and lack of interpreters did not allow our men to learn more about other customs of the islanders. The peaceful people still feed on roots similar, in size and shape, to our turnips, but tasting like tender chestnuts. They call them *ages*; there is another kind of roots which they called *yuca*: with this they also make bread. In fact, they use *ages* either roasted or boiled, besides making bread. They also ground into flour the *yuca*, after they cut and smash it (since it is juicy), and then bake it into cakes. What is peculiar is their claim that *yuca* juice is more poisonous than aconite: anyone drinking it would die immediately. However, all our people after tasting it agree that the bread made from this dough is tasty and wholesome. They do make a slightly different bread, also with the type of italian wheat greatly abundant among Lombards and Spaniards of Granada, namely millet. The millet-cob is longer than a palm and ends in a point, almost the size of an arm; its grains, remarkably arranged by nature resemble in shape and size those of a pea. When growing are white, but once ripened, they are very black; and, broken in half, whiter than snow. They call this type of wheat maize. Gold too is also of some value for them: indeed they wear it wrought in very fine leaves, on ear lobes and perforated nostrils. Nevertheless, our men, when they found out that no merchants were doing business with them and the natives did not know any lands other than their own, began to ask them through signs where they obtained the gold. As nearly as they could understand from their gestures, it had been gathered without much difficulty from the sands of the rivers flowing from the high mountains: they compress it in small balls before beating it into leaves, but not in that part of the island over which that king ruled (this became clear later on, through experience). By chance, after leaving that place,

alii similes Indicis, torquati minio, uti Plinius[4] ait, quadraginta
tulerunt, sed coloribus vivacissimis et laetis maximopere: alas
habent versicolores, viridibus enim et flavis pennis quasdam
habent ceruleas et purpureas mixtas, quae varietas parit delec-
5 tationem. Haec volui de psittacis, illustrissime Princeps, recitasse, quoniam, quamvis huius Christophori Coloni opinio ma-
gnitudini sphaerae et opinioni veterum de subnavigabili orbe
videatur adversari, psittaci tamen, inde asportati, atque alia
multa, vel propinquitate vel natura, solum Indicum has insulas
10 sapere indicant, cum praecipue Aristoteles circa finem libri *De
coelo et mundo*[5], Seneca[6] et alii, non ignari cosmographiae, ab
Hispania Indica littora per occidentem non longo maris tractu
distare attestentur. Masticis, aloes, gossampii atque aliarum
huiuscemodi rerum copiam suapte natura tellus illa producit;
15 ex arboribus, veluti apud Seres[7], vellera colliguntur. Grana
quaedam rugosa diversorum colorum, Caucaseo pipere acutiora,
ramalia etiam ex concisis arboribus, cinnamomi forma, gustu
autem et odore acrem zingiberim[8] et medulla et superiore libro
imitantia tulerunt. His igitur inventae novae telluris et inauditi
20 alterius terrarum orbis signis contentus, prospero reditu, flan-
tibus zephyris[9] iam propter nostrum ver propinquum, redire
constituens, octo et triginta viros apud eum regem, de quo
supra memoravimus, reliquit qui locorum et temporum naturam, donec ipse reverteretur, inquirerent. Is rex ab incolis
25 dicebatur *Guaccanarillus*. Cum quo icto singularis amicitiae foedere, de vita et salute ac tutela eorum quos ibi relinquebat,
quibus potuit modis, egit. Misericordia contactus rex erga no-

[4] Pliny's description of a parrot shows it to be a bird with green plumage and
a red collar, original to India (*nat. hist.* X 117: *India hanc avem mittit, siptacen vocat,
viridem toto corpore, torque tantum miniato in cervice distinctam*). See also Aristot. *hist. an.*
VIII 12, 597b.

[5] See Aristot. *de coel.* II 14.

[6] See Sen. *nat. quaest.* I 13: *quantum est enim quod ab ultimis litoribus Hispaniae usque
ad Indos iacet? Paucissimorum dierum spatium si navem suus ferat ventus.* See also Eratost. *ap.*
Strabo. I 6.

[7] An East Asian population with Sera as capital city, renowned for the making
of silk. See Verg. *georg.* II 121; Plin. *nat. hist.* VI 54; Strabo XV 20; Paus. VI 26,6.

[8] A Plant native to tropical Asia, see Plin. *nat. hist.* XII 28. The latin term is of
a neutral gender.

[9] Westerly wind, mild and warm, See Plin. *nat. hist.* XVIII 337; Sen. *nat. quaest.*
V 16, 5.

they ran into a river whose sand when they went for some fresh water and fish and noticed a lot of gold in it. They say they never saw any quadruped with the exception of three kinds of rabbits. The islands are full of snakes of the harmless kind; they found wild geese, turtle-doves, ducks bigger than ours, white as swans, with a red head. Forty parrots were brought back, some green, some yellow all over the body, and others similar to those from India with a red collar, as Pliny says, but with very bright and cheerful colors: these parrots have multicolored wings, showing some blue and red feathers mixed in with green and yellow ones, a delightful combination. Most illustrious Prince, I wanted to give you these details about the parrots because, although the opinion of this Christopher Columbus seems to be in conflict with the size of the earth and the ancients' ideas concerning the navigable world, nevertheless, these birds found there and many other objects as well, prove that these islands' proximity and nature have the same characteristics of the Indian soil, especially since Aristotle, at the end of his book *De coelo et mundo* [of Heaven and Earth], Seneca and others who studied cosmography affirm that the shores of India are separated from Spain, to the West, only by a short stretch of sea. The island produces spontaneously an abundance of gum, aloe, cotton and similar products; from the trees are gathered thin threads of silk, as done at Seres. They also brought some rough-looking seeds of different color, spicier than the Caucasian pepper, and dried twigs from trees which had been cut, resembling cinnamon in shape, but more like spicy ginger, in taste, smell, bark and pith. Therefore, satisfied with these proofs of his discovery of a new land and world up to now unheard of, Columbus planned on making a safe return voyage, since the zephyrs were blowing with the approaching spring; he left thirty-eight men with that king, of whom we spoke before, so that they might go on exploring the nature of those places and climate until he would come back. That king was Guacanagarí to the islanders. After reaching an agreement of special friendship with him, Columbus made arrangements, as best he could, for the life, health and safety of those he was leaving behind. The king, moved to compassion for those being left behind in foreign lands, was seen shedding tears: he pledged full assistance. So, after embracing each other, Columbus, meaning to return to Spain,

stros, quod alienis terris desererentur, lachrymas effudisse visus
est atque omnem opem pollicitus. Sic, alter alterum complexi,
ad Hispaniam Colonus rediturus, vela dari imperat, secum decem viros ex illis, abducens a quibus posse omnium illarum
5 insularum linguam nostris litteris Latinis, sine ullo discrimine,
scribi compertum est. Vocant enim coelum *turei*, domum *boa*,
aurum *cauni*, virum bonum *tayno*, nihil *mayani*. Reliquave omnia
vocabula non minus liquide proferunt atque nos Latina nostra.
Haec habes quae de prima eius navigatione memoratu digna
10 existimaverim. Rex autem et Regina, quorum omnes cogitatus
vel dormientium in religionis nostrae augmento sunt siti, sperantes ad Christi legem tot nationes et simplices gentes facile
trahi posse, iis auditis, commoventur. Colonum advenientem
honorifice, uti pro talibus ausis merebatur tractant; sedere illum
15 coram se publice, quod est maximum apud Reges Hispanos
amoris et gratitudinis supremique obsequii, signum fecerunt.
Praefectum marinum vocari deinceps Colonum imperant. Is *Almirantus Colonus* apud Hispanos nuncupatur. Fratrem etiam ipsi
Bartholomaeum Colonum rei marinae et ipsum peritum prae-
20 fecturae insulae Hispaniolae titulo ornarunt (hunc magistratum
vulgo *adelantatum* appellant). Almirantum igitur et adelantatum
ac navigiorum praesentia nomina, caetera etiam huiuscemodi
data opera, suis aliquando vulgaribus appellabo nominibus, quo
apertius intelligar. Nunc ad institutum redeamus. Ex insulis,
25 uti in initio Colonus ipse, iam Praefectus marinus, pollicebatur,
maxima eorum, quae mortales omnes totis viribus sequimur,
commoda proventura creditum est. Duabus igitur his causis
commoti, sanctissimi hi duo Consortes, septemdecim ad secundam expeditionem navigia parari iubenti tria oneraria caveata
30 magna duodecim (id genus navium quas dici apud Hispanos
caravelas scripsimus sine caveis) eiusdem generis duas aliquanto
grandiores atque ad sustinendas caveas propter malorum magnitudinem aptas. Huius classis parandae curam Ioanni Fonse-
cae, viro genere nobili, decano Hispalensi, ingenio atque animo
35 pollenti, tradunt, ultra ducentos et mille armatos pedites illi
imperant conduci, inter quos omnium mechanicarum artium
fabros et opifices innumeros stipendio accersiri iubent; equites
quosdam caeteris armatis immiscent. Ad foetus procreandos
equas, oves, iuvencas, et plura alia cum sui generis masculis,
40 legumina, triticum, hordeum, et reliqua iis similia, non solum
alimenti, verum etiam seminandi gratia Praefectus apparat. Vites

gave the order to set sails taking with him ten islanders, thanks to whom it became clear that the language spoken in all those islands could be transcribed, without difficulty, into our Latin characters. Thus, they call heaven *turei*, house *boa*, gold *cauni*, an honest man *tayno*, nothing *mayani*. They pronounce all the other words not any less distinctly than we do our Latin words. This is what I deem worthy to be remembered of his first voyage. The King and the Queen, then, whose thoughts even in their sleep are always focused on the spreading of our religion, in the hope that many nations and simple peoples may be easily led to the law of Christ, were touched as they heard these reports. Upon Columbus's return, they received him with the honor he deserved for his accomplishments; they had him publicly seated in front of them which at the Spanish court is a most important gesture of affection, gratitude and highest esteem. Thus they ordered that he be appointed Admiral i.e. *Almirante Colón* in Spanish. They also named his brother Bartholomew, he too an expert seaman, governor of the island of Hispaniola (this position's common title is *Adelantado*). For clarity sake I occasionally add the terms more frequently used (*Almirante* and *Adelantado*), or the ships' current names and other recurring terms. But now let us go back to our narrative. As Columbus himself, now Admiral, predicted at the beginning, everyone believed that all of those advantages, which we mortal men seek out with all of our energies, would come from those islands. Therefore, this most holy Couple, convinced by these two arguments, ordered that seventeen ships be equipped for a second expedition, that is, three large square-rigged vessels and twelve lateen-sail vessels (of the type called caravels by the Spaniards, as we said earlier) and two more of this type but larger and suited, for the height of the masts, to support sails. They entrusted the task of equipping the fleet to Juan de Fonseca, a nobleman by birth, dean of Seville, a man of great ability and courage; they ordered him to enlist more than 1,200 foot-soldiers with among them workers representing all the work fields and numerous craftsmen, including some cavalry-men. The Admiral also procured mares, sheep, cows and many other female animals with males of the same species for procreation; legumes, wheat, barley and other similar products, not only for eating but also for sowing. Vines and shoots of various trees from our land were

et aliarum nostratium arborum plantaria, quibus terra illa caret, ad eam important; nullas enim apud eas insulas notas arbores invenere praeter pinus palmasque et eas altissimas ac mirae duriciei et proceritatis ac rectitudinis, propter soli ubertatem
5 atque etiam ignotos fructus alias plures procreantes. Terram aiunt esse terrarum omnium, quas ambiunt sidera, uberrimam. Instrumenta omnia fabrilia ac demum alia cuncta, quae ad novam civitatem in alienis regionibus condendam faciunt, unicuique artifici imperat. Ex fidis regiis clientibus plures hanc
10 navigationem et rerum novarum studio et Praefecti autoritate promoti, sua sponte, aggressi sunt. Secundis igitur velis, vii Kalendas Octobris anni tertii et nonagesimi supra quadringentesimum et millesimum a salute nostra, a Gadibus movit. Fortunatas in Kalendis Octobris tetigere; ex Fortunatis ultima
15 dicitur ab Hispanis *Ferrea*: in qua nulla est alia potabilis aqua praeterquam ex rore de arbore unica, in insulae supremo dorso, stillante assidue et in lacunam manufactam cadente. Ab hac insula, vela in altum oceanum tertio Idus eiusdem coepit protendere. Haec nobis intra paucos dies ab eius discessu renun-
20 ciata fuerunt. Quicquid succedet accipies. Vale, felix!

Ex Hispana curia, Idibus Novembris 1493.

taken there where they didn't exist. Known trees in those islands were only the pines and palms, with the latter being extremely tall, exceptionally hardy and very slender on account of the fertility of the soil. They found also many plants that produced unknown fruits. They state that the land is the most fertile of all the lands around which the stars rotate. The admiral ordered each man to procure all the tools needed for his craft and, in addition, all the implements useful for the founding of a city in foreign lands. Many loyal servants of the Crown, attracted by the desire to know new things and by the reputation of the Admiral, spontaneously joined in this voyage. With favorable winds, on September 25, 1493 A.D., he sailed from Cádiz. On October 1, they reached the Fortunate Isles. The farthest one is called by the Spaniards Hierro island: it has no potable water other than that which comes from the dew constantly dripping from a tree, located on its highest peak and falling in a man-made hollow. On the 13th of the same month Columbus set sail from this island for the high sea. These reports were given to us a few days after his departure. You shall learn whatever happens. Take care and be happy!

From the court of Spain, 13 November 1493

I 2: ad Ascanium Sfortiam Vicecomitem, cardinalem, vicecancellarium

Repetis, illustrissime Princeps, cupere te quae accidunt in Hispania de orbe novo cognoscere placuisseque tibi, quae hactenus de prima navigatione scripserim, insinuasti. Accipe quae successerunt. Methymna Campi celebre oppidum est in
5 Hispania respectu vestri ulteriore et in ea parte, quae *Castella Vetus* dicitur, a Gadibus circiter quadringenta millia passuum distans. Ibi cutia commorabatur, cum circiter nono Kalendas Aprilis huius anni nonagesimi quarti, cursores ad Regem et Reginam missi, adventasse. Duodecim ex insulis navigia ret-
10 tulerunt, Gadesque prospero reditu appulsa esse. Sed nihil aliud se velle Regi et Reginae ductor ipsarum navium per nuncios significare ostendit, praeterquam Praefectum mari-num, cum quinque navigiis et nongentis hominibus, vesti-gandi causa in Hispaniola permansisse; caetera se coram re-
15 citaturum scribit. Pridie igitur Nonas Aprilis dux ipse classis, frater nutricis primogeniti regii, a Praefecto marino legatus advenit. Ab eo caeterisque simul fide dignis hominibus, quae mihi per ordinem interroganti fuerunt enarrata, ut tibi gra-tum faciam, recensebo; accepi etenim ego quae dederunt,
20 quae autem dederunt cognoscito. Tertio Idus Octobris, ex insula Ferrea, Fortunatarum ultima, ab Hispanis littoribus discedentes cum classe navium septemdecim, in altum unum et viginti aequos dies, priusquam insulam ullam attingerent, consumpserunt. Ad laevam, multo magis quam itinere primo,
25 aquilonem[10] secuti data opera vertere proras, propterea in Canibalium sive Caribium insulas, de quibus fama tantum apud nostros erat noticia, inciderunt. Insulam arboribus ita consitam quod neque ulnam quidem aut nudi aut lapidei soli conspicere licuerit, primum viderunt. Hanc, quoniam die do-
30 minico sors obtulerat, *Dominicam* placuit vocari. Nulla ibi mora contracta, quod desertam esse praesenserunt, progre-diuntur. His uno et viginti diebus octingentas et viginti le-quas sese arbitrati sunt percurrisse, adeo prosperi illos venti

---

[10] A violent, polar wind blowing from the North also called tramontane or boreas. Ancients identified it with Aquilo because of its violence (see Paul. Fest. 20, 14 L.; Isid. XIII 11, 13).

I 2: To Cardinal Ascanio Sforza, Vice-Chancellor

Most illustrious Prince, you repeatedly express your desire to know the events taking place in Spain, concerning the new world, and you led me to believe that what I wrote to you about the first voyage was well received by you. Listen now to the events that followed. Medina del Campo is a famous city of Spain, a little farther away from you, located in the region called Old Castile, about 400 miles from Cádiz. The Court was staying there when, around March 24 of this year, 1494, some messengers sent to the King and Queen reported that twelve ships had returned from the islands and had landed at Cádiz after a successful voyage. But the commander of the vessels indicated through the messengers that he did not want to say anything to the Sovereigns other than this: that the Admiral, with five ships and 900 men, had remained at Hispaniola to explore; he added that he would relate the rest of the events in person. Then, on April 4, the commander of the fleet himself, who was a brother of the nurse of the King's first-born, came as ambassador of the Admiral. In order to please you, I will relate exactly what was told to me by him and other trustworthy witnesses, when I kept asking questions, one after the other. I learned of events which they related, so now you too will know them. On October 13, the sailors left from Spanish Hierro, the last of the Fortunate Isles, with a fleet of seventeen ships; they spent 21 days in high seas before landing on any island. After following the North wind, they turned the prow to the left, much more so than during the first voyage thus coming upon the islands of the Cannibals (or Caribs), of whom our sailors had heard only by hearsay. At first they saw an island so densely wooded that they could not see a single parcel of bare or stony land. Since chance had them run into this island on a Sunday, they decided to call it *Domínica*. Waisting no time there, given its clearly deserted condition, they went on. They thought that in 21 days the distance traveled was 820 leagues with the North wind blowing favorably from behind until then. After a small stretch of sea, they discovered islands rich with trees whose limbs, trunk, roots and leaves were different and gave off sweet, aromatic

aquilones a puppi secuti sunt. Post breve spacium aequoris occurrerunt insulae diversis arboribus, vimine, trunco, radicibus et foliis, aromaticos et suaves odores ernittentibus, refertae; neque homines neque ulla se ibi animalia vidisse prae-
5 terquam inauditae magnitudinis lacertos referunt qui in terram, scrutandi gratia, descenderant. *Galanam* hanc appellant. Ex eius insulae promontorio, quodam monte a longe viso, discessere; a triginta millibus passuum, ab hoc monte fluvium descendentem, magni fluvii latitudinis signum, prospexisse
10 visi sunt. Hanc primam a Fortunatis terram habitatam inveniunt; obscoenorum esse Canibalium, de quibus fama prius acceperant, nunc experimento et his interpretibus quos primo itinere ad Hispaniam Praefectus duxerat, cognoverunt. Insulam peragrantes, innumeros sed viginti tantum aut triginta
15 domorum singulos vicos inveniunt: ordinem plateae, tuguriis in gyrum circa plateam constructis, servant. Quandoquidem de illorum domibus in sermonem incidimus, haud absurdum mihi fore videbitur si, quales eas esse audiverim, enarravero. Ligneas omnes et sphaerali forma fabricatas esse aiunt. Ex
20 arboribus sublicibus altissimis terrae affixis circumferentiam primum domus construunt, aliis postmodum ab interiore parte curtis trabibus appositis, quae exteriores altas, ne labantur, sustineant, altarum cacumina in tentorii castrensis forman coniungunt, ita ut acuta culmina domus illae omnes habeant.
25 Tegunt deinde palmarum et quarundam aliarum similium arborum foliis contextis modo tutissimo a pluvia. A trabibus curtis postmodum ad trabes interius deductis funibus gossampinis aut ex quibusdam radicibus, sparto similibus, contortis lodices ex gossampino super imponunt. Gossipium namque
30 nutrit insula suapte natura, sic lectis pensilibus ex rudi gossipio quod Hispanum vulgus *algodonum*, italum *bombasium* appellat vel stramine superiniecto utuntur. Atrium habent quod vulgares aliae domus circumeunt in quod omnes lusuri conveniunt. Domos vocant *boios*, media acuta. Duas ligneas sta-
35 tuas, rudes tamen, singulis anguibus ipsis inhaerentibus elevatis conspicati simulacra quae colerent arbitrati sunt; sed ad decorem ibi posita postmodum didicerunt. Nam, uti supra memoravimus, nihil adorare praeter coeli numen creduntur, quamvis ex gossipio texto larvas in pictorum lemurum quos
40 se noctu videre praedicant, similitudinem conficiant. Sed unde digressi sumus, redeundum est. Adventare nostros incolae

fragrances. The men who landed to explore did nor report seeing either people or animals, with the exception of giant lizards. They call this island *Galana*. Having seen a far-away mountain, they set off from the promontory of that island; 30 miles or so into their march they saw a river flowing from the mountain, apparently an impressive sizeable body of water. This was the first inhabited land they found since the Fortunate Isles; they knew it was inhabited by the ferocious Cannibals whom they had earlier heard of by hearsay, but now by experience, through interpreters the Admiral had taken to Spain during his first voyage. Walking on the island, they discovered numerous villages, with only 20 or 30 houses each, shaped like a square, with small houses built around it. On the subject of their dwellings, it does not seem to be out of place for me to describe what they are like, based on what I heard. They claim all are round and built of wood. First, they draw the circumference of the house with logs of very tall trees, set in the ground like piles; then shorter beams are placed inside to prevent the taller ones, from falling in; finally they join the ends of the taller posts much like a military tent, thus all the houses have pointed roofs. Next, interwoven leaves from palm trees and some other similar trees are used to protect them very ingeniously from the rain. Across, from the short planks and the inside posts, are then strung cotton ropes or of certain twisted roots similar to esparto, on top of which they lay cotton blankets. Since the island spontaneously produces cotton, they make use either of suspended beds made of raw cotton that Spanish people call *algodón* and Italians *banbaso*, or of heaps of leaves. The courtyard surrounded by these ordinary dwellings is used for gathering and play. They call the houses *boíos*, with the stress on the middle vowel. Having noticed two wooden, roughly hewn statues, each with climbing snakes on top, they thought that might be of worshipped gods; later they learned that the statues were merely ornamental. As mentioned earlier, we believe they venerate nothing but some heavenly deity, although they make puppets of interlaced cotton that resemble those depicted ghosts which they claim to see at night. But now let us go back to where we left off. As the natives realized that our people were approaching, men and women alike left their huts and fled. About 30 children and women prisoners, which had been captured from other islands

sentientes, domibus derelictis, tam viri quam foeminae pro-
fugerunt. Ex pueris et mulieribus captivis, quos ex aliis insulis praedati fuerant, vel obsequii vel epularum gratia ser-
vatis, ad nostros circiter triginta confugiunt. Domos ingressi,
5 habere vasa fictilia omnis generis, fidelias, orcas, cantharos
et alia huiuscemodi a nostris non multum dissimilia atque in
eorum coquinis elixas cum psittacis et anserinis carnibus carnes humanas et fixas verubus alias assandas comperere. Pe-
netralia et domorum latibula quaeritando, tibiarum et bra-
10 chiorum humanorum ossa accuratissime apud omnes, ad cuspides sagittarum conficiendas, servari cognitum est: ex
ossibus enim illas, quod ferro careant, fabrefaciunt. Caetera
ossa, exesis carnibus, proiiciunt; invenere etiam caput nuper
occisi iuvenis trabi appensum sanguine adhuc madidum.
15 Quaeritando vero insulam interne, septem alia flumina praeter
id grandius, quod esse Baeti ubi Cordubam lambit, nostro
autem Ticino latius aiunt, descendere per insulam, mira ri-
parum amoenitate, invenerunt. Hanc vocant *Guadalupeam* insulam, a montis Guadalupi similitudine ubi Intemeratae Vir-
20 ginis mirabile colitur simulacrum. *Carucueriam* incolae appellant, est Caribium primaria habitatio. Tulerunt ab hac insula
septem psittacos phasianis grandiores: qui ab aliis psittacis
colore longissime absunt, habent enim totum corpus et ven-
tre et tergo purpureum; ex longioribus plumis illis ab hu-
25 meris lena dependet super purpureas breves, modo quo apud
nostros ruricolas saepenumero capones habere ego ipse ani-
madverti. Alarum autem pennas versicolores tenent: sunt
enim earum glaucae aliae, aliae purpureae, flavis immixtae.
Psittacorum non minor est in omnibus insulis copia quam
30 apud nos passerculorum aut aliarum avium nostratium. Uti
nostri picas, turdos et alia huiuscemodi ad delicias nutriunt,
ita illi quamvis eorum nemora psittacis plena sunt, psittacos
educant, illos tamen deinde comedunt. Mulieres, quas ex captivis ad nostros concessisse supradictum est, munusculis do-
35 natas ad Canibales adducendos ire per signa Praefectus imperat: nec enim illae ubi laterent ignorabant. Hae, apud viros
illa nocte commoratae, mane sequenti, Canibalium plurimos
spe munerum commotos adducunt. Hi, nostris visis, vel terrore vel scelerum conscientia permoti, inter sese exorto mur-
40 mure, alter in alterum oculos flectentes, cuneo facto, ex insperato, celerrime, ut multitudo avium concitati, ad nemoro-

and were kept as slaves or to be eaten, took refuge with our men. Upon entering these huts, they found clay vessels of all kinds, vases, cruets, cups and other containers of the kind, not very different from ours, but in their kitchens discovered boiled human flesh mixed in with parrot and goose meat as well as on spits with other meats ready to be roasted. Searching deep inside hidden areas it was learned that they all preserved human leg and arm bones with great care in order to make pointed arrows: indeed, these are made of bones, as there is no iron. They discard the other bones after they strip the flesh off of them; also discovered was the head of a young man recently slain, hanging from a beam and still dripping blood. Continuing to explore the island's interior, seven rivers with wonderful and pleasant banks were counted flowing through it, beside the one which they say is bigger than the Guadalquivir as it goes through Cordoba, and larger than our Ticino. They named this island *Guadalupa* [Guadeloupe] because it resembled mount *Guadalupa*, where we honor a beautiful statue of the Immaculate Virgin. The natives called it *Caracueria*, it is the main Carib location. From this island they brought seven parrots bigger than pheasants, very different in color from the other parrots for their breast and back are purple all over, and from the junction of the wings, a tuft of longer feathers hangs over the red short ones, much the same way the capons — I myself often observed — raised by our farmers. However, the feathers of their wings are multicolored: some blue and others red mixed in with yellow. Parrots are as numerous in all the islands as sparrows or other such birds in our towns. Just like our people raise magpies and thrushes and other birds of the kind for mere pleasure, so do natives keep parrots, although their forests are so full of them, but for the fact they eat them. The Admiral, through gestures, pushed the women who, as we said earlier, had taken refuge with other prisoners to try and attract the Cannibals with token presents since, indeed, knew where they hid. These women spent the night with the men and the following day they brought several Cannibals who hoped to receive gifts. When they saw our men, either out of fear or possible awareness of their crimes, murmured among themselves and, looking in each other's eyes, suddenly formed a wedge, and with the swiftness of a flock of birds, headed for the wooded valleys. And so our sailors, who

sas valles pedem referunt. Nostris igitur qui insulam, inquirendi gratia, aliquot dies pererraverant in unum collectis sine ullo Canibale, fractis eorum lintribus uniligneis, pridie Idus Novembris ex Guadalupea anchoras elevant. Visendorum comitum, qui primo itinere in Hispaniola, vestigandae telluris gratia, superiore anno relicti fuerant, desiderio Praefectus permotus a dextra laevaque plures insulas navigando cotidie postergabat. Apparuit a septentrione grandis quaedam insula: et qui prima navigatione in Hispaniam vecti fuerant et qui a Canibalibus redempti, vocari insulam ab incolis *Madanino* affirmarunt quam solae mulieres inhabitant. Ad nostrorum aures primo itinere de hac insula fama devenerat. Ad eas haud secus Canibales certis anni temporibus, concedere creditum est atque ad Amazonas Lesbicas transfretasse Thraces rettulit antiquitas et, eodem modo, filios ad genitores mittere, ablactatos, foeminas autem apud se retinere. Has mulieres subterraneos grandes cuniculos habere aiunt, ad quos, si alio quam constituto tempore quisque ad eas proficiscatur, confugiant. Unde, si aut per vim aut per insidias tentare aditum sequentes audeant, sagittis sese tueantur quas certissimas iacere creduntur. Haec dant, haec accipito! Ad hanc insulam propter Boream[11] ab ea flantem non licuit pervenire: Vulturnum[12] enim iam sequebantur. Inter navigandum a conspectu Madaninoe, ad quadraginta millia passuum, non longe ab alia quam vecti indigenae populosissimam et rerum omnium victu necessariarum copia pollentem esse aiebant, praeterlabuntur, quoniam altis montibus instructa esset, *Montem Serratum* illam vocant. Inter caetera, quae ab iis quos vehebant, tum verbis, tum signis, colligere inter loquendum potuerunt, isse Canibales plerunque venatum, vescendorum hominum gratia, supra mille millia passuum a suis littoribus didicere. Altero die quandam aliam vident cui, quod sphaerica esset, *Sanctae Mariae Rotundae* nomen indidit Praefectus. Ne moram traherent, aliam iterum sequenti ab isto die quam *Sancti Martini* nomine placuit vocitari praetermisit. In tertium

---

[11] Greek name for the North wind, Aquilone for the Romans; see Serv. *ad Aen.* X 350; Verg. *georg.* I 93; Manil. IV 591; Ov. *met.* I 65; Plin. *nat. hist.* XVIII 333; Gell. II 22,9.

[12] South and Southeasterly, i.e. sultry, wind. So named after Mount Vulture. See Plin. *nat. hist.* II 119; Sen. *nat. quaest.* V 16, 4; Gell. II 22, 11.

had explored the island wandering for several days without encountering any Cannibals, gathered together and set sail from Guadeloupe on November 12 after destroying their canoes made from single tree-trunks. The Admiral, driven by the desire to see the companions who, during the first voyage the year before had been left at Hispaniola to explore the territory, sailed on, leaving behind every day several islands to the right and to the left. A large island appeared to the North: both, the natives who during the first voyage had been taken to Spain and those who freed from the Cannibals said that this island, inhabited only by women, was called *Madanino* by the islanders. The sailors had heard of this island during the first voyage. It was surmised that the Cannibals at set times of the year would go to those women, not any differently than the ancients' claim that Thracians crossed the sea to reach the Amazons of Lesbos [ancient name of Mytelene], and that, similarly, women sent male infants back to their fathers after weaning them, but kept the girls. They claimed these women live in huge underground tunnels, where they withdraw in case of unexpected visits. From there they defend themselves with arrows, they are believed to be sharp shooters that do not miss their mark, whenever someone dares to chase them or force their way either with violence or deceit. This is the story I am told so I pass it own! They could not reach that island because of bobeas, [North wind] blowing from it: and now they were following Volturnus [Eurus, the South or S.E. wind]. As they sailed, at about 40 miles off Madanino island, they came close to another island which the natives said was very populous and rich with all the foods necessary for living; they went by and, since it had high mountains, called it Montserrat. Among the information which, in talking with words or gestures, they were able to gather from the people with them, they learned that the Cannibals would often reach farther than 1,000 miles away from their shores looking for humans to eat. The next day, another island appeared, which the Admiral named *Santa María la Redonda*, because it was round. The day after again, in order not to loose time, he passed by another island which he named *San Martín*. Then, on the third day, they saw yet another, whose East-to-West width they estimated to be 150 miles, just by looking; they later learned that all these islands possess an extraordinary beauty and fertil-

inde diem aliam cuius diametrale latus ab oriente in occidentem centum et quinquaginta millia passuum esse iudicarunt, extrinsecus conspexere; esse has insulas omnes mirae pulchritudinis et fertilitatis accipiunt. Hanc ultimam *Beatam Virginem*
5 *Antiquam* dixerunt a qua pluribus aliis relictis, ad quadraginta millia passum caeteris omnibus grandior alia quaedam occurrit quam *Ay Ay* ab indigenis vocitatam, *Sanctae Crucis*, nomine appellari voluerunt. Anchoras e proris iacere Praefectus aquandi gratia in hac imperat triginta ibi viros in
10 terram descendere navi qua ipse vehebatur iubet qui loca tentarent. Ibi canes invenere; quattuor in littore iuvenes ac foeminae totidem statim protentis, in supplicum modum, lacertis quasi auxilium et a manu gentis nefandae libertatem expetentes, obvii nostris efficiuntur, multo meliorem sortem
15 sese consecuturos, quaecunque illa foret, existimantes. Canibales autem, eodem quo apud Guadalupeam modo, se fugientes ad silvas receperunt. Biduum ibi commorati et stantibus interea nostris triginta viris in insidiis, ecce venientem a longe canoam e caveis specularibus conspexere qua octo
20 viros cum totidem foeminis vectari advertentes, dato signo, canoam nostri adoriuntur. Appropinquantes nostros, viri simul et mulieres sagittis, mira celeritate, et crudelibus ictibus, transfigere coeperunt, ita priusquam sese scutis contegere potuerint, unum ex nostris, qui Cantaber erat, quaedam
25 ex mulieribus peremerit atque alium illa eadem alia sagitta, acri vulnere, transegerit. Venenatas sagittas medicamenti quodam genere illinitas esse adverterant, acie ipsarum circumcisa, qua medicamen, ne discurreret, retineretur. Erat inter eos foemina quaedam cui, uti per coniecturas percipere
30 fas erat, caeteri obtemperabant atque veluti reginae assurgebant. Hanc filius iuvenis torvus, robustus, ferocissimi intuitus, leoninae faciei, comitabatur. Nostri ergo, ne gravius malum a longe vulnerati perferrent, multo satius esse manum conserere ducentes, remis agitata nostra navicula qua
35 vehebantur, canoam impetu maximo invertunt. Ea in profundum missa, neque pigrius neque rarius natando, tam viri quam foeminae spicula in nostros dirigebant. Ad saxum quoddam aqua coopertum recepti, strenue dimicantes, tandem capiuntur, uno interempto et reginae filio duobus vul-
40 neribus confosso. In Praefecti navim adducti non magis feritatem ac vultus atrocitatem deponebant quam Libyci leo-

ity. They called this last one *Beata Virgen de la Antigua*. Left several others behind, 40 miles farther on, they reached another island, bigger than all the previous ones, and wanted this one named *Santa Cruz*, whereas the natives called it *Ay Ay*. The Admiral gave orders to drop the prow anchor in this island, so as to get a fresh supply of water, and ordered thirty of his men, off ship and start to explore it. Here the men found some dogs; four men and as many women, their arms outstretched in supplication, as if looking for help and freedom from the hands of wicked people, immediately approached our sailors certain to meet a much better fate, no matter what. The Cannibals, however, fled, as they did at Guadeloupe, taking shelter in the woods where they remained two days; in the meantime, 30 of our sailors as they lay in ambush saw from their places of observation a canoe coming from far away: realizing that there were eight men and as many women, at the given signal our men attacked it. Both men and women at the same time began to shoot with remarkable rapidity at our approaching men, delivering arrows and unrelenting blows; and so, before the men could protect themselves with shields, one of the women wounded one of them, a Cantabrian, and struck another with a different arrow, fatally wounding him. They realized the arrows were smeared with some type of poisonous substance, because the poison-laden tips had been notched in a way to preserve the liquid. Among them stood out a woman whom, as one could guess, the others obeyed and respected as their queen. Her son, a fierce and robust young man, with a ferocious look and the appearance of a lion, was next to her. And so, our men, who had been wounded from far away, in order to avoid further casualties, decided it would be better to engage them, rowed their boat next to the cannibals' canoe and overturned it with the greatest fury. Even with their canoe capsized, both men and women kept shooting arrows at our sailors while swimming with intense vigor. Having retreated to a reef, while still fighting bravely, they were finally captured, after one of them was killed and the queen's son wounded twice. Even after being taken on board the Admiral's ship the natives did not lose their fierceness and ferocious looks, not unlike African lions once they feel trapped. There is no one who would look at them and not admit to their heart shuddering in horror, so frightful and disgusting is

nes, cum sese in vincula detrusos esse praesentiunt. Hos
nullus est qui videat quin scalpi sibi horrore quodam prae-
cordia fateatur, adeo atrox Tartareusque est illis a natura
et immanitate insitus prospectus. A me ipso et reliquis qui
5 una mecum plerunque ad illos intuendos Methymnae confluxerunt coniecturam facio. Ad iter redeo. In dies, magis
atque magis procedentes iam ultra quinque et quingenta
millia passuum ad Africum [13] prius, deinde ad Favonium, [14]
postea ad Argestem, [15] protenderant, cum pelagi quandam va-
10 stitatem immensam, insulis innumeris et miris modis inter se
differentibus passim contextam, intrarunt. Harum alias nemo-
rosas atque herbidas et amoenas, alias siccas et steriles ac la-
pidosas, altissimorum montium saxeorum, transeundo videbant. Quarum aliae purpureos in nudis saxis colores, aliae
15 violaceos, aliae candidissimos ostendebant: metallis et gemmis
esse conditas non desunt qui existiment. Sed ne illic naves
firmarent et obstitit maris intemperies et frequentiae insularum
metus, ne forte naves maiores saxo aliquo illiderentur. In aliud
igitur tempus harum insularum vestigatione dilata, quas ob
20 multitudinem et confusam intermixtionem numerare non licuit,
iter suum prosequuntur; sex tamen et quadraginta cum levioribus quibusdam navigiis quibus non magno opus erat fundo,
intersecuerunt maioribus navibus ab alto, scopulorum metu,
iter peragentibus; *Archipelagus* contecturam hanc insularum
25 vocavere. Ab hoc tractu procedentes itinere in medio iacet
insula, dicta ab indigenis *Burichena*: hanc *Sancti Ioannis* insulam
appellavit. Inde sese plures ex iis qui a Canibalibus liberati
fuerant oriundos aiebant. Populosissimam, cultam, portuosam
nemorosamque esse insulam fatebantur eiusque incolas summa
30 cum Canibalibus odia atque inimicitias semper exercuisse. Non
habent ipsi navigia quibus a suis finibus ad littora Canibalium

[13] The *Libeccio* is a South-Westerly wind that blows from Africa bringing rain
along. Its name is used often as a synonym for any violent or stormy wind. See Plin.
nat. hist. II 119; Sen. *nat. quaest.* V 16, 5; Verg. *Aen.* I 86; Hor. *carm.* I 3, 12.

[14] Zephyrus, i.e. Favonius, is the personification of Zephyr, the west wind that
blows in springtime at equinoctial time and stimulates plant sprouts (Isid. XIII 11, 8).
See also Plin. *nat. hist.* II 119, 122; Sen. *nat quaest.* V 16, 5. For ancient Greeks on the
other hand it brought gale force winds i.e. storms.

[15] The North West "maestro" wind. See Serv. *ad Aen.* VIII 710; Ov. *fasti* V 161.
According to Seneca (*nat. quaest.* V 16, 5) it does not cause flashing (*Caurus* or *corus* in Latin
as claimed by others (See Plin. *nat. hist.* II 119, 120; Gell. II 22, 12; Isid. XIII 11, 10).

the appearance imparted to them by nature and their ferocity. I say this on the basis of my experience and that of others, who often came with me to see them at Medina. I go back to the narrative. Advancing farther each day, our men had by now sailed more than 505 miles, driven first by the *Libeccio* [southwest wind], then by Favonius [i.e. Zephyrus, West wind], and finally by the North-West wind, when they came into a very wide stretch of sea, dotted with numerous islands, different from each other in amazing ways. As they sailed by, they saw that some of these islands were richly wooded, green and delightful, while others were barren, sterile, and stony because of rocky and lofty mountains. Some of the mountains' exposed rock showed a reddish color, others bluish-purple, others still very white. Some claim it is so being rich in metals and precious stones. Yet, the ships were kept from stopping on account of the unfavorable conditions of the sea and fear that the bigger ships, with so many islands, would crash against some shallows. They postponed, then, to another occasion the exploration of these islands, which they were not able to count because of their number and confusing position and continued their voyage. However, with other ships that were lighter and did not require deep water, they encountered 46 islands, while the heavier ships kept sailing way out for fear of the reefs; they named this group of islands *Archipélago*. Proceeding from this place half way into the sea there is an island called *Burichena* by the natives: Columbus named this the island of *San Juan*. Many of those who had been freed from the Cannibals said that they came from it and reported the island to be very populous, cultivated, with many ports and forests, and that its inhabitants had always fostered deep hatred and hostility toward the Cannibals. These natives have no boats with which to sail from their land to the shores of the Cannibals. Given the uncertain outcome of war sometimes it happens that they defeat the Cannibals, during their frequent and plundering raids thus even the score a bit by cutting their victims to pieces under each other's eyes, roasting them and angrily tear them to shreds and devour them. They had learned all these details from the native interpreters while taking them to Spain during the first voyage. In order not to waste any time, they bypassed this island. However, when they reached the westernmost corner, a few sailors landed to get a supply of water. There they

possint transfretare; sed si Canibales eorum terras, praedae
gratia, incursionibus infestantes, profligaverint, ut interdum
contingit, quod belli eventus sint incerti, vices reddunt easdem. Alterum enim ante oculos alterius secant, assant et ra-
biosis dentibus lacerant et vorant. Haec omnia per interpretes
indigenas vectos in Hispaniam primo itinere discebant. Hanc
insulam, ne moram traherent, praetermisere. Attamen in eius
ultimo ad occidentem angulo, aquandi solum gratia pauci in
terram descendere. Ubi more gentis eius, domum invenere
magnam et conspicuam quam vulgares aliae duodecim, sed
desertae, circuibant. An quod pro anni temporibus, nunc ad
montana, ratione caloris, nunc ad planities, quando frigescit
aer, transmigrent, an Canibalium timore domos penitus dere-
liquerint, non plane constitit. Regem habet unicum universa
insula, cui imperanti mira parent reverentia. Circiter ducenta
millia passuum huius insulae meridionale latus quod abrase-
rant, protenditur. In mare, noctu, duae mulieres et unus ado-
lescens ex liberatis a Canibalibus transilicntes, sese natando ad
natale solum receperunt. Cum reliquis deinde optatam Hispaniolam, a prima insula Canibalium quingentas lequas distantem, intra paucos dies attingunt, sed infoelici eventu quod
omnes socios ibi relictos interemptos repererint. Est, in huius
insulae Hispaniolae initio, regio *Xamana* ab incolis nuncupata.
Ab ea ad Hispaniam prima navigatione Praefectus rediturus,
cum decem illis indigenis, quos supra memoravimus, vela tetendit e quibus tres tantummodo superstites erant, reliquis
contraria terrarum, aeris, et ciborum, mutatione defunctis. De
tribus, cum primum *Santheremus* Xamanae latus, ab eo sic appellatum, attigit, unum solvi iubet. Alii duo, noctu, sese in
mare, furtim, deiiciunt, natando profugiunt. Id Praefectus octo
et triginta hominum, quos superiore anno paulo interius in
insula reliquerat miserandae necis ignarus, non multum aegre
tulit, interpretes sibi non defuturos existimans, quam ob causam hos non magnifaciebat. Ulterius advectis nostris parumper,
canoa oblonga multorum remigum occurrit. In ea frater Guaccanarilli eius regis quem sibi, astricto foedere, discedens ab
insula, devinctum amicitia Praefectus reliquerat, cui etiam nostros maximopere commendaverat, uno tantum comitatus, vehebatur. Is ad Praefectum duas imagines aureas, nomine fratris,
dono ferens de nostrorum morte, uti postea per rei eventum
cognitum est, suo idiomate egit, sed quoniam interpretes de-

found a big house, built acording to the customs of those people and well in sight, surrounded by twelve other ordinary houses, which had been abandoned. It was not clear whether the inhabitants move with the seasonal cycle to the mountains to avoid heat, or to the lowlands when it is cooler, or if they had run away for good for fear of the Cannibals. The whole island has only one king, whom they obey with unusual reverence. The south side of this island along which they sailed, is about 200 miles long. During the night, two women and a young man, from among those who were freed from the Cannibals, jumped in to the sea and swam to their homeland. A few days later, then, they all reached the much desired Hispaniola, 500 leagues away from the first island of the Cannibals, but with a sad discovery: all the companions left behind were dead. As you enter this island of Hispaniola, there is a region called by their inhabitants *Samana*. From there the Admiral had set sail during his first voyage to return to Spain, taking with him the ten natives of whom we spoke earlier; of them, only three survived, the others died due to the harmful change of environment, climate and food. As soon as Columbus reached the coast of Samana, named by him *San Teremo*, he ordered that one of the three be let go. The remaining two, at night, stealthily jumped into the sea and escaped by swimming. The Admiral, unaware of the slaughter of the 38 men whom he had left on the island, a little farther in the mainland the preceding year, did not miss them much, thinking that he would not lack interpreters and therefore did not worry greatly. Our men sailed a little farther and met a long canoe with many rowers. Travelling on that canoe, accompanied only by another person, was the brother of that king Guacanagarí to whom the Admiral, upon leaving the island, had left our men, after exchanging with him a promise of friendship, with a special recommendation to care for our men. Bringing two gold statues to the Admiral as a gift from his brother, in his own language he reported the death of our men, as it was later learned from the sequence of events but lacking the interpreters they did not understand his words. When our men reached the blockhouse and the cabins the Spaniards had built for them together with a rampart all around, they realized that most everything was reduced to ashes in an eerie silence. The Admiral and all the other leaders deeply troubled by this did

fuerant, eius colloquia non perpenderunt. Cum autem ad castellum ligneum et casas quas sibi, aggere circunducto, nostri
construxerant pervenissent, omnia in cinerem versa et silere
omnia cognoverunt. Ea res Praefectum marinum caeterosque
5 viros graves deturbavit. Vivere tamen aliquem, etsi male co-
niectarent, existimantes, tormenta et ballistas, igni supposito,
una omnes exonerant ut gravibus tonitruis littoribus et altis
montibus late concussis, si qui inter homines aut inter ferarum
latebras forte metu perculsi degant, adventasse nostros per
10 haec signa persentirent. Id incassum: vivebat enim nullus.
A Praefecto post haec missi ad regem Guaccanarillum nuncii
haec dicta, quantum potuere percipere, rettulerunt: esse in ea
insula maiores se reges quod mirae sit magnitudinis, plures
ait. Horum duos, maximis copiis suo more comparatis, fama
15 novae gentis commotos, adventasse belloque victos nostros
omnes trucidasse repagula casasque simul et eorum supellectilia
combussisse et se, quod nostris esse auxilio conatus fuerit, ab
eisdem fuisse sagitta vulneratum crus vitta gossampina ligatum
ostendens, rettulit, propterea non ivisse ad Praefectum, quod
20 maximopere cupiebat. Varios ibi esse reges hosque illis atque
illos his potentiores inveniunt, uti fabulosum legimus Aeneam
in varios divisum reperisse Latium, Latinum puta Mezentium-
que ac Turnum et Tarchontem, qui angustis limitibus discri-
minabantur et huiuscemodi reliqua per tyrannos dispartita. Sed
25 Hispaniolos nostros insulares illis beatiores esse sentio, modo
religionem imbuant, quia nudi, sine ponderibus, sine mensura,
sine mortifera denique pecunia, aurea aetate viventes, sine legibus, sine calumniosis iudicibus, sine libris, natura contenti,
vitam agunt, de futuro minime solliciti. Ambitione et isti ta-
30 men imperii causa torquentur et se invicem bellis conficiunt;
qua peste auream aetatem haudquaquam credimus vixisse im-
munem quin et eo tempore "cede, non cedam", inter mortales
pererraverit. Ad rem a qua digressi sumus, redeamus. Altero
die, missus a Praefecto Melchiorius quidam Hispalensis vir,
35 apud Pontificem Summum pro Rege et Regina functus oratoris officio, quo anno Malaca venit in eorum potestatem, neque
vulnus neque vulneris ullius cicatricem, vitta sublata, se vidisse
rettulit. Lecto illum tamen, adversa valitudine simulata, iacen-
tem reperit; cuius cubiculo septem concubinarum pellicum
40 lectuli adhaererent. Unde peremptos eius consilio nostros su-
spicari coepit. Re tamen dissimulata, cum Guaccanarillo egit

nonetheless, hope that some might still be alive — but were wrong — and so fired and discharged at the same time all the crossbows and the mortars, so that if any companion had by chance been hiding among the islanders or in the lairs of animals out of fear, upon seeing the beach and high mountains shaken by the loud roar would understand from these signals that our men had arrived. All this in vain, for no one was alive. Later on, some messengers sent by the Admiral to chief Guacanagarí related the following, as far as they could understand: the King said that in that island of extraordinary vastness there were kings more powerful that he. He said that two of them, after assembling huge armies, according to their custom, driven by the reputation of the newcomers, had come and, after defeating our men in battle, had slain all of them ransacking and burning at the same time their defenses, cabins and possessions; and, showing a leg still dressed with cotton bandages, he claimed to have been wounded by them with an arrow, because he attempted to help our men: for that reason he could not come to see the Admiral, although he desired it very much. Our people realized the presence of several kings, some more powerful than others, just as we read that the mythical Aeneas found Latium divided among the kingdoms, of Latinus, Mezentius, Turnus and Tarchon, separated by narrow borders, with the remaining territories shared by tyrants. But I feel that our natives of Hispaniola are happier than they, — more so were they converted to the true religion — because naked, without burdens, limits or death-inducing currency, living in a golden age, free, without fraudulent judges, books, and content of their natural state, they live with no worries about the future. However, even these men are troubled by the desire to rule and waste each other away with wars; we think that not even this golden age was immune from such plague, i.e. the overriding principle of "*you give in, as I shall not.*" But now let us go back to our original narrative. The following day a certain Melchior of Seville, who had once been appointed ambassador to the Sovereign Pontiff by the King and Queen in the year when they captured Malaga, and had been sent by the Admiral, declared that once the bandage had been removed he had not seen a wound nor a scar of it. Instead he had found Guacanagarí feigning ill health in bed, near which there were seven small beds of concubines. Therefore, he began

Melchiorius ut postero die ad visendum Praefectum sese ad
naves conferret. Naves igitur, uti pactus fuerat, ingressus, nostris salutatis atque auro donatis primoribus, ad mulieres a Canibalibus ereptas conversus, in unam, quam *Catherinam* nostri
vocabant, oculos semifractos coniicere visus. Eam blande al-
locutus est atque sic urbaniter ac lepide a Praefecto veniam
petens, aspectu equorum et aliarum rerum illis incognitarum
admiratus, discessit. Fuere qui Praefecto consulerent Guaccanarillum detinendum fore uti, si eius consilio nostros peremptos fuisse comperirent, poenas daret. Sed irritandi animos
indigenarum non esse tempus Praefectus ratus, eum dimisit.
Postridie eius diei regis frater ad naves se conferens, vel suo,
vel fratris nomine, mulieres seduxit. Nam, sequenti nocte intempesta, Catherina ipsa ut sese et quascunque posset in libertatem vendicaret, aut regis et fratris eius pollicitationibus
subornata, multo maius facinus aggressa est quam Cloelia [16]
Romana, quae Tiberim, ruptis vinculis, Porsenae imperium
fugiens, cum reliquis obsidibus virginibus enatavit. Illa enim
fluvium equo, haec cum septem aliis mulieribus suismet lacertis confisa circiter tria millia passuum atque etiam maris non
bene tranquilli, traiecit: tantum enim a littore classis omnium
opinione distabat. Illas insecuti cymbis levioribus nostri, eodem lumine, quo in littore viso mulieres regebantur duce, tres
assecuti sunt. Catherinam cum quattuor reliquis ad Guaccanarillum evasisse creditum est. Nam, ubi eluxit, missi a Praefecto
nuncii aufugisse cum omni supellectile Guaccanarillum simul
et foeminas ipsas cognoverunt. Id non iniuria fuisse nostros
eius consensu interemptos suspitionem adauxit. Hunc deinde
Melchiorius, de quo supra, tribus armatis centuriis acceptis,
quaeritans (*centuriam* centum virorum numerum appello, licet
me non lateat constare centuriam ex viris centum viginti octo
quindecimque decuriam), in fauces quasdam retortas utrinque
collibus erectis munitas incidit. Fluvii alicuius grande ostium
arbitratus, portum ibi valde commodum ac tutum adinvenit,

[16] A Roman noble young woman (see Dion. Hal. V 33, 2; 35, 2; Liv. II 13,
6 ss.; Flor. I 4, 7-8), claimed to have been the protagonist of a courageous episode
during the early republic. Turned over to Porsena Lars in sign of peace with nine [sic]
other young girls, Cloelia escaped from the Etruscan camp *ruptis... vinculis*, see Verg.
Aen. VIII 649 ff.) Out of admiration Porsena claimed her back and sent her to Rome
full of honors. Other literary sources, except Livy, introduced variations to this story.

to suspect that our men had been murdered by his will. However, Melchior, concealing his doubts, made arrangements with Guacanagarí to go aboard the ships and visit the Admiral the next day. And so he went aboard ship as agreed and greeted our men handing out some gold to the officers, and then, turning to the women who had been saved from the Cannibals, he was seen gazing and leering at one of them, named Catalina by our men. He spoke to her sweetly and, after asking permission of the Admiral with good manners and courtesy he took leave, still amazed at the sight of horses and other things never seen before. There were those who advised the Admiral to keep Guacanagarí so that he could be punished if they learned that our men had been murdered by his order. But realizing that this was not the time to irritate feelings, the Admiral let him go. The following day, his brother went on board the ships and corrupted the women both in his own name and his brother's, the king. In the middle of the following night, Catalina herself, perhaps to regain her own freedom and that of as many companions as she could, or maybe allured by the promises of the king or of his brother, risked a more heroic undertaking than Cloelia who, escaping from Porsena, broke her chains and swam across the Tiber with seven other virgins equally taken hostages. Whereas, Cloelia crossed the river on horse back Catalina, with seven other women, relying only on the strength of her arms, swam about three miles in a not very calm sea: indeed, that was the distance of the fleet from the shore, according to everyone's opinion. Our sailors pursued them with the smaller boats, using the same light which guided the women from the shore, and they captured three of them. It was thought that Catalina and four other women had escaped to Guacanagarí. As a matter of fact, at daybreak the messengers sent by the Admiral found out that Guacanagarí had left with those women, taking all his possessions. That, justifiably, increased the suspicion that our men had been murdered with his consent. So Melchior, whom I have mentioned earlier, taking with him three centuries of armed men (I call century a company of 100 men, although I realize that it had 128 and a decury of fifteen men), went to search for him and ended up in some tortuous gorges, with steep hills on both sides. He thought this could be the large outlet of a river and saw in it a favorable and safe harbor; the

Portum Regalem propterea nominandum censuerunt. Falcatum eius ingressum atque adeo in arcum dispositum ferunt, quod sive in laevam sive in dextram introductas naves flectant, unde, donec ad ostium revertantur, ingressi fuerint non facile
5 dignosci possit, quamvis tribus simul paribus proris onerariae naves procedere valeant. Hinc atque inde sublati colles, littorum loco, vemientes frangunt ventos. In eius medio sinu promontorium nemorosum psittacis atque aliarum volucrum ibi nidificantium multis generibus suavissimeque concinentium eri-
10 gitur. Duo in portum hunc flumina non mediocria defluere cognoverunt. Dum inter utrunque terram explorant, altam a longe domum vident. Ibi latere Guaccanarillum rati, accedunt: adeuntibus nostris, vir quidam, fronte rugosa et elato supercilio, centum hominibus comitatus, efficitur obvius; arcu,
15 sagittis et lanceis praeacutis fundalibus omnes armati minantibus similes accurrunt, se *tainos*, id est nobiles, esse, non Canibales inclamitant. Signo pacis a nostris dato, arma simul et feritatem illam deposuere et singulis accipitreis tintinnabulis acceptis, statim cum nostris adeo strictain imicitiam iniere, ut
20 in nostrorum potestatem sese, sine ulla mora, in naves ex altis fluvii ripis demiserint et suis postea muneribus nostros donaverint. Domum illam, qui eam dimensi sunt duorum et triginta magnorum passuum, a circumferentia ad circumferentiam (erat enim sphaerica), iacto diametro, fuisse afferunt triginta
25 aliis popularibus circunseptam, lacunaribus harundineis versicoloribus, super inductis, mira arte intertextis. Interrogati quibus modis melius dabatur de Guaccanarillo responderunt non esse Guaccanarilli regionis huius sed eius qui aderat imperium. Sensisse sese fatebantur quod Guaccanarillus a littoribus ad
30 montana secesserit. Icto igitur cum hoc *cacico*, id est rege, fraterno foedere, ad Praefectum quae viderant renunciaturi rediere. Diversos interea centuriones exploratum longius suis centuriis comitatos Praefectus emittit, inter quos Hoiedam et Gorvalanum, nobiles iuvenes et animosos ambos. Horum alter
35 quattuor flumina, alius, alia parte, tria ab iisdem montibus collabentia comperere. In quorum omnium arenis, aurum, nostris praesentibus, indigenae qui eos comitabantur, hoc modo colligebant: arena manibus effossa ad scrobem usque lacerti profunditate, ex imo scrobis plenas arena sinistras dehinc ex-
40 trahentes, dextra, auro delecto, sine ulteriore industria, in manus nostrorum grana porrigebant. Quorum se vidisse multa,

men decided, therefore, to call it Puerto Real. Our men report that its opening is in the shape of a crescent so arched that, once a ship has entered and keeps going right or left, one cannot easily determine whence it has come, until it returns to the opening, that can simultaneously accommodate with three cargo-ships prows of equal size. Here and there lofty hills, instead of beaches, offer resistance to the blowing winds. In the middle of the bay there rises a wooded promontory full of parrots and many other nesting birds that sing so melodiously. Two medium-sized rivers noticeably flowed into this bay. While they explored the territory in between, they saw from far away a big house. Thinking that it may be the hiding place of Guacanagarí, they approached it: a man with a wrinkled forehead and thick eyebrows, accompanied by 100 men, met the approaching men; armed with bows, arrows, painted lances and poles, they all hastened toward our men with a threatening look shouting they were *tayno*, that is, noble people, not Cannibals. After our sailors gave a peace signal, they abandoned their arms and their fierceness at the same time. After each received a hawk's bell, they quickly became such good friends that, from the steep banks of the river they slid on board the ships without hesitating, in the hands of our men; and then they offered our men their gifts. Those that measured that house say that, from side to side (it was round), it was 32 long paces in diameter and was surrounded by 30 other huts with, overhead, multicolored reeds, layered with singular ability. Questioned, as much as they could be, about Guacanagarí, they answered that this region was not under Guacanagarí's rule, but under a chief that lived there, and admitted hearing that Guacanagarí had left the beach to go to the high lands. After negotiating a friendly treaty with this cacique, that is, a king, our men went back to the Admiral to report what they had seen. In the meantime, the Admiral sent several commanders to explore the interior farther, including Hojeda and Gorvalán, both noble and courageous young men, accompanied by their centuries. One of them discovered four rivers, and the other three more on the opposite side of the island, flowing from the same mountains. The natives who accompanied them gathered gold from the sand of these rivers, under the eyes of our men, in this fashion: first they would dig out the sand with their hands, until the hole was an arm's length deep;

ciceris crassitudine, plures fatentur. Vidi ego ipse postea allatum rudem fluviali petrae similem globum ponderis unciarum novem, ab ipso Hoieda repertum. His signis contenti rem ad Praefectum referunt. Iusserat enim Praefectus, ut mihi relatum
5 est, poena etiam praeposita, ne quid ulterius praeterquam de locis et locorum signis curarent. Fama etiam increbuit esse quendam regem montium a quibus flumina illa decidunt, quem cacicum *Caunaboam* vocant, id est dominum domus aureae. *Boam* enim domum dicunt, *cauni* autem aurum et *cacicum* re-
10 gem, uti iam dictum est. Nullibi aquarum pisces inveniri posse illis praestantiores, saporosiores aut minus noxios et aquas illorum omnium fluminum esse saluberrimas aiunt. Diem esse apud Canibales, mense Decembri, noctibus aequalem Melchiorius ipse mihi rettulit, sed id sphaerae ratio non patitur, quam-
15 vis eo mense avium aliae nidificarent, aliae filios iam natos in nidis haberent et calor vigeret non mediocris. Abscondi totum plaustrum sub arctico polo atque occidere Custodes[17] Canibalibus, mihi de altitudine poli ab horizonte diligentius scrutanti enarravit. Cui de iis maior sit fides quam huic adhibenda nul-
20 lus hoc itinere rediit. Si ergo fuisset astronomiae peritus, diem fere noctibus aequalem dixisset: nullibi enim terrarum aequa est versus solstitia nox diei. Ipsi vero aequinoctialem nunquam tetigere, quandoquidem arcticum polum semper habuere ducem et ab horizonte semper elevatum. Sunt enim alii neque
25 litterarum aut rerum experientia periti. Propterea brevibus nunc et incomposita epistola quae colligere potuerim accipito; propediem, uti spero, a me caetera quae detegentur habiturus. Scripsit enim ad me Praefectus ipse marinus, cui sum intima familiaritate devinctus, sese mihi latissime quaecunque sors
30 ostenderit significaturum. Ipse propinquum portui cuidam editum locum ad civitatem condendam elegit ibique intra paucos dies domibus, ut brevitas temporis passa est, et sacello erectis eo die quo *Trium Regum* solennia celebramus, divina nostro ritu, in alio, potest dici, orbe, tam extero, tam ab omni cultu
35 et religione alieno, sacra sunt decantata, terdecim sacerdotibus ministrantibus. Tempore quo iam sese ad Regem et Reginam missurum fuerat pollicitus appropinquante et prospera navigatione se offerente, non ultra cunctandum ratus Praefectus,

---

[17] Peter Marty's reference here is to the entire 53-star constellation of Ursa Major and Boötes (see Ov. *met.* X 447; *ep. ex Pont.* IV 10, 39).

then, from the bottom of the hole would pull out the left hand full of sand, picking out the gold with the right; and in no time they would place the nuggets in the hands of our men, who claim to have seen many nuggets, several as big as chick-peas. I myself have later seen a rough chunk coming from there, similar to a river stone, weighing nine onces, that had been found by Hojeda himself. Satisfied by these clues, our men reported it all to the Admiral. As I was later told, the Admiral had really forbidden them, threatening punishments, to do more than to inquire about the places and their characteristics. The news also spread that there was a king in those mountains, whence the rivers flow: they call that cacique *Caunaboa* [Caonabó], that is "lord of the golden house". In fact, they call the house *boa*, the gold *cauni*, the king *cacicco*, as has already been said. They also say that in no river can you find better looking fish or tastier and less harmful, and that the water of all the rivers is very wholesome. Melchior himself related to me that among the Cannibals, in the month of December, days are as long as nights, but the spherical nature of the earth contradicts it, regardless of the fact that birds were nesting, or their chicks had already hatched, and that there was considerable heat. When I asked more specific questions about the height of the pole on the horizon, he replied to me that where the Cannibals live Ursa Major i.e. the full Great Bear was hidden by the arctic pole and Boötes was less brilliant. No one who came back from this voyage deserves more trust than he on these facts. Had he been expert in astronomy, he would have said that the day is almost as long as the night: the fact is that there is no place in the world where the night is as long as the day during the solstices. In truth they never reached the equator, because they always followed as a point of reference the arctic pole star, always high on the horizon. There are others who really have neither literary knowledge nor personal experience. Therefore, learn, now, although succinctly and in a hurried way, the details that I have been able to gather; soon, I hope you will be able to receive from me more news that will be revealed. The Admiral himself, to whom I am tied in close friendship, just wrote to me saying that he will inform me amply of all that Fate will show him. He himself chose an elevated place near a port to found a city, and there, in a few days, built some houses and a chapel as the

duodecim has caravelas, quas adventasse diximus, commeavit,
non mediocri molestia nostrorum internicione confectus; quorum morte multa, quae iam de illorum locorum natura co-
gnosceremus, adhuc nos latent. Ut pharmacopolis, syrophoenicibus et aromatariis accitis possis, quid regiones illae ferant,
quam calida sit earum superficies dignoscere, ex granis, omnis
generis ex libro et medulla earum arborum quas cinnami esse
autumant, ad te mitto. Sive ex granis, sive ex animulis quibusdam, quas ex ipsis granis decidisse conspicies, sive ex ligno
gustare volueris, illustrissime Princeps, tenuiter admoto labello,
pertingito: sunt enim quamvis non noxia, ob nimiam tamen
caliditatis acuitatem acria et linguam, si in ea diu morentur,
expungunt; sed statim, si forte eius degustatione lingua concoquatur, epota aqua, asperitas illa tollitur. Ex frumento etiam,
quo panem conficiunt, grana quaedam alba et nigra tabellarius,
meo nomine, dignationi tuae dabit. Ligni quod *aloes* esse dicunt truncum affert, quod si iusseris scindi suavem senties ex
eo odore-1m emanare. Vale!

Ex Hispana curia, tertio Kalendas Maii 1494

short time allowed. On the day when we commemorate the feast of the Three Kings [Epiphany], the sacred functions were celebrated according to our rite, with thirteen priests attending as ministers, in a world, it could be said, so different, so far away, so alien to all civilization and religion. As it was time to send news to the King and Queen, as he had promised, and circumstances favorable to sailing presented themselves, the Admiral, quite saddened by the murder of our men but being of the opinion that he should not delay any longer, ordered these twelve vessels, which, as we said, have arrived, to return. Because of their death we now lack many details concerning the nature of those places which we might have had by now. So that you may see the contributions those regions bring to apothecaries, grocers and perfumers whom have been summoned, and how hot their surface is, I send you samples of seeds of every kind, bark, and pith from those trees they think may be cinnamon. Were you to wish to taste either the seeds or the crumbs which you see fall from the very seeds or the bark, most illustrious Prince, barely touch them when you draw them near your lips: indeed, although not harmful, they produce excessive heat that can irritate and sting the tongue, if you leave them on it a long time. If by chance you feel the tongue burning after tasting them, the hot sensation is quickly eliminated by drinking water. The bearer will also offer to your Eminence, on my behalf, some white and black wheat grains, the kind they make bread from. He also brings a piece of wood, which they claim to be aloe: if you have it split, you will smell the ensuing delicate perfume. Take care!

From the court of Spain, 29 April 1494.

I 3: ad Ludovicum Aragonium cardinalem

Petis iterum ut Phoebaeos currus ineptus Phaeton guber-
net, ex nudo silice suaves liquores exhaurire contendis. Novum,
ut ita dixerim terrarum orbem, Catholicorum Fernandi et Helisabeth Regum tibi patruorum ductu, ab occidente qui hactenus
5 latitabat, repertum, ut ego describam Federici regis inclyti patrui tibi mihi litteras de hac re ostendens, imperas. Preciosum
hunc lapillum plumbo inepte circundatum ambo accipietis. Sed
cum eruditos amice, detractores invide, mordaces rabide, in
nostras formosas Nereides oceaneas spumantia tela detorquere
10 praesenties, quam brevi spacio, inter rerum angustias et valitu-
dinatium, hos me conscribere coegeris, ingenue profiteberis.
Scis namque me tanto celeriter ex Praefecti ipsius marini Coloni
archetypis pauca haec delegisse quanto tuus a manu famulus,
qui, me dictante, scribebat, poterat exarare. Infestabas namque
15 me cotidie, tuum discessum obiicens ut nostri Regis sororem
Parthenopaeam reginam, tibi amitam, quam huc fueras comitatus, in patriam reduceres. Singulis interdum diebus singulos
me libellos cudere adegisti. Duos in prima fronte alieno com-
peries nomine signatos; quod, dum ista quaerebantur, ad in-
20 foelicem ego Ascanium Sfortiam, tibi affinem, cardinalem, vicecancellarium, scriptitare incoeperam. Quo cadente, cecidit et
mihi animus a scribendo, quem tu nunc tuique inclyti patrui,
regis Federici, litterae ad me directae, excussistis. Rem, non
picturam degustate! Vale!

Ex Granata .ix. Kalemdas Maii anno 1500

25 Canibalium littora Colonum Praefectum marinum percurrisse ad Hispaniolamque insulam cum integra classe quarto
Nonas Februarii anni tertii et nonagesimi appulsum fuisse superiore libro descripsimus. Nunc autem quid de insulae natura
explorans repererit, quidve postea finitimam insulam, continen-
30 tem uti credit terram, percurrens invenerit enarremus. Insula

250

I 3: To Cardinal Ludovico of Aragon

You ask again that an inexperienced Phaethon drive the chariots of Phoebus [Apollo sun]; you expect to draw sweet liqueurs from a barren rock. Showing me a letter from your illustrious uncle, King Federico, on this topic, you order me to write about the new western world, up to now kept hidden, which was discovered, so to speak, under the auspices of the Catholic Sovereigns, your uncle Ferdinand and aunt Isabella. You both will receive this precious stone so inconveniently set in lead; but when you realize that the learned out of benevolence, the accusers out of envy, and the critics out of rage throw frothing arrows against our beautiful oceanic Nereids, you will shall honestly acknowledge to have forced me to write these books in a short time, amid worries and troubles of ill health. You know, indeed, I chose these accounts from the originals of Admiral Columbus himself, as rapidly as your copyist could write under my dictation. Yes, each day you nagged me, using the pretext of your departure to take back home the queen of Naples, sister of our King, your aunt, whom you had accompanied here. Thus, you forced me to write some pamphlets every day. You will find two of them with a different dedication on the title page, because, as I was doing this research, I had started to write for the unfortunate cardinal Ascanio Sforza, vice chancellor, your relative. When he died, my will to write also passed away, but which you and the letter from your illustrious uncle, King Federico, have now rejuvenated. Appreciate the effort, if not the narrative. Fare well!

From Granada, 23 April 1500

In the preceding book I told how Admiral Columbus sailed along shores inhabited by Cannibals and of his safe landfall with all his vessels on the island of Hispaniola on 2 February 1493. Now instead, I would like to write about what he found while exploring its configuration and what he finally did discover next traveling through the nearby island, that he believes to be a continent. This island of Hispaniola,

haec Hispaniola, quam ipse *Ophiram* de qua legitur Regum
tertio esse asseverat, latitudinis est graduum australium quinque: elevatur enim a septentrione gradus septimus et vigesimus
a meridie vero, ut ipsi referunt, vigesimus secundus; longitudo
5 autem ab oriente in occidentem passuum millia octoginta super
septingenta. Ex ipsius Praefecti Coloni comitibus non desunt
qui utranque insulae mensuram producant ab oriente ad occidentem. Distare a Gadibus insulam gradus praedicant aliqui
novem et quadraginta, alii amplius; neque enim certam adhuc
10 rationem reperere. Insulae forma castaneae folium aemulatur.
Super edito igitur colle a septentrione civitatem erigere decrevit, quod huic loco mons eminens et saxifodinis ad aedifican-
dum et calcem concoquendam aptissimus adiaceat. Inhaeret
praeterea huius montis radicibus vasta planities longitudinis
15 millium passuum circiter sexaginta, latitudinis vero duodecim
alicubi, alibi, ubi angustior sit sex, ubi vero amplior viginti.
Planitiem salubrium aquarum flumina interluunt plura, sed
eorum maius et id navigabile in portum, qui urbi subiacet, ad
stadium dimidium cadit. Quanta sit eius vallis ubertas, quanta
20 soli benignitas, eorum relatu, adverte. In huius fluminis ripa
hortos colendos limitibus concluserunt, ex quibus de omni
holerum genere ut puta raphanorum, lactucarum, caulium, bo-
raginum et aliorum huiuscemodi, intra diem a iacto semine
sextum decimum, vulgo matura evulsa sunt; melones, cucurbi-
25 tas, cucumeres et alia id genus, in diem sextum et trigesimum
carpserunt, sed nusquam se meliores unquam comedisse aiebant: haec hortensia toto anno habent recentia. Cannarum radices, ex quarum succo saccarum extorquetur, cubitales cannas
(sed non coagulatur succus), intra quindecimum etiam diem
30 emiserunt. De plantatis propaginibus aut sarmentis itidem aiunt
et secundo a plantatione anno suaves ex eis uvas comedisse,
ast ex nimia ubertate, racemos edunt perpaucos. Rusticus praeterea quidam tritici parumper circiter Kalendas Februarii semi-
navit: res miranda, in omnium conspectum, maturum spicarum
35 manipulum tertio Kalendas Aprilis, qui eo anno erat vigilia
Resurrectionis Dominicae, secum ad urbem tulit. Legumina
quaeque quotannis maturescunt bis. Scripsi quae omnes uno
ore,inde redeuntes, de eius terrae foetura rettulerunt; nonnulli
tamen ferunt tritici non esse terram feracem in universo. Inte-
40 rea, dum ista agerentur, triginta viros qui Cipangi, alias *Cibavi,*
regionem explorarent per diversa dimisit Praefectus. Est autem

identified by him as Ophir, of which we read about in the 3rd Book of Kings, spreads over five degrees: that is from 27° South latitude to the north, and 22° to the south, as they themselves report; its East to West length is 780 miles. Among the companions of Admiral Columbus there are those who would extend the East-West dimension of the island. Some claim it is 49° off Cádiz, but other say more; the exact distance has not yet been determined. The shape of the island resembles a chestnut leaf. Hence, the Admiral decided to found a city on the northern side over an elevated site, since in its vicinity there is a high mountain, very convenient for construction and for kilning lime, given its stone quarries. Moreover, at the foot of this mountain there is a large but irregular plain about 60 miles long and six to 12 wide, in some places, reaching twenty miles at its widest. Several rivers of wholesome waters flow through the plain, with the largest, also navigable, emptying into the port below the city at a distance of half a stadium. From their narrative, consider how fruitful that valley is and how fertile the soil. On the banks of this river they parceled out gardens to cultivate, and from them, sixteen days after sowing, they gathered all kinds of fully ripe vegetables, such as radishes, lettuces, cabbages, borage [burridge] and so on; they also picked, after 35 days, melons, pumpkins, cucumbers [or watermelons], and other similar products. Above all they claimed no tastier food had ever been eaten anywhere: they enjoy these vegetables fresh from the garden throughout the year. The roots of canes too, from whose juice sugar is extracted (although the juice does not crystalize), sprouted gigantic tops in fifteen days. They claim the same is true for planted vine shoots whose branches yield tasty sweet grapes two years after planting, yet because of their excessive leafiness the vines produce very few bunches of grapes. In addition, a farmer sowed a bit of wheat the first part of February: what a surprise — on March 30, which that year fell on the vigil of Easter Sunday, he carried a ripe sheaf of wheat with him to the city for everyone to see. All vegetables are harvested twice a year. I have written to you that all those returning from there have unanimously agreed on the fertility of that land, with some even claiming there is no land on earth as fertile in producing wheat. In the meantime, while these things were being done, the Admiral sent 30 of his men in different direc-

17

haec regio montosa, saxea et medium totius insulae dorsum; in qua maximam esse auri copiam incolae signis ostendebant. Missi a Praefecto de regionis opibus mira referentes revertuntur. Ex illis montibus quattuor ingentia flumina defluunt, quae totam insulam, reliqua suis alveis suscipiendo, memoranda naturae industria, in quattuor fere partes aequales dividunt. Tendunt enim, unus recta ad orientem qui ab accolis *Iunna* vocatur, ad occidentem alius, huic terga vertens qui *Attibunicus*, tertius ad septentrionem, quem *Iachem* appellant, ultimus ad meridiem, quem *Naibam*. Sed redeamus ad condendam urbem. Fossis et aggeribus urbe circumvallata, ut si, eo absente, praelium incolae tentarent, sese qui relinquebantur tutari possint, pridie Idus Martii cum omnibus equitibus, peditibus autem circiter quadringentis, ipsemet ad auriferam regionem recta ad meridiem proficiscitur; fluvium praeterlabitur, transgreditur planitiem, montem, qui aliud planitiei latus cingit, superat. In aliam convallem, quam flumen priore maius aliaque multa mediocria interluebant, incidit; exercitum traducit. Hac valle, quae priore nulla parte inferior est, superata, tertium montem facit pervium qui hactenus fuerat invius descenditque in aliam convallem quae iam *Cibavi* est initium. Per hanc flumina et ex omni colle rivi currunt in quorum omnium arenis aurum reperiebatur. Cum iam secundum et septuagesimum ab urbe lapidem intra regionem auriferam profectus fuisset, in magni cuiusdam fluminis ripa, eminenti super colle, condere arcem instituit ut interioris regionis secreta inde tuto paulatim scrutarentur. Hanc arcem *Sancti Thomae* nomine insignivit. Dum interea arcem aedificaret, eius regionis incolae tintinnabulorum et aliarum rerum nostratium cupidi, cotidie moram trahentem adibant. Praefectus vero marinus se illis quae peterent libentissime daturum, si aurum ferrent, insinuat. At illi, dato tergo, ad haec promissa ad ripam propinquiorem currentes, intra breve temporis spacium onustis auro manibus redibant. Grandaevus incola duos auri calculos ponderis unius fere unciae, tintinnabulum tantum modo petens, attulit. Qui, cum nostros calculorum magnitudinem admirari conspiceret, eorum admiratione admiratus, eos esse parvos ac nullius momenti calculos innuebat captisque manu quattuor lapidibus quorum minor nucem, maior autem grande aureum aequabat malum, adeo magnos auri globos in solo natali suo, quod ad dimidiam inde dietam distabat, passim reperiri aiebat, nec apud vicinos suos magnae curae esse aurum colligere.

254

tions to explore the region of Cipango, otherwise called *Cibavo*. This is a mountainous and rocky region, the main divider of the whole island; the natives gave to understand through gestures that this area had great quantities of gold. The men sent by the Admiral come back bringing wonderful news of the riches of the region. From those mountains flow four large rivers that divide the whole island in four parts nearly equal and fed by tributaries, thanks to a remarkable work of nature. One of them, the natives call it *Iunna*, winds in an easterly direction; another, the *Attibunico*, flows west in the opposite direction; the third named *Iache*, lies to the north, and the last, *Naiba*, to the south. But let us go back to the founding of the city. After having surrounded the city with ditches and ramparts, so that, had the natives attacked during his absence, those who were left there could defend themselves, Columbus heads due south on 14 March, with all his cavalrymen and about 400 foot-soldiers, toward the region of the gold; he crosses a river, a plain and climbs a mountain that borders the other side of the plain. He reached another valley bathed by an even larger river and several others of lesser size; he makes the army go on. He crosses this valley, which is in no way less than the other one, crosses over a third mountain, up to that time inaccessible, and descends into a third valley, which is the beginning of the *Cibavo* region. Through it flow down from every hill rivers and streams, whose sands yield gold. After advancing almost 72 miles from the city into the gold region, Columbus decided to build a fortress on the bank of a large river on a high hill, so that from there they could gradually and safely explore the region's hidden places of the interior. This fortress he named *Santo Tomás*. In the meantime, while he was building the fort, the inhabitants of that region, wanting to have bells and other objects from our country, were coming to him daily as he lingered. The Admiral indeed made them understand that he was very willing to give them what they wanted, if they brought him gold. They, would turn around, go running because of his promise to the nearest stream and return shortly with their hands full of gold. An elder native brought two golden nuggets, each weighing almost an ounce and asked for only a bell. In return, seeing our men looking with astonishment at the nuggets and amazed at their surprise, tried to explain with gestures that those nuggets were small

Cognitum enim est illos aurum in quantum est aurum non magnifacere, sed tanti illud aestimare quanti artificis manus in formam cuique gratam diducere aut conflare didicerit. Quis rude marmor aut ebur incultum comparat magno? Nullus equi-
5 dem, sed si Phidiae aut Praxitelis dextra fabrefactum in coma-tam Nereidem aut Hamadriadem pulchre formatam prodierit, nusquam emptores deerunt. Praeter hunc senem, accesserunt et alii plures qui decem et duodecim drachmarum calculos attulerunt ausique sunt fateri, ubi aurum illud collegerant, auri
10 globos pueri caput, quem ostendebant, aequantes fuisse aliquan-do repertos. Dum ibidem dies aliquot moraretur, Luxanum quendam iuvenem nobilem cum paucis armatis, regionis partem exploratum, misit. Hic etiam maiora sibi ab incolis fuisse dicta rettulit, nihil tamen attulit. Ex Praefecti putant mandato ita
15 fieri. Aromatibus, sed non iisdem quibus nos utimur, habent plena nemora quae pari modo colligunt ut aurum; tantum scilicet unusquisque quantum permutando, aliquid sibi gratum a finitimarum insularum incolis assequantur, ut puta paropsides, sedilia et huiuscemodi, quae in aliis insulis ex nigro quodam
20 ligno, quo ipsi carent, conficiuntur. Rediens ad Praefectum, Luxanus circiter Idus Martii labruscas in silvis maturas invenit optimi, ut ait, saporis, sed nulla est insularibus de his cura. Est haec regio, quamvis saxea (nam eorum lingua *Cibavum* id quod saxosum sonat), arborifera tamen et herbida. Immo et aiunt
25 herbam eorum montium, quae solum gramen est, si scindatur, quattuor dierum intercapedine, tritico altiorem crescere. Fre-quentes in ea pluvias cadere referunt, hinc esse rivos et flumina adeo crebra, quorum cum sit arena ubique auro commixta, ex montibus illud aurum detrahi per torrentes autumant. Gentem
30 constat esse ociosam: nam interdum, hyeme urgente, tremunt in montibus frigore nec, quum sint illis nemora gossipio[18] refertissima, vestes sibi laborare student. In vallibus autem vel campestribus locis, minime, frigescunt. His ita, in initio regionis Cibavi, diligenter perquisitis, Kalendis Aprilis, quem diem Re-
35 surrectio sequebatur, ad *Isabellam* (id est urbis nomen), reverti-tur. Unde in eius et totius insulae gubernationem fratre suo et

---

[18] Peter Martyr's reference is to the cotton plant known since antiquity in Egypt and India. The name was first reported by Pliny (*nat. hist.* XIX 14: *gossypion*; XII 39: *gossypinus*), who distinghishes between the plant and its product i.e. *arbor* e *frutex*.

and of little value; he then took in his hand four stones, the smallest of which was the size of a nut and the largest a big quince, saying that gold nuggets that size could be found here and there in his native land, half a day's journey away, and that his neighbors were not interested in gathering gold. In fact, it was found out that those natives did not value gold as such, but prized it only inasmuchas the hand of the craftsman that moulded or shaped it into an admirable object. Who appreciates rough marble or unworked ivory? Certainly, no one; but once chiselled by the hand of Phidias or Praxiteles, into a shapely long-haired Nereid or a beautiful Hamadryad, in no place will buyers be lacking. In addition to this old man, several others also came bringing nuggets weighing ten and twelve drachmas, and who dared claim that where they had gathered that gold, they had sometimes found nuggets as big as the head of the child to whom they were pointing. While spending a few days here, Columbus sent a young nobleman by the name of Luján with few armed soldiers to explore a section of the region. He related that the natives had told him even more amazing stories, but did not bring anything back. It is believed he acted in this way on orders from the Admiral. The natives have woods full of spices, but not the same we use, and they harvest them in much the same way they do gold; trading obviously as much as each gathers, they obtain from their neighboring islanders something that pleases them, such as cups, seats and other similar products manufactured in the other islands from a kind of wood they lack. Around the 15th of March, upon returning to the Admiral, Luján found in the woods ripe grapes of a most sweet taste, as he reports, but the islanders do not care about them. This region, although covered by rocks (indeed, *Cibavo* in their language means rocky), is nevertheless full of trees and grasses. It is even said that the couch or dog grass of those mountains, really weeds, if cut, grows taller than wheat in the span of four days. It is related that in that region frequent rains fall and thus streams and rivers are so numerous; and, since their sand is everywhere mixed with gold, it is asserted that gold is removed from the mountains by the torrents. It seems that people are given to idleness: in fact, when the winter season presses, they sometimes shiver with cold in the mountains and, although there are very abundant groves of cotton, they are

Petro quodam Margaritaeo, regio antiquo familiari, relictis, ad discurrendam quam arbitrabatur continentem terram, quae inde septuagesimum tantum lapidem distabat, sese accingit Regum imperii memor, qui illum admonuerant ut percurrere
5 nova littora festinaret, ne rex alius quisquam prius suae dicioni terras illas subdere studeret. Rex enim Portugaliae publice sua interesse latentia illa detegere aiebat. Summus vero Pontifex Alexander sextus Regi et Reginae Hispaniarum per plumbatas concessit bullas ne quis princeps alius incognitas illas regiones
10 pertingere auderet, a septentrione ad austrum linea recta extra parallelum insularum, quae dicuntur *Caput Viride*, proiecta, ut dissidii causa, tollatur lequas centum, ex composito, demum ter centum. Credimus has insulas esse *Hesperides*. Hae sunt regis Portugaliae et inde sui nautae nova littora quotannis
15 detegentes semper in laevam a tergo Africae, per Aethiopum maria, ad orientem vertebant proras (neque ab Hesperidibus unquam ad meridiem aut ad occidentem Portugalenses adhuc navigaverant). Cum tribus igitur navigiis discedens ad eam regionem, quam prima navigatione, insulam existimans, *Ioan-*
20 *nam* vocitarant, brevi tempore pervenit vocavitque eius initium *Alpha Omega*, eo quod ibi finem esse nostri orientis, cum in ea sol occidat, occidentis autem, cum oriatur, arbitretur. Instat enim esse ab occidente principium Indiae ultra Gangem, ab oriente vero terminum ipsius ultimum. Neque enim absonum
25 penitus est, cum Gangetidis Indiae terminos indiscretos co- smographi reliquerint nec desint qui ab Hispanis oris non longe Indica littora discedere sentiant. *Cubam* incolae hanc partem vocant; in cuius prospectu, in Hispaniolae angulo extremo, portum reperit commodissimum: sinum enim in se
30 recipit latum in ea parte ipsa insula. Hunc portum *Sancti Nicolai* nomine insignivit; a quo vix viginti lequas recedit Cuba. Transfretat igitur et, Cubae meridionale latus capiens, ad occidentem vergit. Incipiunt illi, quo ulterius procedebat tanto magis littora in latum protendi et ad meridiem curvari.
35 In Cubae latere ad meridiem primam reperit insulam, quam incolae *Iamaicam* vocant; hanc insulam Sicilia longiorem la- tioremque praedicat, uno tantum monte contentam, qui ab omnibus sui partibus, a mari incipiens, paulatim usque ad insulae medium elevatur atque ita leniter sese in dorsum ex-
40 tendit ut ascendentes vix se ascendere sentiant. Tam in littore, quam in internis feracissimam et populis plenam esse asseverat

258

not concerned with weaving clothes for themselves. In the valleys, however, and in the fields, they do not at all suffer from cold. Having examined with such diligence these places at the entrance of the *Cibavo* region, on April 1, the day before Easter, the Admiral returned to *Isabela* (that is the name of the city). After entrusting the government of that city and of the whole island to his brother and to a certain Pedro Margarit, an old courtier, he set out to explore that land which he thought was a continent, only 70 miles away, mindful of the Sovereigns' instructions who had urged him to hurry and discover new shores before others might attempt to impose their rule over those lands. Indeed, the king of Portugal had publicly stated he was very much interested in discovering those unknown lands. But the Supreme Pontiff Alexander VI, with bulls sealed with lead, in order to eliminate the cause of confrontations, had granted the King and Queen of Spain that no other Sovereign might dare touch those unknown regions from North to South along a straight line drawn 100 leagues beyond the parallel of the Cape Verde islands, a line which was later moved by mutual accord to 300 leagues. We think that these islands are the *Hesperides*. They belong to the king of Portugal, from here his seamen, discovering new coasts every year, kept turning their prows always to the left, leaving behind the coasts of Africa, to cross the Ethiopian seas to the East (up to then the Portuguese had never sailed South or West from the *Hesperides*). And so, leaving with three ships, Columbus reached that land which during his first voyage he considered an island and named *Juana*, and called its tip *Alpha Omega*, because he thought it represented the end of our East as the sun set, and the end of the West, when, instead the sun rose. Indeed, he insisted that India begins to the West, beyond the Ganges and that it ends to the East. And this opinion is not incongruous, since the cosmographers have left the boundaries of India beyond the Ganges undetermined, and there are those who believe that the coasts of India are not too far away from the coasts of Spain. The natives call this country Cuba. Within sight of it, in the farthest corner of Hispaniola, Columbus discovered an excellent port for in that section, the island itself formed a bend. He named this port *San Nicolás*; Cuba is almost twenty leagues away from it. He went beyond this stretch of sea and, touching the southern coast of Cuba, he

incolasque eius caeteris insularibus ingenio acutiores ac me-
chanicis artibus magis deditos bellicosioresque finitimi fatentur. Nam pluribus in locis, volenti Praefecto terram capere armati ac minitantes occurrerunt pugnasque saepius
attentarunt, sed victi semper, amicitiam omnes cum Praefecto
iniere. Iamaica igitur relicta, ad occidentem prospero ventorum flatu septuaginta dies navigavit seque non longe ab
Aurea Chersoneso, nostri orientis ultra Persidem initio, per-
rexisse per inferiorem nobis terrae ambitum arbitratur; credit
enim se duas tantum solis horas de duodecim quae nobis
erant incognitae reliquisse. Dimidium enim solis cursum
veteres intactum reliquerant, cum eam tantum terrae super-
ficiem quae a Gadibus usque ad Gangem vel ad Auream
usque Chersonesum discussam habeamus. Hoc itinere in cur-
rentia more torrentis maria, in vadosos gurgites, in angustias
innumeras propter insularum adiacentium multitudinem cotidie incidebat; omnia tamen haec pericula parvi faciens,
tantum procedere instituit donec an insula esset Cuba an
terra continens certior fieret. Navigavit igitur eius semper
littora abradens ad occidentem duas lequas et viginti supra
bis centum, ut ipse ait, hoc est millia passuum circiter tercentum et mille septingentisque insulis nomen imposuit, in
laevam plusquam tribus millibus passim, ut ipse dicere audet,
relictis. Sed ad ea quae memoratu digna inter navigandum
reperiebat revertamur. Cum iam per Cubae latus locorum
naturam adnavigans perquireret, ab Alpha Omega, id est ab
eius initio, non magno tractu portum multarum navium capacem reperit. Falcatus enim est eius introitus, promontoriis
utrinque venientes undas recipientibus inclusus. Intus autem
ingens spacium et immensa profunditas. Portus littora ambiens, casulas vidit, non procul a littore culmeas duas pluribusque in locis ignem accensum; demittit e navibus viros
quosdam armatos qui casulas adeant. Descendunt, neminem
reperiunt; verubus tamen ligneis appositas ignibus piscium
libras circiter centum duosque octipedales serpentes cum
piscibus ipsis invenere. Admirati, si quos incolas videant,
circunspiciunt; cum nemo illis in toto prospectu sese offerret
(venientibus enim nostris sese ad montana piscium domini
receperant) discumbunt et captis alieno labore piscibus laeti
fruuntur; serpentes relinquunt quos nihilo penitus ab Aegyptiis crocodillis differre affirmant praeterquam magnitu-

changed course to the West. The farther he advanced, the wider the shoreline began to appear to him and more bent to the South. Next to Cuba, South of it, he found the first island, which the natives call Jamaica; he goes on stating that this island was longer and broader than Sicily, with a single mountain, that, from all sides out at sea is seen slowly rising in the center of the island, with slopes so gentle that in climbing it one hardly notices. He asserted that, on the coast and in the interior, the island was very fertile and populous, and its neighbors realized that its inhabitants are sharper in intelligence and more dedicated to the mechanical arts and more bellicose than all the other natives. In fact, in several places they confronted the Admiral who intended to land, all armed and threatening, and more than once they attacked, but, having been defeated every time, they all made peace with him. Then, after leaving Jamaica, he sailed West for seventy days with favorable winds thinking he had reached the land not far from the Golden Chersonese, which is the beginning of our East, beyond Persia, through that part of the earth below us. As a matter of fact, he believed that of the twelve hours [distance] unknown to us he had not covered the last two. Indeed, the ancients had left unexplored half of the sun's course, since we only know that portion of the globe which extends from Cádiz to the Ganges, or to the Golden Chersonese. During this voyage, he daily ran across seas that resembled torrents with deep vortexes and innumerable difficulties caused by the great number of neighboring islands; yet, underestimating all these dangers, he decided to advance only until he could ascertain whether Cuba was an island or a continent. So he sailed West always bordering its coasts, for 222 leagues, that is 1,300 miles, as he gives to understand, and named 700 islands, leaving behind to the left more than 3,000 here and there, as he himself dared to say. But let us return to what the Admiral thought worthy of being remembered of his voyage. Sailing by now along the coasts of Cuba to explore the nature of the places, he discovered a port capable of holding many ships, not too far away from *Alpha Omega*, that is, its tip. Clearly, its entrance is in the shape of a sickle, shut on both sides by promontories against which the incoming waves break. In addition, there is much space and enormous depth inside. Coasting the shores of the port he saw, not far from it, two huts and fires burning in

dine: nam crocodillorum ait Plinius[19] aliquot fuisse repertos duodeviginti cubitorum, horum autem maiores octipedales. Propinquum nemus postmodum iam saturi ingredientes, ex iis serpentibus arboribus funiculis alligatos plures comperere, quo-
5 rum ora alii funibus astricta, dentes alii evulsos habebant; cum deinde portus vicina scrutarentur, circiter septuaginta homines in cuiusdam altae rupis culmine viderunt, qui, nostris adeunti-bus, profugerant ut inde quid sibi vellet haec nova gens perdi-scerent. Nutibus et signis blanditiisque nostri illos adducere
10 conabantur. Munerum oblatorum a longe spe motus accessit unus, sed in propinquam rupem, tamen timenti similis. Almi-rantus, autem qui secum habebat Didacum quendam Colonum, inter suos educatum iuvenem, prima navigatione abductum ex insula Cubae vicina, nomine *Guanahaini*, Didaco interprete
15 (cuius lingua patria fere horum linguae quadrabat), insularem qui propius venerat alloquitur; metu deposito, adit incola cae-terisque ut tuto venirent nec vererentur persuadet. Nuncio habito, ex rupibus ad naves circiter septuaginta descendunt, amicitiam ineunt, muneribus a Praefecto donantur. Esse pisca-
20 tores a rege suo, qui solenne convivium alteri regi parabat, piscatum missos Praefectus cognovit. Quod pisces ignibus ap-positos Praefecti gens comederit aequo libentique animo passi sunt, quandoquidem serpentes reliquere: neque enim quicquam est, inter edulia, quod tanti faciant quanti serpentes illos. Po-
25 pularibus eos comedere minus licet quam apud nos phasianos aut pavones. De piscibus autem se totidem ea nocte capturos dicunt. Interrogati cur pisces, quos regi suo laturi erant, co-quere pararent, ut recentiores et incorruptos illos afferre possent responderunt. Ita dextris in amicitiam iunctis, ad sua quisque
30 proficiscitur. Sequitur Almirantus, ut instituerat, solem occi-dentem, a principio Cubae, quod *Alpha Omega* vocatum ab Almiranto diximus. Littora ad hunc portum media, quamvis arboribus consita, aspera tamen et montosa. Ex arboribus, floridae erant aliae et ad mare suaves ex se odores emittebant,
35 aliae vero fructibus onustae. Ultra portum autem terra est feracior populosiorque cuius incolae caeteris mitiores rerumque novarum cupidiores; nam ad littora omnes, visis nostris navi-

[19] See Plin. *nat. hist.* VIII 89: …*magnitudine excedit plerumque duodeviginti cubita.* The C[1] reading *duorum et triginta* is viewed as an exaggeration already in Nebrija's 1516 edition (p. 125).

several places; he ordered some armed men to land and approach the huts; they landed, but they did not find anybody; however, about 100 pounds of fish was left roasting on the fires on wooden spits including two snakes about eight feet long. Surprised, they looked around to see if there were any people; when no one showed up (as they saw our approach, the owners of the fish fled into the mountains), they sat down and gladly fed themselves on the fish caught by someone else's hard work. They left the snakes, which they claimed were not substantially different from the crocodiles of the Nile, except in size; indeed, Pliny says that some crocodiles reached eighteen cubits in length, whereas the biggest of these measured eight feet. Once full, as they entered the nearby woods, they found several of these snakes tied to trees with rope, again, some had their mouth tied with a rope while others had their teeth pulled out; then, while scouting the neighborhood of the harbor, the Spaniards saw at the top of a high cliff about seventy men who had fled at their approach but curious to discover from a safe location what these new people wanted. Our men attempted to attract them by motions, signals and friendly gestures. One of them, driven by the alluring gifts offered from a distance, came forward but only to a nearby cliff, still acting fearfully. Then, the Admiral, who had with him a certain Diego Columbus — a young man whom he kept with his children, after bringing him back in the first voyage from an island near Cuba named *Guanahainí* [Guanahani, i.e. San Salvador] — spoke to the native who had come closer using Diego as interpreter (his native language was similar to theirs); having set aside his fears, the native approached and persuaded others to come and have no fear. At the signal, about seventy men climbed down from the cliffs toward the ships, made friends and accepted gifts from the Admiral. He found out that they were fishermen sent by their king to fish as he was preparing a solemn banquet for another king. They didn't seem to mind much that the Admiral's men had eaten the roasted fish, since they left the snakes: there is nothing edible that they truly appreciate more than those snakes. Common people are allowed to eat them less often than we would pheasants or peacocks. For the fish on the other hand, they claimed they could catch as many that very night. Asked why they were cooking the fish to be brought to their king, they answered that in this

bus, certatim concurrebant, panem, quo ipsi vescuntur, et cucurbitas aqua plenas nostris offerentes, ut in terram descenderent, invitabant. Habent hae insulae omnes arboris quoddam genus ulmos aequans magnitudine, quae cucurbitas gignit pro fructu. Ad aquae usum illis utuntur, ad esum minime. Medullam namque ipsius felle amariorem esse aiunt, sed cortice testudineam aequante duriciem. Idibus Maii, ex altiori cavea in laevam ad austrum speculatores prospicientes, densam insularum multitudinem viderunt inter navigandum, herbidas, virides, arboriferas, uberes et habitatas esse animadverterunt. In continenti littore in fluvium incidit navigabilem aquarum adeo calidarum quod manum in ipsis ferre diu nemo posset. Altero vero die, piscatorum canoam a longe videns, ne, nostris visis, piscatores aufugerent veritus, ut illos tacitis cymbis intercipiant imperat. Illi autem intrepidi nostros expectant. Audi novum genus piscationis: non aliter ac nos canibus Gallicis per aequora campi lepores insectamur, illi, venatorio pisce, pisces alios capiebant. Piscis erat formae nobis ignotae: corpus eius anguillae grandiori persimile, sed habens in occipite pellem tenacissimam in modum magnae crumenae. Hunc vinctum tenent in navis sponda funiculo, sed tantum demisso quantum piscis intra aquam carinae queat inhaerere: neque enim patitur ullo pacto aeris aspectum. Viso autem aliquo pisce grandi, aut testudine, quae ibi sunt magno scuto grandiores, piscem solvunt; ille, quom se solutum sentit, sagitta velocius, piscem aut testudinem, qua extra conchile partem aliquam eductam teneat, adoritur pelleque illa crumenaria iniecta, praedam, raptam ita tenaciter apprehendit, quod exolvere ipsam, eo vivo, nulla vis sufficiat, nisi extra aquae marginem paulatim, glomerato funiculo, extrahatur. Viso enim aeris fulgore, statim praedam deserit. Praeda igitur iam circa aquae marginem evecta, in mare saltat piscatorum copia tanta quanta ad praedam sufficiat sustinendam; donec e navi comites eam apprehendant. Praeda in navim tracta, funiculi tantum solvunt, quantum venator possit ad locum suae sedis intra aquam redire. Ibique de praeda ipsa per alium funiculum escas illi demittunt. Piscem incolae *guaicanum*, nostri *reversum* appellant, quod versus venetur. Quattuor testudines eo modo captas quam naviculam illis fere implebant nostris dono dant: cibus est enim apud eos non illautus. Nostri autem, e converso, gratis muneribus donatos alacres eos reliquere. Interrogati nautae de terrae illius ambitu non habere finem ab

manner they would deliver them fresher and unspoiled. And so, after shaking their right hands as a sign of friendship, they all went their separate ways. As he had already decided, the Admiral followed a route West from the tip of Cuba which we said he had named *Alpha Omega*. The shores along this port, although full of trees, were nevertheless rough and mountainous. Some of the trees were in bloom, their sweet perfume spread onto the sea, others were loaded with fruits. Beyond the port, however, the land is more fertile and populated, and its inhabitants are of milder nature and more keen to novelties; indeed, at seeing our ships they raced to the shore, offering our sailors the bread which they eat and gourds full of water, signaling to come ashore. On all these islands grows a kind of tree about the size of the elm, which bears gourds as fruit. They use those gourds for water and do not eat them. In fact, they say that the pulp is more bitter than gall, but its bark is as tough as a turtle shell. On 15 May, the watches, looking left in a southerly direction from a higher maintop, saw a dense multitude of islands: grassy, green, rich in trees so fertile and clearly inhabited. On the shore of the continent, he ran into a navigable river whose water was so warm that no one could keep the hands in it for long. The next day, seeing far away a canoe of fishermen, and fearful that upon seeing our people they would leave, he ordered to quietly surround them with two boats. Instead, those fishermen awaited our men without fear. Hear now about a different way to fish: those people were catching other fish with a hunting fish, not very unlike our giving chase to hares with beagles through the fields. From its look the fish is unknown to us; its body was much like that of a very large eel, but with a very tough skin on the occipital area, resembling a big leather pouch. They kept this fish tied to the side of the boat with a string, but slack enough for the fish to remain under water, near the edge: it really cannot tolerate air at all. When they see some big fish or turtles — larger than big shields around here — they loosen the rope on the fish that as he feels free, attacks more swiftly than an arrow its fish or turtle, choosing an exposed part, i.e. outside the shell, using its suctorial circular mouth borring so tightly into the prey that no force can separate them as long as it is alive, except after being slowly pulled out of the water into the brightness of the light which causes it to let go of its prey

occidente significarunt. Institeruntque ut Almirantus aut descenderet aut suo nomine salutatum suum cacicum, id est regem, cum eis mitteret, cacicum nostris multa munera daturum, si adirent, pollicentes. Praefectus autem, ne ab incepto detine-
retur, morem illis gerere recusavit, petiere tamen nomen eius suique cacichi nomen nostris dederunt. Ulterius inde procedens ad occidentem semper, intra paucos dies monti adhaesit altissimo, habitatoribus ob ubertatem referto. Ad naves panem, gossipium, cuniculos et volucres ferentes incolae confluebant. Ab
interprete an e coelo gens ista descenderet miro affectu sciscitabantur. Rex horum et alii plures qui illi astabant, viri graves, non esse insulam terram illam innuebant. Aliam insulam postmodum ex his quae in laeva huic terrae adhaerebant, ingressis, comprehendere quemquam non licuit: fugere enim omnes viri
foeminaeque nostris adeuntibus. Quattuor canes in ea, sed non latrabiles, aspectus foedissimi, quos comedunt uti nos haedos, comperere. Anseres, anates, ardeas haec insula gignit innumeras. Gurgites demum inter insulas et continentem adeo angustos ingressus est quod vix vertere retro navigia fas esset adeoque
vadosos quod arenam carina interdum verrerent. Horum gurgitum, per quadraginta milliaria, erat aqua lactea spissaque ac si farinam toto illo pelago sparsissent. In amplum aequor, quom tandem evasissent, ad octogesimum milliare, mons alius altissimus sese illi obtulit. Aquandi lignandique gratia hunc adit, inter
palmeta pinetaque altissima fontes nativos dulcium aquarum duos reperit. Interea, dum ligna scinduntur, cadi implentur, ex nostris sagittariis unus venatum silvam ingreditur. Ibi vir quidam alba tunica amictus, adeo improvisus sese illi offert quod, prima facie, esse quendam fratrem ordinis Sanctae Mariae Mer-
cedis quem secum Almirantus pro sacerdote habebat, existimaverit. Sed hunc statim ex nemore alii duo sequuntur; deinde a longe vidit agmen veniens circiter triginta hominum vestibus contectorum. Tunc vero terga vertens ac proclamans ad naves, quam celerrimo potest cursu, profugit. Tunicati autem illi ap-
plaudere et, ne vereretur, persuadere omnibus modis nitebantur, sed nihilominus noster fugiebat. His Praefecto renunciatis, alacer quod gentem cultam invenerit, statim armatos in terram misit cum mandatis ut, si opus fuerit, quadraginta milliaria intra insulam pergerent, donec aut tunicatos eos aut alios incolas,
omni studio quaesitos, inveniant. Nemus transgressi, vastam planitiem herbidam in qua nec semitae vestigium unquam ap-

right away. With the prey at water level, a proportionate number of fishermen sufficient to hold it get in the water until their companions pull it aboard. Once the prey is in the boat, they loosen the string enough to allow the "Lamprey" to go back to its place under the water where they feed it by lowering with another string morsels taken from its prey. The natives call this fish *guaicano*; our men call it *reverso*, because it hunts on its back. The islanders gave our men, as a gift, four turtles caught by the fish and which almost filled their boat; it certainly is a delicacy for them. Our men, satisfied as well, left them after exchanging friendly gifts. The sailors, questioned about the size of the land, said it was endless to the West. They insisted the Admiral either land or send someone in his name to greet their cacique, that is, the king, promising that the cacique would give our men many gifts if they went to him. The Admiral, however, in order not to be diverted from his undertaking, refused to comply with their request; nevertheless, they asked him his name and gave our men the name of their cacique. Advancing farther from there, still heading East, in a few days the Admiral reached a place near a very lofty mountain, crowded with people because of its fertility. The natives flocked to the ships, carrying bread, cotton, rabbits and birds. With amazement, they asked the interpreters if those people had come from heaven. Their king and many others, standing near him with a very dignified look, indicated by signs that the land was not an island. Later, when our sailors landed in another of those islands near this land, to its left, they could not capture anyone: indeed all, men and women, had fled at their arrival. They found four, most horrible looking dogs, that could not bark; the natives eat them as we do young goats. In this island live innumerable geese, ducks and herons. Lastly, the Admiral ventured trough channels, between the islands and the mainland, so narrow that it was hard to tack, and so shallow that at times they were scraping bottom with the keels. The water of these channels was milky and thick for 40 miles, as if they had sprinkled flour all over the sea. When they finally exited into the open sea, 80 miles away, another very lofty mountain appeared. He approached it to stock up on water and wood; among palm groves and very tall pine forests he found two freshwater springs. In the meantime, while the men cut wood and filled their barrels, one of

paruit, offenderunt. Per herbas proficisci conantes, adeo sese implicuerunt quod vix milliare processerint: erat enim herba nostris segetibus spicatis nihilo minor. Fessi igitur revertuntur, non reperta semita. Postero die quinque et viginti armatos dimittit, quibus imperat ut, quae gens terram incolat, diligenter explorent. Hi, cum non longe a littore magnorum animalium vestigia, quaedam recentia, comperissent, inter quae leones esse arbitrati sunt, metu perculsi redeunt. Inter veniendum, silvam reperiunt, serpentibus per altas arbores, passim vitibus suapte natura productis arboribusque aliis plurimis aromaticos fructus parturientibus consitam. Racemos tulere ponderosos ac succi plenos in Hispaniam; de fructibus autem aliis quos ferebant, cum in navibus passari non commode possent, nullus allatus est: putruerunt enim omnes et corrupti in mare proiecti sunt. In pratis eorum nemorum gruum agmina nostratibus duplo grandiorum se vidisse rettulerunt. Inter navigandum, cum ad alios quosdam montes vela dirigeret, in duabus casulis in littore visis unum tantum reperit hominem. Hic, ad naves ductus, terram quae trans illos montes iacebat esse populatissimam capite, digitis et quibus aliis poterat modis, signifcabat. Applicanti se ad ea littora Praefecto multae canoae obviam prodeunt; invicem se placidissime, per signa, compellarunt. Neque Didacus ille, qui in Cubae initio incolarum linguam intellexerat, hos intelligebat. Varia enim esse idiomata in variis Cubae provinciis perpenderunt. Incolereque regionis interna potentissimum regem, qui se indueret ostendebant. Hunc tractum omnem summersum et aquis coopertum littoraque coenosa, arboribus referta, ut nostras paludes, ait. Ibi tamen, cum aquandi gratia in terram descendisset, conchilia, ex quibus uniones habentur, vidit. Nec eo magis moram traxit: erat enim eius intentus non alius tunc, ex praecepto Regum, quam, quotquot posset maria, discurrere. Ulterius igitur procedentibus, omnia littorum culmina usque ad alium montem, qui se ad octoginta millia passuum ostendebat,fumigabant. Nulla erat specularis rupes ex qua fumus non egrederetur, nec an incolarum essent ignes bene constitit ad necessitatem parati an, uti suspectis bellorum temporibus fieri solet, per eos fumos signa vicinis darent, ut se in tutum reciperent aut ut in unum convenirent, si quid nostri contra eos moliri tentarent aut forte, quod magis consonum videtur, uti tanquam ad rem mirandam, nostra navigia inspecturi concurrerent. Littora iam Praefecto modo ad austrum,

our archers went hunting in the woods. Here, a man dressed in a white tunic appeared so suddenly that at first sight he thought it was a friar of the order of Santa María de la Merced, whom the Admiral had brought along as a priest. But suddenly from the woods, two more followed this one; then, from far away, he saw a whole group of about thirty so-clothed men coming. He then, turned around shouting and ran as fast as he could toward the ships. These men dressed in tunics, then, clapped their hands at him and attempted to persuade him with all means not to be so fearful, but he kept running. As the Admiral learned of this incident was happy to have found civilized people and instructed armed men to go ashore and advance for 40 miles into the interior of the island, if necessary, until they found either those men dressed in tunics or other natives: they were to look for them with the greatest care. After marching through woods, they came upon a vast plain covered with grass, where there was not even a trace of a path. Trying to advance through the grass, they got themselves so entangled that they hardly made a mile; the grass in fact was as tall as our wheat when the ears are ripe. Thus, they came back tired, without having found a trail. The following day the Admiral sent twenty-five men with the order to explore carefully what kind of people might live in that land. These men, having found not far from shore some rather fresh footprints of huge animals, imagined there could be lions and turned back terrified. On their way back, they discovered a forest full of vines that grew spontaneously here and there winding up tall trees, as well as other trees bearing aromatic fruits. The men brought back to Spain some heavy bunches of grapes, full of juice; but they could not show any of the other fruits they had carried, because they did not adequately ripen on the ships, did spoil and were thrown into the sea. They also reported having seen in the clearings of those woods flocks of cranes, twice as big as ours. Continuing his voyage, the Admiral sailed toward some other mountains, but found only one man in the two huts he had sighted on shore. When the man was brought on board the ships, he indicated, using his head, hands and other means, that the land which lay beyond those mountains was very populous. Several canoes came to meet the Admiral as he approached those shores; by means of gestures, the natives called each other very gently. And our Diego,

modo ad Africum sive Libym[20] curvabantur; mare vero ubique
insulis implicitum. Hinc igitur carinae, quae terram saepius
propter vadosa maria verrerant quassatae, rudentes, vela et
reliquum amplustre[21] iam putrida alimentaque, per rimas male
stipatarum navium madefacta, sed praecipue panis bis coctus,
corrupta vertere retro proras Praefectum coegerunt. Hanc ultimam existimati continentis oram, quam ipse attigit, vocavit
Evangelistam. Retro vela vertens inter alias insulas continenti
non ita finitimas, in pelagus incidit testudinibus magnis adeo
condensum quod naves aliquando detardarent, gurgitemque
postea ingressus est albidarum aquarum, uti alium reperisse
supra scripsimus. Ad crediti continentis tandem littora, qua
venerat, reversus est insularum vada pertimescens. Ad eumque
cum neminem veniens molestia affecisset, hilari vultu, posito
omni timore, utriusque sexus incolae dona ferebant: psittacos
alii, alii panem, aquam, cuniculos, sed praecipue palumbes,
nostris grandiores, quos sapore et gustu perdicibus nostris
meliores fuisse Praefectus ait; quare cum sensisset inter come-
dendum spirare ex eis aromaticum quendam, iussit de recenter
interemptis quibusdam ingulos aperire. Plena illis odoratis floribus reperit guttura inde gustum eum in palumbibus novum
emanare arguerunt: nutrimenti enim naturam sorbere carnes
animalium aequum est credere. Dum in littore rem divinam
Praefectus audiret, ecce primarium quendam octogenarium,
virum gravem, nec eo minus nudum, multis illum comitantibus.
Hic, donec sacra peragerentur, admiratus, ore oculisque intentus, assistit; dehinc Praefecto, canistrum quem manu gerebat,
plenum patriae fructibus dono dedit sedensque apud eum, per
interpretem Didacum Colonum, qui id idioma, cum propius
accessissent, intelligebat, orationem habuit huiuscemodi: "Terras omnes istas, hactenus tibi ignotas manu potenti te percurrisse renunciatum nobis fuit populisque incolis metum non
mediocrem intulisse, quare te hortor moneoque ut itinera duo,

[20] A wet, very violent wind generally blowing from the west or south-west
almost always with gales. Also referred to as *africo* (S) and *garbino* (SW) wind.

[21] A mariner's term for the ornament on Greek or Roman ships, high above
the stern, made of curved planks arranged in a fan-like manner on a single base. See
Paul. Fest. 9, 11 L.: *aplustria navium ornamenta, quae quia erant amplius, quam essent
necessaria usu, etiam amplustria dicebantur.* See also Lucr. IV 436: *in portu clauda videntur
navigia aplustris fractis obnitier undae;* Iuv. X 133: *bellorum exuviae... victaeque triremis
aplustre.*

who earlier at Cuba had understood the language of those islanders, could not understand them and realized then the existence of different languages in the various provinces of Cuba. The natives explained that a very powerful king, who wore clothes, was living in the more interior parts of the island. The Admiral said that this whole strip of beach was submerged by water and that the coast-line was muddy and full of trees, like our swamps. However, when they landed here to get a supply of water, he saw the shells that yield pearls. Nevertheless, he did not stay any longer; clearly, his intention at that time in obedience to the Sovereigns' orders was to explore as many seas as he could. Then, those who proceeded farther saw smoke rising all along the heights off shore, and another mountain eighty miles away. There was not a single cliff to be seen from which smoke did not rise, and it was not clear whether these were fires lighted by the natives out of necessity, or, as it usually happens during the distrustful times of war, smoke signals sent to their neighbors, warning them to seek safety or assemble in one place, in case our men were to plot some action against them; or, finally, which seems more probable, they were just inducing others to watch our ships as an extraordinary sight. By now, the coast-line in front of the Admiral was bending Southward, either South or South-West; all around the sea was full of islands. As a result, because the keels, which so often sailed near bottom, were by now ruined by shallows and because the ropes, sails, and whatever was left of the stern had in the meantime rotten, and because the food, ill-stowed and soaked through the cracks of the ships — especially the toasted bread — had spoiled, the Admiral was forced to turn back. *Evangelista* is the name he gave this last coast explored by him, a shore of the land he thought was a continent. Reversing his course through other islands not so close to the continent, he reached a sea so crowded with turtles that the ships had to slow down somewhat; then he crossed currents of whitish water — we wrote earlier he had already found another. Finally, he returned to the coasts of that land which he thought was a continent whence he had departed, fearing the shallows. Since he had not mistreated anybody before, when he arrived, smiling natives of both sexes, showing no fear, brought him gifts: some parrots, others bread, water, rabbits and especially pigeons, bigger that ours, which the

cum e corpore prosiliunt, animas habere scias, tenebrosum unum ac tetrum, his paratum qui generi humano molesti infensique sunt, iucundum aliud et delectabile illis statutum qui pacem et quietem gentium viventes amarunt. Si igitur te mor-
5 talem esse et unicuique pro praesentibus operibus futura merita obsignata memineris, neminem infestabis". His et aliis pluribus, per interpretem insularem, Praefecto, admiranti tale hominis nudi iudicium relatis, respondit compertissima sibi esse quaecunque dixerit de animarum e corpore exeuntium variis itineri-
10 bus ac praemiis, immo et existimasse hactenus illa ipsi et reliquis earum regionum incolis fuisse ignota, cum ita vivant, natura contenti. Ad caetera, vero se a Rege et Regina Hispaniarum ut eas omnes orbis oras hactenus incognitas pacaret missum respondit, ut scilicet Canibales et reliquos scelestos
15 homines indigenas debellaret debitisque suppliciis afficeret, innoxios autem ob eorum virtutes tutaretur et honoraret; quare ne ipse aut alius quisquam cui non sit animus nocendi, vereantur. Immo si quid forte a vicinis iniusti sibi aut aliis bonis illatum fuerit, aperiat. Seni Praefecti dicta adeo placuerunt ut
20 se iturum, quamvis aetate iam gravescentem, cum Praefecto libentissime praedicaret confectumque id fuisset nisi uxor et filii obstitissent. Attamen quod alterius impetio hic subiaceret summopere admiratus est, sed tunc multo magis quando relatum illi fuit, per interpretem, qualis et quanta essent Regum
25 pompa, potentia, ornatus, bellorum apparatus, quantae urbes, qualia oppida, obstupuit. Subtristis igitur, prostratis ante pedes eius, obortis lachrymis, uxore et filiis, honoratus senex permansit, iterum atque iterum an coelum esset ea terra quae tales tantosque viros gigneret interrogans. Compertum est apud eos,
30 velut solem et aquam, terram esse communem neque "meum aut tuum"[22], malorum omnium semina, cadere inter ipsos. Sunt enim adeo parvo contenti, quod in ea ampla tellure magis agri supersint, quam quicquam desit. Aetas est illis aurea: neque fossis neque parietibus aut sepibus praedia sepiunt, apertis
35 vivunt hortis, sine legibus, sine libris, sine iudicibus, suapte natura rectum colunt. Malum ac scelestum eum iudicant qui inferre cuiquam iniuriam delectatur. Maizium tamen et iuccam

[22] Peter Martyr implies recollection of an expression from a manuscript (ms Matr. BN Vitr. 25-6, f. 15 v.): *Meum et tuum incitant omne bellum*. See J. Gil y Consuelo Varela, *Cartas de particulares a Colón y Relación coetáneas*, Madrid 1984, p. 77 n. 115.

Admiral found to be better than our partridges for taste and flavor; and so, since he noticed that, when eaten, they exhaled a certain aromatic smell, he asked that the gullets of some of them, recently killed, be opened. He found their gullets filled with aromatic flowers, thus understanding the aroma of the pigeons: it makes sense to think that the flesh of the animals absorb also the flavor of the food they eat. While the Admiral was attending Mass on the beach, there came an eighty-year-old man, a leader of all respect, though naked, with many followers. During the service, this man remained still, looking surprised, face and eyes still; then, he gave the Admiral a local basket full of fruits which he was holding in his hands, and, sitting next to him, with the help of interpreter Diego Columbus who being now closer could hear his words, made a speech of this tenor: "It has been reported to us that you have travelled through all these lands, previously unknown to you, with a powerful army stirring up a great fear among the native populations; therefore, I admonish you and warn you so that you may know that the souls, once they leave the body, follow one of two paths, the first dark and gloomy, set for those who are troublesome and harmful to the human race, the other pleasant and enjoyable, reserved for those who in this life loved men's peace and tranquillity. Were you then to remember you are a mortal and that future rewards will be bestowed based on actual deeds, you shall harm no one." With the help of the native interpreter, these and many other words were reported to the Admiral, who was surprised at the wisdom of a "naked" man, and replied that what he said about the different ways and rewards of the souls when they leave the body was very well known to him, and that actually he thought, up to that time, that those truths were unknown to the old man and the inhabitants of those regions, since they lived content in a natural state. Concerning other matters, he answered that he was sent by the King and Queen of Spain to bring peace in all those regions of a world uncharted until then, in other words, to subdue the Cannibals and all the other criminal natives inflicting on them the rightful punishments and, on the other hand, to defend and honor the innocents for their virtues; therefore, neither he nor anybody else who did not want to harm anyone should fear him. Moreover, he said that if by chance any injustice had been done to him or to any of his

agesque isti colunt, uti diximus in Hispaniola fieri. Inde igitur
rediturus discedens, in Iamaicam iterum ab ipsius latere meridionali incidit ab occidenteque ad orientem totam percurrit.
Ex cuius ab oriente ultimo angulo, cum a septentrione montes
5 altos ad laevam sibi conspiceret, novit tandem esse meridionale
latus Hispaniolae insulae quod nondum percurrerat. Quare,
portum eius insulae in Kalendas Septembris, qui *Sancti Nicolai*
dicitur ingressus, navigia reparabat hoc animo ut iterum Canibalium insulas devastaret canoasque eorum omnes combureret,
10 ne nocere ulterius lupi rapaces finitimis ovibus possint. Sed
obstitit ne id exequeretur adversa valitudo, quae illum prae
nimia vigilia oppresserat. Semianimis igitur a nautis ad Isabel-
licam civitatem ductus, inter fratres, quos ibi duos habebat et
reliquos familiares, pristinam tandem valitudinem recuperavit.
15 Nec eo magis Canibales infestare, ob exortas inter Hispanos,
quos in Hispaniola reliquerat, seditiones licuit. De quibus infra
dicemus. Vale!

neighbors, he should reveal it. The words of the Admiral pleased the old man so much that, although by now up in years, he would have very willingly joined the Admiral; and he would have done so if his wife and children had not objected. However, he was very surprised that the Admiral was subject to the authority of another man; but, he was even more amazed when he was told, through the interpreter, how great were the pomp, power, and magnificence of the Sovereigns and their wars, how big their cities and how strong their fortresses. Then, while the wife and the children bowed down at his feet in unrestrained weeping, the old man, remaining respectful, asked many times if that country which gave birth to such great men was not indeed heaven. It was learned that for them earth was a shared asset, like sun and water, and that among them the "mine and yours" concepts, which are the seed of all evils, do not apply. Indeed, they are satisfied with little, and in that land there are more available fields to cultivate than there is need. For them this is the golden age: they do not surround their properties with ditches, walls, or hedges; they live in open fields, without laws, books or judges; they behave naturally in a just manner. They consider evil and wicked anyone who delights in harming others. The natives also grow maize, yuca, and *ages*, as we said is also done in Hispaniola. When he left this place with the intention of returning to Hispaniola, he again reached the southern coast of Jamaica and skirted through all of it from West to East. From the lower eastern corner of the island he saw to his left some high mountains to the North, and finally realized that it was the southern coast of Hispaniola, which he had not yet explored. Therefore, upon entering the port of that island, which is called *San Nicolás*, the first days of September, he repaired his ships with the clear purpose of ravaging again the islands of the Cannibals and burning all their canoes, so that these rapacious wolves would not injure the neighboring sheep any longer. But his health, which he had weakened with frequent watches, prevented him from accomplishing this project. And so, taken back by the sailors, more dead than alive, to the city of Isabela, with the help of his two brothers and other friends which he had there, he recovered his good health. For this reason he could not attack the Cannibals and because of the revolts which had arisen among the Spaniards he had left in Hispaniola. On these topics we will comment later. Fare well!

I 4: ad cardinalem Ludovicum Aragonium, nostri Regis nepotem

Ex continenti, ut ipse arbitratur, Indico Colonus Praefectus
marinus rediens, fratrem Boilum et Petrum Margaritem veterem
Regis familiarem, virum nobilem atque alios plures, ex iis quos
ad regionis gubernationem reliquerat, ad Hispaniam corrupto
5 animo discessisse, comperit. Quapropter, ut apud Reges si quid
horum relatu male sentirent se expurgaret, nec non ut viros
peteret alios eorum loco, qui redierant, sufficiendos, tum etiam
ut provideret alimentorum penuriae, ut puta, tritici, vini, olei
et aliorum huiuscemodi, quibus Hispani vesci solent, cum in-
10 sularibus cibis non facile assuefieri possent, redire ad curiam,
quae tunc Burgis, urbe celebri in Castella Veteri morabatur
constituit. Sed quae prius confecerit, breviter enarrabo. Insulares reguli, qui hactenus suo parvoque contenti tranquille quie-
teque vitam duxerant, cum nostros in eorum solo natali pedem
15 figere conspicerent, graviter id ferebant: nihil magis quam
funditus eos inde detrudere aut evertere penitus et omnem
eorum memoriam abolere cupiebant. Nam ea gens, quae Praefectum in ea navigatione secuta fuerat, maiori ex parte indomita, vaga, cui nihil pensi esset, libertatem sibi, quoquo modo
20 posset, quaeritans, ab iniuriis minime se abstinere poterat. Insularum foeminas ante parentum, fratrum et virorum oculos
raptans stupris rapinisque intenta animos omnium incolarum
perturbarat. Quam ob rem pluribus in locis, quotquot impara-
tos e nostris incolae reperiebant, rabide et tanquam sacra offe-
25 rentes deo, trucidaverant. Pacandos igitur perturbatorum animos eosque, qui nostros interfecerant, puniendos esse priusquam inde discederet ratus, eius convallis regem, quam esse
in radicibus montium *Ciguavorum* superiore libro descripsimus,
in colloquium adducit. Hic vocabatur *Guarionexius*; cui, ut
30 Praefecti amicitiam arctius sibi conciliaret, placuit Didaco Colono, homini apud Praefectum a teneris educato, quo interprete
in Cubae discursu usus fuerat, sororem dare in uxorem. Ad
Caunaboam deinde Cibavorum montium, id est aureae regionis,
dominum, cuius ditionarii Hoiedam cum quinquaginta armatis
35 intra arcem Sancti Thomae obsessum triginta dies tenuerant,
nec obsidionem unquam solverant donec adventare Praefectum
ipsum cum magna manu persenserint, Hoiedam ipsum oratorem

I 4: To Cardinal Ludovico of Aragona, Nephew of our King

When Admiral Columbus returned from what he thought was the Indian continent, he found out that Friar Boyl and Pedro Margarit, a nobleman and long-time friend of the King, and many others whom he had left behind to govern the region had gone to Spain with wicked intentions. He thus decided to go back to Court, which now resided at Burgos, a famous city of Old Castile, in order to justify himself before the Sovereigns, in case they disapproved of anything related by his enemies, and to ask for other men to replace those who had come back as well as securing provisions of food stuffs, such as wheat, wine, oil and other staples of the kind, which Spaniards regularly eat since they could not easily get used to those of the natives. However, I will report briefly on what he did before leaving. The chieftains who up until then had lived peacefully, satisfied with little, when they saw our men settle on their soil, took this very hard: they desired nothing more than to drive the Spaniards out or destroy them altogether erasing all memory of them. In truth, the crew that had followed the Admiral in that voyage, being for the most part unruly, lawless without values and seeking personal freedom any way it would come to them, could not keep from committing injustices. Kidnaping women of the islands under the eyes of their parents, brothers and husbands, and prone to rape and robberies, they could not refrain from committing injustices. Therefore, in many places, with anger and as if offering sacrifices to a god, the natives slaughtered as many of our unprepared men as they could catch. The Admiral, thinking then that the spirits of the victims had to be appeased and those who had killed them punished, before departing summoned to a meeting the king of that valley, located near the feet of the mountains of *Ciguavi*, which we described in the preceding book. His name was Guarionex and he decided to secure closer friendship with the Admiral by giving his sister in marriage to Diego Columbus, by now an adult, educated since his childhood in the Admiral's house and whose services as an interpreter he had used during the raid in Cuba. Afterwards, the Admiral sent Hojeda as an ambassador to Caonabó, lord of the Cibao mountains, the gold

mittit. Hoieda apud Caunaboam moram trahente, a diversis
regionis regulis legati mittuntur, qui Caunaboae persuadere
nitantur, ne figere pedem in insula Christianos patiatur, servire
nisi malit quam imperare. Fore enim ut nisi Christicolae ab
5 insula penitus eliminentur, insulares omnes servi sint illorum
futuri; alia parte, Hoieda cum Caunaboa agebat ut ad Praefectum ipsemet proficisceretur cum eoque foedus et amicitiam
iniret. Regulorum legati, ad eam regionem capessendam, se
suaque omnia offerebant. Hoieda caedem perniciemque suorum,
10 si bella quam pacem cum Christianis mallet, minitabatur. Caunaboa igitur, hinc atque inde tanquam scopulus diversis fluctibus in medio mari conflictatus, etiam conscientia scelerum
agitatus, quod viginti ex nostris hominibus per dolum incautos
obtruncasset, quamvis pacem cupere videretur, adire tamen
15 Praefectum verebatur. Tandem, fraude pensitata, Praefectum
et reliquos, sub pacis specie, si sors offerret, perempturus, cum
omni familia sua pluribusque aliis, suo more, armatis ad Praefectum movet. Interrogatus cur adeo magnas hominum catervas
secum duceret, respondit tantum regem, quantus ipse sit, per-
20 gere iter domoque incomitatum exire non decere. Sed aliter
longe quam cogitaverat evenit, decidit namque in laqueos, quos
paraverat. Blanditiis enim et pollicitationibus sui erroris inter
eundum quod domo discessisset pertaesum Hoieda tandem ad
Praefectum illum ducit. Capitur, in vincula coniicitur, nec no-
25 strorum animae, diu inultae, sine corporibus quieverunt. Caunaboa cum omni familia eius capto, insulam percurrere Praefectus instituit, sed significatum ei fuit tanta fame insulares
urgeri ut quinquaginta millia hominum amplius iam perierint
cadantque cotidie passim tanquam morbosi gregis pecudes.
30 Quod illis sua pervicacia accidisse scitum est. Cum enim videbant nostros in insula velle sibi sedem eligere, existimantes
posse eos inde propellere, si insulares commeatus deessent, non
modo non seminare plantareque ulterius statuerunt, sed etiam
utrunque panis genus, de quo primo libro mentionem fecimus
35 seminatum, perdere evellereque, in sua quisque regione coepit,
sed inter Cibavos sive Cipangos montes praecipue cum urum,
quo ea regio abundabat causam esse potissimam quae nostros
in insula detineret, cognoscerent. Decurionem interea cum armatorum turba, qui latus meridionale insulae exploraret, dimi-
40 sit. Tunc omnes regiones, quas percurrerat, panis penuria adeo
laborare fassus est quod nihil unquam sexdecim dierum spacio

region, whose subjects had held Hojeda and 50 soldiers in a state of siege for 30 days inside the fortress of *Santo Tomás*, and did not lift the siege until they realized the Admiral himself was coming with a huge army. While Hojeda was delayed with his mission to Caonabó, messengers were sent by the various chiefs of the region in an attempt to persuade Caonabó not to allow the Christians to take over the island, unless he wished to be a slave instead of a leader; for if the Christians were not completely eliminated from the island all the natives would become their slaves. Hojeda, on the other hand, was pleading with Caonabó that he himself meet with the Admiral and sign a pact of friendship with him. The messengers of the chiefs, in order to retain that territory, were offering themselves and all of their possessions. Hojeda was threatening Caonabó with the massacre and ruin of his people, if he would choose war rather than peace with the Christians. Understandably, Caonabó was like a reef in the middle of the sea, tossed this way and that by opposite currents, distressed also by the memory of the crimes he had committed, since he had deceitfully murdered twenty of our defenseless men; although he seemed to desire peace, he was nevertheless afraid to go to the Admiral. Finally, after elaborating a plot with the intention of killing the Admiral and the others when the opportunity presented itself and pretending to want to make peace, he set out to meet the Admiral with all his retinue and many others, armed according to their custom. Asked why he would take with him such a great number of men, he answered that it was not becoming for such an important king as he was to undertake a trip and leave his house without escort. Things, however, turned out far differently than he thought, because he fell victim to the very trap he had planned. In fact, Hojeda, with enticements and promises, in the end managed to bring Caonabó, by now exhausted for having wandered away from home, to see the Admiral. He was taken and put in chains; and the souls of our men, unavenged for too long away from their bodies, found peace. Once Caonabó and all his household were captured, the Admiral decided to travel throughout the island, but it was pointed out to him that the natives had been vexed by a famine so widespread that already more than 50,000 men had died and that every day they fell everywhere like sickened flocks. It became known that it so happened to them because of their

comederint aliud quam herbarum palmularumque radices aut arborum nativos montanos fructus. Guarionexius, cuius regnum non aeque ac reliqua premebatur, nostris edenda quaedam impartitus est. Intra paucos dies, ut breviora essent itinerum spacia utve crebriores ac plures nostri receptus haberent, si qua vis insularium aliquando ingmeret, ab Isabella urbe ad arcem Sancti Thomae, in finibus regni huius Guarionexii, intra Cibavi terminos, super clivo salubrium aquarum scaturientium celebri, arcem aliam erexit, quam *Conceptionem* appellavit. Tum vero, cum nova in dies insulares aedificia surgere, cum in portu nostras naves iam putridas ac semifractas conspicerent, ab omni spe libertatis decidere coeperunt; subtristes an essent ex insullis Christiani discessuri sciscitabantur. Ex arce demum Conceptionis Cibavorum montium interna vestigantes, auri rudem massam, in tofi nativi similitudinem, concavam pugillo grandiorem, ponderis viginti unciarum a quodam regulo non in amnis illius ripa, sed in sicco tumulo repertam habuerunt. Hanc ego ipse in emporio Castellae Veteris Methymna Campi, ubi tunc curia hyemabat, vidi; manibusque captam admirans, libravi attrectavique. Vidi et electri puri [23] quo campanae pharmacopolarumque mortaria possunt et alia huiuscemodi, veluti ex aere corinthiaco [24], constari, frustum adeo magni ponderis, ut illud vix non modo non elevare ambabus manibus e terra, sed aut laevorsum aut dextrorsum movere sufficerem. Librarum octuncialium tricentarum pondus superasse massam aiebant. Eam in cuiusdam reguli atrio a maioribus relictam repererant. Sciebant tamen ipsi, quamvis nullius insularis viventis aetate electri quicquam eductum fuisset, ubi electrifodina esset, sed ab eis locus eius vix potuit extorqueri: adeo iam stomacho pleni in nostros vivebant. Ostenderunt tandem, sed dirutam et lapidibus ac terra super iniecta obcaecatam: tametsi levius quam in ferrifodinis [25] ferrum fodiatur, eam electrifodinam, si opifices fossoresque ad id ministerium apti adeant, reduci posse arbitrantur. Non longe

[23] A silver and gold alloy for precious objects. On account of its color and brilliance amber was also called electrum. See Plin. *nat. hist.* XXXIII 81; XXXVII 31.

[24] Corinthian bronze was an alloy highly regarded by the ancients who made vases and statues with it. See Plin. *nat. hist.* XXXIV 7-8.

[25] See Varro *de ling. Lat.* VIII 62; Prob. *ad Verg. georg.* I 56 ff.

own stubborness. Indeed, when they saw that our men wanted to set up residence for themselves on the island, hoping to be able to drive them away if they noticed a lack of provisions, they decided not only not to sow or plant, but each began to destroy and tear up both kinds of bread which, as I mentioned in the first book, had already been sown in his own territory, but especially in the *Cibao* and *Cipangu* mountains, for the natives knew that gold, abundant in that region, was the main reason keeping our men on the island. In the meantime, the Admiral sent an officer with a troop of armed men to explore the southern coast of the island. He reported that all the areas he traveled through suffered so much from lack of bread that, in a span of sixteen days, our men did not eat anything other than roots of plants and palm trees or fruits of mountain trees. Guarionex, whose territory had suffered less than the others, gave our soldiers something to eat. In a few days, in order to shorten the length of the journeys or so that our men might have more numerous retreat sites in case some native forces would attack them, the Admiral built another fortress, which he named *Concepción*, on a hill rich with wholesome spring waters, between the city of Isabela and the fortress of *San Tomás* on the borders of the realm of Guarionex, in the territory of *Cibao*. Then the natives, upon seeing new buildings rise every day and that our anchored ships rotted and shattered, began to lose all hope of freedom; being troubled, they asked whether the Christians were planning on leaving the islands. It was only then, while exploring the interior of the *Cibao* mountains from the fortress of *Concepción*, that our men came into possession of a raw cluster of gold that looked like native tufa, roundish, bigger than a fist, weighing 20 ounces, which was found by a native chief, not on the bank of that river, but on a dry, small mound. I myself have seen this lump in the market of Medina del Campo, in Old Castile, where the court was then spending the winter, and, admiring it, I took it in my hand, weighed and handled it. I also saw a piece of pure electrum, out of which bells and mortars of chemists and other such things could be made, just as from Corinthian bronze, of such weight that I could hardly lift it from the ground with both hands or even move it right or left. They said it weighed more than 300 pounds of eight ounces each. They had found it in the dwelling of a chief where it had been left by his

ab eadem arce Conceptionis, in eisdem montibus, succini copiam non parvam alibique stillare in speluncis glaucum colorem, quo pictores utuntur, non vulgarem invenerunt. Nemora praetergradientes, silvas immensas, quae arbores nullas nutrie-
5 bant alias praeterquam coccineas, quarum lignum vestri mercatores Itali *verzinum*, Hispani *brasilum* appellant, reperere. Hic forte, Princeps illustrissime, tecum ipse anceps contemplaberis dicesque tecum veluti ex coccineis arboribus naves quasdam onustas Hispalim advexerunt, veluti ex auro parum, ex gossipio
10 modicum, ex succino aliquid, ex aromatibus pauca, cur non auri caeterarumque rerum eam copiam quam, uti tu praedicas, polliceri tellus illa videtur attulerunt? Ad haec quae dederunt, respondebo. Praefectus ipse Colonus, super his interrogatus, Hispanos, quos secum duxit, sommo ocioque magis fuisse
15 quam laboribus deditos seditionumque ac novarum rerum studiosiores quam pacis aut quietis aiebat. Ab eo enim pars maior defecit; praeterea non potuisse prius insulares vinci aut domari refert eorumque vires frangi ad imperium insulae libere capessendum. Hispani se impetia eius saeva iniustaque ferre nequi-
20 visse multaque in eum commenti sunt; propter quos obiices hactenus vix impensae lucrum respondisse voluit. Hoc tamen anno primo et quingentesimo quo haec, tuo iussu, scribo, intra duorum mensium spacium, circiter ducentas supra mille octunciales libras auri collegerunt. Sed ad inceptum redeamus. Haec
25 enim, quae per digressionem leviter tetigimus, suo loco diffusius aperientur. Quum amxios igitur perturbatisque animis incolas Praefectus videret nec a vi et rapinis, donec inter eos versarentur, prohibere nostros posset, pluribus ex finitimarum regionum primoribus convocatis, convenerunt ut Praefectus
30 vagari per insulam suos non sinat: sub praetextu enim auri et aliarum insularium rerum quaerendarum nihil intactum aut impollutum relinquebant. Ipsi vero incolae Praefecto se daturos viritim, a quarto decimo anno usque ad septuagesimum, de suae quisque regionis proventibus tributum quod vellet serva-
35 turosque quod ille statueret omnes pollicentur. Id foedus ita ictum est: Cibavomm montium incolae ut singulis tribus mensibus (quos illi a luna *lunas* denominant) mensuram quandam illis obsignatam plenam auro ad civitatem mittant; qui vero terras incolunt ubi aromata aut gossipium suapte natura orian-
40 tur, quantitatem quandam per capita tribuant. Placuit foedus confectumque esset ut pars utraque promissa servasset, sed

forefathers. Although no electrum had been brought to light during the islanders lifetime, nevertheless they knew where the electrum mine was; yet we barely did obtain from them its location, so strong was their indignation against our men. They finally pointed out the mine, but its site was ruined and hidden by stones and dirt thrown over it; despite that, our men thought that it could be reactivated, if workers and miners skilled for that task were available, more easily than iron could be extracted from iron mines. Not far away from the same fortress of *Concepción*, in the same mountains, they discovered no small quantity of amber and, elsewhere in caves, the light blue kind, pretty rare, which painters use. In going through the woods they discovered vast sections where only scarlet-colored trees grew, that wood our Italian merchants call *verẕino* and the Spanish merchants brazil. At this point, o Most Illustrious Prince, you may wonder and ask: if the Spaniards brought to Seville several shiploads of scarlet wood and a little bit of gold, a modest quantity of cotton, some amber and a few spices, why did they not transport an abundance of gold and the other products which, as you say, that land seems to be full of? To these questions I give the answers they gave. Admiral Columbus himself, asked about these things, said that the Spaniards whom he led had been more given to sleep and idleness than to work, more desirous of rebellions and novelties than of peace or tranquillity; as a matter of fact, most of them deserted him. Moreover, he reported that before the natives were conquered and subdued and their forces weakened, it was not possible to establish uncontested rule over the island. On the other mand, the Spaniards argued they could not endure his cruel and unjust orders, and invented many accusations against him; because of these difficulties, the Admiral accepted that up to now the gain had barely met the cost. However, for this year 1501, during which, following your orders, I am writing these comments, the Spaniards collected in two months about 1,200 pounds of gold of eight ounces each. But let us return to our task. For, these issues, upon which we have touched rather lightly in our digression, will be better clarified at the right time. Since the Admiral saw the natives worried and upset and since he could not keep our sailors from violence and robbery as long as they circulated among them, he assembled several chiefs from the nearby areas and an agreement

fames improba haec omnia rescidit. Vix enim illis satis corpora ad victum per nemora quaeritandum sufficiebant, herbarum radicibus et silvestrium arborum fmctibus longo tempore contenti. Plerique tamen cum ditionariis suis reguli, inter eas egestatis
5　angustias, promissi vectigalis partem attulerunt, petentes a Praefecto supplices ut aerumnae eorum misereretur ignosceretque, donec insula ad statum pristinum restitueretur, fore ut quae nunc deficerent reintegrentur in duplum. Ex Cibavensibus pauci foedera servarunt: laborabant enim acriore fame quam caeteri. Hos
10　moribus et lingua non aliter ab incolentibus plana differre aiunt ac in caeteris regionibus ruricolae montani sunt a curialibus diversi; licet eodem genio vivant omnes, rudi scilicet ac simplici agrestique, aliquod tamen est inter eos discrimen. Ad Caunaboam captum redeamus. Ille, cum se coniectum in vincula videret,
15　tanquam leo Libycus [26] dentibus frendens, die noctuque quomodo se inde liberaret animo versans, suadere Praefecto coepit ut, quandoquidem Cipangi regionem sibi assumpsit in dicionem, praesidia Christiana, quae ab incursibus veterum hostium suorum finitimorum eam tueantur, mitteret. Significatum enim sibi fuisse
20　ferebat eam quoto die grassationis infestari in praedamque bona suorum cuncta trahi, sed, hoc excogitato dolo, existimavit fore ut frater eius, qui erat in regione cum caeteris propinquis, aut per vim aut per insidias, tot ex nostris caperent quot ad se redimendum permutatione suppeterent. Praefectus autem, intellec-
25　ta fraude, Hoiedam mittit, sed cum ea armatorum copia quae Cibavensium arma, si arma noverint, superare posset. Vix intra regionem nostri venerant, cum Caunaboae frater, convocatis circiter quinque millibus suo more armatorum (nudi enim, sagittis sine ferreis cuspidibus sudibusque et clavis quibusdarn bella
30　gerunt) intra quandam domunculam eos circunsepsit obseditque. Hic Cibavus, tanquam vir disciplinae bellicae non ignarus, ad unius stadii distantiam exercitum in quinque acies dividit cuique in gyrum, per aequos tractus locum statuens, suam autem aciem e regione nostris opponit. Inde, cum diligenter omnia instituisset,
35　ex acie sua ut omnes aequis passibus una gradiantur paulatim, signa dari iubet pedetentimque ut una omnes, vocibus sublatis, pugnam undique ineant manusque conserant; imperatum omnibus ordinibus reliquerat ne nostrorum quisquam ita circumvalla-

---

[26] See Sil. VII 401; Sen. *Oed.* 919.

was reached that the Admiral would not allow his men to wander about the island, because, under the pretext of looking for gold and other local products, they did not leave anything intact or unpolluted. In exchange the natives themselves, between 14 and 70 years of age, pledged to each give the Admiral the tribute he wanted of the products of their respective region, with everyone promising they would carry out what he had established. The agreement was struck as follows: every three months (which they call "moons," from the moon) the inhabitants of the *Cibao* mountains would send to the city the set amount of gold agreed with them; those who lived in lands where spices and cotton grow naturally would give a certain amount per head. The agreement was approved and it would have been realistic for each party to maintain its promise, but for the famine, which makes everybody wicked, rendered all of the resolutions void. In fact, the natives hardly had enough strength to hunt for food in the forest, having for a long time had to be content with roots of grasses and fruits of wild trees. Nonetheless, most of those chiefs, with their subjects, even amid that difficult time of poverty, brought part of the promised tribute, begging the Admiral to have pity on their misfortune and be lenient, until the island might return to its earlier good times; what was now shorted would be doubled in the future. Few of the inhabitants of *Cibao* kept the agreements; they truly were afflicted by the famine more severely than the others. They say these people differ in customs and language from those who live in the plains, just as in other regions mountain folk differ from those who are associated with the Court; even if they all live the same way, rough, simple, and in the open, there is, nevertheless, some diversity among them. But let us now return to the story of Caonabó, who had been captured. When he saw himself in chains, gnashing his teeth like a Libyan lion, night and day thinking how to gain his freedom from there, he began to convince the Admiral that he should send garrisons of Christians, who, since he had subdued the region of *Cipangu*, would have to defend it from raids of his neighbors, longtime enemies, claiming it was reported to him that every day the region was infested by robbers and all the property of his people had been looted. But, in devising this scheme he thought that his brother, who was in the region with other relatives, would be able to cap-

tus posset evadere. Sed nostri, cum una acie confligere satius esse rati quam eum impetum expectare, in aciem grandiorem per apertos agros venientem irruunt, eo quod, equestri praelio committendo, ea pars commodior esset. In eos igitur sese equites

5 praecipitant, equorum pectoribus eos prosternebant; leviter profligantur, perimuntur quicunque expectarunt. Caeteri, metu perculsi, in fugam convertuntur ad montanasque rupes asperas, relictis domibus, se recipiunt indeque ut eis ignosceretur precabantur se quodcunque imperatum libenter subituros, si intra

10 natales suos eos vivere patiantur, attestantes. Caunaboae fratre tandem capto, popularium quemque in sua remiserunt. His actis, regio illa pacata est. Inter eos montes vallis, quam Caunaboa incolebat, *Magona* vocatur, amnibus auriferis et fontibus fortunatissima fertilisque maiorem in modum. Eo anno, mense Iunio,

15 inauditum ab euro turbinem, elevatis usque ad sidera rapidis vorticibus, exortum fuisse praedicant qui quascunque maximas arbores offendebat, radicitus everteret. Is tipho, quum ad civitatis portum iam pervenisset, tres naves quae solae in anchoris stabant, ruptis rudentibus, sine ulla maris procella aut fluctu, circumactas

20 ter aut quater, in profundum mersit. Crevisseque eo anno praeter solitum intra terram et extendisse se mare pusquam cubiti mensuram ferunt. Gentem hanc perturbasse elementa atque portenta haec tulisse immurmurabant insulares. Has aeris procellas, uti Graeci τυφῶνες, *furacanes* isti appellant. Crebro namque surgere

25 in ea insula inquiunt, sed furacanes nunquam aeque violentos aut furibundos: neque enim viventis ullius aetate aut memoria maiorum extabat similem unquam turbinem qui et grandiores arbores evelleret ad eam insulam ruisse. Neque mare ibi tempestatem ullam fuisse unquam perpessum constat, immo neque maris

30 aestuatia pati; ubicunque enim littora planitiem aliquam attingunt, prata florida littoribus proxima reperiuntur. Caunaboam repetamus. Caunaboa rex et frater eius, cum ad Reges in Hispaniam ducebantur, dolore animi confecti, in itinere moriuntur. Praefectus autem, summersis fero turbine navigiis, se interceptum videns, duas statim

35 caravelas iussit fabrefieri: omnium enim artium magistros secum habebat. Interea, dum haec fierent, fratrem suum Bartholomaeum Colonum ipsius insulae, more Hispano, Adelantatum cum metallariis quibusdam armata manu ad aurifodinas[27], quas ad lequas

---

[27] See Plin. *nat. hist.* XXXIII 78; Gaius *dig.* III 4, 1.

ture, either by force or by deceit, as many Spaniards as were needed to ransom him in exchange. However, the Admiral, anticipating his plot, sent Hojeda with a supply of armed men, so great as to overcome the arms of the *Cibao* soldiers, should they seek combat. Our men had just arrived in the region when Caonabó's brother, gathering 5,000 men armed their way (they really fight naked, using arrows without iron points, slings and clubs), surrounded the Spaniards and besieged them in a little house. Here, the Cibao chief, acting as an expert in the art of war, divided his army into five troops distanced about a stadium, and distributed in a circle at equal intervals, then put his troop right in front of our soldiers. Having arranged everything with care that all soldiers would advance slowly in step from their place, he ordered that the signal for battle be given, and that all together shouting more and more from all sides, would begin the battle and engaged in combat. All the troops had instructions not to let any of our men escape their concerted all-side attack. Our soldiers, however, thinking that it would be better to confront one troop than to wait for their attack, rushed into the larger troop, which was advancing across open fields, because that section of the front was more suited for the cavalry. The cavalrymen charged and knocked them down head on with their horses. The natives were put to flight easily, with the slow ones being killed. The other troops, frightened, turned to flight and, abandoning their camps, took refuge on steep, mountainous cliffs from which they begged to be spared, swearing that they would quickly comply if allowed to live with their families. Eventually, when Caonabó's brother was captured, the Spaniards sent all of the people back to their homes. After these events, that region was pacified. Among those mountains, the valley in which Caonabó lived, is called *Magona*; it is very rich with gold-bearing rivers and springs, very fertile. They tell us that in the month of June that year came a terrible storm from the East, with violent whirls reaching the skies, that uprooted any tall tree it encountered in its path. That typhoon, when it reached the port of the city, sank the three ships that stood there at anchor, breaking their cables and spinning them around three or four times, even though there was no storm or tidal wave at sea. They say the sea that year grew more than usual, pushing into the land and extending itself in length

ab Isabella sexaginta antecipangas, ductu insularium, repertas, ire tentatum iubet. In eis effossos veterum tempestate profundos puteos inveniunt. Praefectus inde ingentes thesauros sibi illos de quibus Veteri Testamento agitur Salomonem Solymo-
rum regem, per sinum Persicum, comparasse contendit. Sit an non non est meum diiudicare, sed longe abest meo iudicio. Metallarii, diversis in locis, superficialem terram aurifodinarum circiter sex millia passuum durantium cribrantes, in sicco tantam ibi auri copiam iacere demersam censuerunt ut mercennarius
quisque fossor ad id conductus tres auri drachmas singulis diebus facile queat effodere. Is ita indagatis, Adelantatus simul et metallarii Praefecto rem per litteras significant. Quibus habitis, quinto Idus Martii anni quinti et monagesimi, naves, quae iam peractae erant, statim ad Reges venturus alacer conscendit,
provinciae gubernandae fratri Bartholomaeo Colono Adelantato omni potestate relicta.

by a cubit. The natives whispered that the Spaniards had upset the elements and brought on these portents. These people call such windstorms *furacanes*, whereas the Greeks called them *typhoos*. They reported that hurricanes are rather frequent in that island, but are never so violent or fierce: actually, no hurricane in their lifetime or in the accounts of their ancestors, ever struck the island with such gales as to uproot even the tallest trees. It is agreed that the sea and the inlets here have never been ravaged by any tempest; indeed, wherever the seashore borders a plain, fields of flowers are found near the coast. Let us return to Caonabó. The chief and his brother, afflicted with grief, died during return crossing to be taken to the Sovereigns of Spain. The Admiral, on the other hand, realizing that he was cut off, since his ships had been destroyed by the violent hurricane, ordered two caravels to be built right away for he had at his disposal artisans of all kinds. In the meantime, while these ships were being built, he ordered his brother Bartholomew, the *Adelantado* of that island according to the Spanish title, to go and explore with some armed miners the gold mines that had been discovered with the help of the natives 60 miles from Isabela, opposite *Cipangu*. In these mines, they found deep pits dug during ancient times. The Admiral claims to have secured from there great treasures just as King Solomon of Jerusalem did, according to the Old Testament, along the Persian gulf. It is not for me to decide whether this assessment is true or false, I abstain judgment. The miners, sifting the dirt in diverse areas on the surface of the mines, which extend for about six miles, think that so much gold lies sunk in the ground there that each worker hired for this job could easily dig up three drachmas of gold every day. After that survey, the *Adelantado* and the miners together informed the Admiral of the discovery by means of letters. Having received them, on March 11, 1495, he immediately set sails on the ships, which had been readied, eager to return to the Sovereigns, having relinquished to his brother Bartholomew, the *Adelantado*, full governing powers over the province.

I 5: ad cardinalem Ludovicum Aragonium, nostri Regis nepotem

Adelantatus autem ipse Bartholomaeus, ex sui fratris
discedentis consilio, arcem in aurifodinis erigit, hanc *Arcem
Auream* appellat, quoniam ex terra, quae ad muros con-
struendos ferebatur, calones et muratores, inter pinsendum,
5 aurum deligebant. Tres menses ad instrumenta, quibus aurum lavari et colligi posset, conficienda consumpsit, sed rem
imperfectam, fame compulsus, reliquit. Ad sexagesimum inde milliare, quo ipse cum armatis pluribus concessit, panis
insularis portionem quandam a provincialibus habuit per-
10 mutatione rerum nostrarum. Attamen morari diutius illic
nequivit. Relictis igitur ad eius arcis praesidium decem hominibus, cum ea panis insularis portiuncula quae supererat,
relictoque illis venatorio cane ad capiendum genus id ani-
malis, quod apud eos esse supra diximus cuniculo nostro
15 simile, nomine *utias*, ad Conceptionem revertitur. Erat praeterea is mensis quo Guarionexius rex et alius illi finitimus
Manicautexius nomine, tributa erant ei laturi. Ibi totum Iu-
nium immoratus, vectigalia in integrum ab his duobus regibus et victui necessaria sibi et iis quos ductabat, qui erant
20 forte quadringenti, exegit. Circiter Kalendas Iulii tres cum
escariis rebus, tritico, oleo, vino, suillis vaccinisque carnibus
salsis, caravelae advenerunt; ea viritim pro constitutione ex
Hispania lata dividuntur, quamvis ex his aliqua madida cor-
ruptaque vecta esse conquererentur. Per has naves a Regi-
25 bus et fratre Praefecto, qui iam multa antea de hac re apud
Reges egerat, ut ad meridionale insulae latus habitationem
traducat, in mandatis Bartholomaeus gubernator habuit: erat
enim ea pars aurifodinis propinquior. Imperatumque etiam
illi est ut regulos eos qui Christianos peremisse reperirentur,
30 cum suis ditionariis errati participibus, vinctos in Hispaniam
mitteret. Tercentum insulares cum suis regulis captos mittit;
post explorata diligentius meridionalia littora transportat
habitationem arcemque ibi super edito colle, apud portum
bene tutum, condidit, quam arcem *Sancti Dominici*, quoniam
35 die Dominico eo appulsus est, vocitavit. Amnis salubrium
aquarum et variis piscium generibus optimis refertissimus
in portum, amoenis utrinque ripis, defluit. Miras esse flu-

The *Adelantado* Bartholomew himself, then, following the advice of his departing brother, built a stronghold on the mines of gold. He named it *Fortaleza del Oro*, because from the ore that was moved and crushed to build the walls, carriers and masons picked out gold. It took him three months to make the tools needed to wash and sift the gold, but famine never allowed him to complete the undertaking. With several soldiers he went to a place sixty miles away, where he obtained from the natives a quantity of local bread in exchange for some of our items. Even so, he could not stay there any longer. Thus, he left ten men to garrison the fort, giving them the small quantity of local bread that was left and a hunting dog to hunt that kind of animal which, as we said earlier, is similar to our rabbit and is called *utia*, and he returned to *Concepción*. Moreover, that was the month during which chief Guarionex and another neighboring chief, named Manicautex, were readying to bring him the tributes. He stayed there the whole month of June and collected the entire tribute from these two chiefs, as well as provisions necessary for himself and those under his command, approximately 400 men. In early July three caravels arrived with such supplies as wheat, oil, wine, salted pork and beef; those provisions were divided among the men in compliance with instructions from Spain, but the recipients still complained that some of the transported goods were spoiled or damp. With these three ships, the *Adelantado* received instructions from the Sovereigns and from his brother the Admiral (who had earlier discussed this project with the Sovereigns) to transfer his residence to the southern coast of the island since this area was closer to the gold mines. He was also instructed to send to Spain as prisoners those chiefs who might be convicted of the killing of Christians, and any of the subjects-accomplices in the crime. He sent 300 prisoners with their chiefs and transferred the colony after having explored more accurately the southern coasts, where he built on a high hill near a safe harbor a fortress which he called *Santo Domingo*, because he landed there on a Sunday. A river of wholesome water, quite rich in excellent varieties of fish, flows into the

minis naturae dotes referunt: quacunque enim fluat, omnia
iucunda, utilia omnia; palmeta frutetaque insularia omnis
generis navigantibus ramos floribus fructibusque onustos in
caput interdum declinabant, aequamque soli eius vel beatio-
rem Isabellica ubertatem praedicant. In Isabella valitudinarios
tantum naviumque magistros quosdam, qui duas quas inceperant caravelas perficerent, reliquit; caeteros ad Sanctum
Dominicum ad meridiem traducit. Post arcem conditam re-
licto in ea viginti hominum praesidio, cum reliquis ipse oc-
cidentales insulae partes internas, hactenus nomine tantum
notas, exploraturus sese accingit. Ad triginta inde lequas, id
est milliaria nongenta, in fluvium Naibam quem a Cibavis
montibus ad meridiem recta, per insulae medium descendere
memoravimus, incidit. Hoc amne superato, cum singulis armatorum hominum quinque et viginti turmis decuriones duos
ad regulorum terras, quorum nemora ex coccineis arboribus
constant, per diversa dimittit. Laevorsum isti tendunt, silvas
inveniunt, ingrediuntur, scindunt, cadunt[28] altae intactaeque
hactenus preciosae arbores; singulas insulares casas decuriones singuli coccineis implent truncis, ubi, donec navigia du-
cantur, quae illos abducant, serventur. Adelantatus autem
dextrorsum iter capiens, non longe a ripa fluminis Naibae,
potentem quendam, nomine *Beechium Anacaucheam*, regem castris positis contra Naibenses incolas in armis esse reperit ut
illos suae dicioni, veluti plures alios insulares regulos, subii-
ceret. Huius potentis regia occidentalem versus insulae calcem
sita *Xaragua* vocatur, a flumine Naiba triginta lequas distans,
montosa, aspera. Sed quicunque reguli medium tenent, huius
imperio parent. Omnis ea regio a Naiba ad ultimam occidentis oram, auri expers est. Nostros, depositis armis datoque
pacis signo placidissime, incertum metu an humanitate susci-
piens, quidnam sibi vellent, interrogavit. Adelantatus inquit:
"Ut quemadmodum et reliqui huius insulae principes Praefecto marino fratri meo, Hispanorum Regum nomine, vectigalia praestes". Cui ille: "Quomodo id a me potestis exigere,
cuius nulla regio de multis quae mihi imperanti auscultant,
aurum gignit?". Audierat enim gentem exteram, quae aurum
avide quaeritaret, ad insulam adventasse, sed quod aliud

---

[28] Peter Martyr's narrative revives at this point a motif typical of epic poems
(see Enn. *ann.* 187 ff. Vahlen²; Lucan. III 440 ff.; Sil. X 528 ff.; Stat. *Theb.* VI 90 ff.).

harbor along charming banks. They reported how its features make things wonderful: wherever it flows everything is pleasant and very enjoyable; native palms and fruit trees of every kind sometimes drooped over the heads of our sailors, their branches weighted with blooms and fruits, and the claim is that the soil appears as fertile as or even more so than at Isabela. The *Adelantado* left at La Isabela only the sick and some carpenters to finish the two caravels they had begun; he took all the others South to Santo Domingo. Once the fortress was completed, he stationed there a garrison of twenty men; with the other Spaniards he set out to explore the western interior, the part of the island unexplored heretofore. Then, at about 30 leagues, that is to say, 900 miles from there, he came to the river Naiba, which, as we mentioned, flows from the Cibao mountains directly South through the middle of the island. Once he had crossed this river, he sent two officers in different directions, each with a troop of 25 armed men, to the lands of the chiefs whose forests have reddish trees. These men went to the left, found the forests, entered and harvested tall, valuable trees, until then untouched; each officer filled with logs a native's huts where they kept them until vessels were built to transport them. The *Adelantado* meanwhile, going to the right, met a powerful chief, not far away from the banks of the Naiba, named *Beechio Anacauchea*, who was camped in battle against the inhabitants of the Naiba region in order to subdue them to his rule, as he had done with many chiefs. The residence of this chief, located toward the southern tip of the island, was called *Xaragua*, a rough and mountainous area about 30 leagues from the Naiba river. All the chiefs living in the central part obeyed his commands. The whole region, from the Naiba to the farthest western shore, lacks gold. As arms were laid down and the sign of peace exchanged, Beechio carefully asked what our men wanted from him, showing some hesitancy, out of either fear or respect. The *Adelantado* said: "That you pay tributes in the name of the Sovereigns of Spain, to my brother, the Admiral, as all the other chiefs of this island have done!" And the chief replied: "How can you ask me that? None of the many regions under my rule produces gold." Indeed, since, he had heard that foreign people had come to the island avidly searching for gold, he did not think for a second that the Spaniards wanted anything but gold. Then

quam aurum cuperet minime arbitrabatur. Tunc Adelantatus: "Absit ut cuiquam tributa iniungamus, quae persolvi facile non possint quibusve regiones careant. Gossampii, cannabi et aliarum huiuscemodi rerum copiam regionem producere compertum habemus: ex quibus proventibus ut nobis liquid impartiaris petimus" At ille, his auditis, hilari fronte, sereno vultu, se quantum voluerint accipere de his daturum pollicetur; dimissoque exercitu ipsemet, praemissis nunciis, Adelantatum usque ad locum ubi ipse regiam habebat ad lequas, uti diximus, triginta, comitatus est. Totoque eo tractu per regulorum ei subditorum dioeceses iter semper fecerunt, aliis cannabi quod non peius nostro lino ad navium amplustre contexendum esse dicunt, panis aliis, aliis gossampii, pro telluris variae natura, tributa imperantes. Ad regiam tandem Xaraguensem veniunt. Hanc priusquam ingrediantur, incolae omnes regem suum Beechium Anacaucheam ac nostros honorifice, suo more, recepturi occurrunt. Inter caetera, spectacula audi duo inter nudas et incultas gentes memoratu digna! Appropinquantibus primum triginta foeminae, regis uxores omnes, ramos palmarum manibus ferentes tripudiis cantibusque ac sonis, ex regis praecepto, nudae toto corpore praeter pudibunda, quae femoralibus quibusdam gossampinis corruptae contegunt, obviam prodeunt. Virgines enim, capillis per humeros sparsis, frontibus tamen vitta ligatis nullam sui corporis partem cooperiunt. Faciem, pectora, mammas manus caeteraque sub albido colore praedicant fuisse pulcherrima. Dryades formosissimas aut nativas fontium nymphas de quibus fabulatur antiquitas se vidisse arbitrati sunt. Palmarum manipulos quos dextris gestabant, chorizantes [29] psallentesque invicem, poplitibus flexis, Adelantato omnes dono dant. Domum deinde regis ingressi, eorum more, laute paratam coenam inveniunt, vires reficiunt. Nocte vero superveniente, pro cuiusque statu, ad hospitia obsignata per regis ministros ducuntur, ubi in paratis pro eorum consuetudine lectis pensilibus, quos alias descripsimus, quieverunt. Altero die ad eam domum, quam sibi loco theatri construunt, nostri ducuntur. Ibi, post multas variasque choreas et saltationes, in latam planitiem duae, ex insperato, ingentes armatorum acies de-

---

[29] A verb form probably created by analogy after the greek aorist tense χορεύω.

the *Adelantado* said: "Be it far from us to impose on anybody tributes that cannot be easily paid or demand products which the region lacks. We know this region produces abundant cotton, hemp and other such products: that you share these crops is what we ask." At these words, the chief readily and cheerfully promised to give as much as they could take; afterwards he dismissed his troops, sent messengers ahead and he himself accompanied the *Adelantado* up to his residence, 30 leagues away as we said. During the journey, they crossed territories of chiefs under his command, ordering tributes that varied according to the nature of each territory, either hemp, which they say is not inferior to our flax for weaving the ropes of ships, or bread, or cotton. They finally reached the chief's house in *Xaragua*. Before they entered it, all the natives came out to meet Beechio Anacauchea and to receive our men with honors, as is their custom. Among other things, hear of two spectacles worthy of being remembered, concerning naked and uncivilized people. First, by order of their chief, thirty women, all his wives, carrying in their hand palm branches — amid dances, songs and sounds — came to meet those who were approaching. The women were all naked, except for their waist shamelessly covered with a cotton loin-cloth, but for the virgins who their hair loose over their shoulders and a ribbon on their foreheads, did not cover any part of their bodies. We are given to understand that the women's face, chest, breasts, hands and all other parts, which were kind of whitish, were most beautiful. They thought they had seen the gorgeous Dryads i.e. the fountain nymphs of ancient stories. They all gave homage to the *Adelantado* with bundles of palms, the ones they carried in their right hands, while taking turns dancing with their knees bent. Next, after entering the house of the chief, the men found a banquet, sumptuously prepared according to the natives' custom, and so regained their strength. As night fell, they were escorted by servants of the chief to their lodgings, assigned according to the status of each, where they slept in hanging beds, a custom we have described earlier. The following day our soldiers were taken to a building that serves the natives as a theater. Here, after many varied choruses and dances, two large troops of armed men unexpectedly appeared into the vast plain, as the chief had ordered for fun and games, just as the Spaniards often set up play for the "Trojan games," with reeds.

scendunt quas, ludi et delectationis gratia, ut apud Hispanos ludus Troicus,[30] id est harundineus, saepius instruitur, rex apparari iusserat. Cominus accedentes ac si hostes collatis signis pro opibus, pro focis, pro natis, pro imperio, pro vita denique ipsa, certaturi concurrerent, ita duae illae acies utrinque manus conserunt. Missilibus, telis et sagittis intra breve horae momentum quattuor cecidere, pluresque vulnerati fuerunt; acrius pugnatum fuisset nisi, rogatu nostrorum, rex, dato signo, pugnam diremisset. In tertium inde diem, consilio regi praebito, ut gossampii plus deinceps in ripis aquarum, quo impositum per focos tributum facilius persolveretur sererent, ad Isabellam valitudinarios et navigia, quae incepta reliquerat, visurus tendit. Variis morbis circiter trecentos reperit cecidisse, quare anxius et quid consilii caperet erat ignarus, cum non modo ad valitudinem resarciendam, sed victui necessaria fere cuncta deessent, neque enim ex Hispania navis ulla adventabat. Sic haesitans, valitudinarios per regiones et castella in ipsis erecta dispartiri constituit. Castella enim ab Isabella recto itinere ad Sanctum Dominicum, id est a septentrione ad meridiem, per insulam, haec erexerunt: ab Isabella ad lapidem sextum et trigesimum *Speranciam* arcem condidit, a Sperancia vero ad lapidem quartum et vigesimum *Divam Catherinam*, a Catherina ad vigesimum *Sanctum Iacobum* arcem, a Divo Iacobo ad alia viginti milliaria turritam condidit munitiorem, quam *Conceptionem* appellavit, quod in radice Cibavorum montium quodque in planitie vastissima ubere et populosa. Aliam deinde mediam inter Conceptionem et Sanctum Dominicum condidit Conceptione munitiorem. Quoniam intra terminos reguli, cui supra quinque incolarum millia parebant, *Bonavum* nomine vocant insulares eius regionis vicum, qui caput est regni, propterea *Bonavum* etiam voluit arcem Praefectus appellari. Per haec igitur castella castellorumque vicina, in insularium domibus infirmis dispartitis, ad Sanctum ipse Dominicum proficiscitur, a regulis, qui medium tenebant, imposita exigens intereundum vectigalia. Ubi cum aliquot dies moraretur rumor exoritur re-

---

[30] An ancient tourney played by children and young men in the amphitheatre (see Paul. Fest. 504, 11 L.: *lusus puerorum equestris*). The most precise and complete description is by Virgil in *Aeneid's* book V (vv. 551 ff.; see also Plut. *Cat. min. 3*; Suet. *Caes.* 39,4; *Tib.* 6,6; *Aug.* 43,5; Serv. *ad Aen.* V 553 ff.; Dio Cass. 54, 26; Tac. *ann.* XI 11; Sen. *Troad.* 777 ff.).

Approaching as if they were enemies in battle to defend their wealth, houses, children, authority, or even survival, those two sides engaged in hand-to-hand combat hurling projectiles, darts and arrows; in a short time, four died and several were wounded. They would have kept up their fierce combat if the chief had not, upon our request, given the signal to end it. The third day, after advising the chief to regularly sow more cotton on the water banks, so that the imposed family tribute could more easily be paid, the *Adelantado* left for La Isabela to visit the sick and see the ships being worked on. Finding that about 300 men had died of various diseases, he grew anxious and did not know what plan to adopt, since all of the means necessary not only to heal from illnesses but just to keep alive were lacking, as no ship had arrived from Spain. Therefore, with hesitation, he decided to distribute the sick among their regional fortresses. These had been built in a straight line from La Isabela to Santo Domingo, that is, from North to South through the island: 36 miles from La Isabela he built the fortress of *Esperanza*, 24 miles from Esperanza that of *Santa Catalina*, 20 miles from Catalina the fortress of *Santiago* and 20 miles yet past Santiago he built a more fortified citadel with towers, which he called *Concepción*, located at the base of the *Cibao* mountains in a vast, fertile and populous plain. Then he built another one half-way between Concepción and Santo Domingo, stronger than the one at Concepción. Because it was within the territory of a chief obeyed by more than 5,000 inhabitants who called *Bonao* this village chief, — the most important of the realm — the Admiral wanted the fortress named *Bonao* as well. So, after he distributed the sick among the fortresses and in the houses of the natives in nearby areas, he himself set out for Santo Domingo, collecting during the trip tributes from the chieftains who ruled over the middle of the island. While there for a few days, rumors came that all the chieftains in the territory of Concepción had feelings of hopelessness in regard to our men and wanted to desert. Upon these reports, he set out advancing against those chiefs at forced march. As he came closer, a rumor spread that Guarionex had been chosen by all as the chief to take back control of this region with enticements or prompting by the others — almost against his will — since he feared the cunning and weapons of our men, from previous experience. They had

gulos omnes finium Conceptionis desperatis in nostros animis vivere studereque defectioni. Ad eos igitur ubi haec nunciata sunt, longis movet itineribus. Cum propius accederet, Guarionexium, provinciae huius capessendae imperatorem ab omnibus
5 fuisse delectum fama increbuit seductumque et sollicitatum, semiinvitum, tamen ab aliis fuisse cum nostrorum astus et arma, iam alias expertus, pertimesceret. Convenerant certo die cum quindecim millibus hominum, suo more, armatorum fortunam belii iterum tentare. Ibi Adelantatus, consilio habito
10 cum arcis praefecto, reliquisve militibus, quos ductitabat, adoriendos esse incautos et palantes regulos in propriis laribus, priusquam exercitum comparent, constituunt. Ad singulos igitur regulos singuli centuriones mittuntur qui, ex insperato, dormientes, priusquam sparsis populis liceat convenire, vicos
15 eorum congressi, quos non moenibus, non fossis, non aggeribus circunseptos habent, impetunt, captant, vinciunt, ducunt quisque, suum uti fuerat imperatum. Ad Guarionexium Adelantatus ipse, tanquam ad potentiorem, perrexerat cepitque sicut et ahi, eadem hora constituta, suos. Quattuordecim, ea
20 nocte, ex eis ad Conceptionem tracti sunt. Paulo post, duobus ex iis, qui Guarionexium reliquosve rerum novarum studiosiores seduxerant ac subornaverant supplicio affectis, ne suorum regum dolore confecti incolae agros desererent, quod summum incommodum propter sementes nostris afferre po-
25 tuisset, Guarionexium et reliquos dimisit Ditionarii ad quinque millium numerum confluxerunt pro suorum regum liberatione inermes. Intonuit aer, contremuit terra prae clamore illorum usque ad sidera elevato. Adelantatus Guarionexium atque alios, pollicendo, donando, minando ut in posterum caverent ne
30 quid molirentur, admonet. Guarionexius apud populum orationem habuit de nostrorum potentia, indulgentia in delinquentes, liberalitate in fidos, ut sedent animos nec quicquam ulterius astruant cogitentque contra Christianos, sed ut illis obtemperent, obsequantur, serviant, nisi se in maiores in dies
35 calamitates trudi cupiant. Oratione habita, pensilem illum humeris captant pensilemque usque ad suae regiae pagum humeris portant. Ita per aliquot dies regio pacata est. Solliciti tamen et tristes nostri, in exteris regionibus deserti, quod quintus decimus iam mensis a Praefecti discessu ageretur, quia
40 cuncta, quibus indui vescique solebant, deficerent, demisso vultu incedebant. Adelantatus eos quam melius poterat, inani

agreed to try their luck in war again on a set day, with 15,000 men armed according to their custom. The *Adelantado*, after consulting with the governor of the fortress and the remaining soldiers which he had with him, decided to attack the chieftains, while still unguarded and scattered in their own houses, before they could gather their army. Thus, he dispatches centurions against each chieftain; they approached one at a time these villages unexpected while the chiefs slept and before the scattered tribesmen could assemble, and attacked the defenseless villages that have no walls, ditches or embankments, and thus captured, tied up and dragged every chief away as per their orders. The *Adelantado* had set out to capture Guarionex himself, as one of the more powerful leaders, and captured him just as the others captured theirs, at the mutually agreed upon time. During that night, fourteen of the chieftains were taken to Concepción. A little later, after punishing two of the ones who, more eager for change had incited and corrupted Guarionex and the others, he let Guarionex and the others go, so that the inhabitants would not abandon the fields broken-hearted in grief for their chiefs; that could have damaged our cause seriously, for it was sowing time. Their subjects, numbering about 5,000, flocked unarmed to free their chiefs. The air resounded with and the earth shook from their shouts that reached the stars. With promises, gifts and threats the *Adelantado* warned Guarionex and the others to be careful in the future not to plot anything. Guarionex spoke to the people about the power of our men, their leniency toward those who made mistakes, their generosity for those who remained loyal, to induce calm in their hearts and prevent further plots or conspiracies against the Christians, in favor of obedience, respect and compliance, thus avoiding daily greater misfortunes. After he finished his speech, the people lifted him up on their shoulders and carried him that way to the village of his royal house. And so, for a few days, the region was at peace. Our men, however, worried, upset and feeling abandoned in a foreign land, kept on being depressed because almost fourteen months had elapsed from the Admiral's departure and there was shortage of all that they were used to wear or eat. The *Adelantado* consoled them as much as he could, generating empty hopes. While these things were happening, Beechio Anacauchea (such was the name of the chief of the western

spe depascendo, solabatur. Dum haec agerentur, Beechius Anacauchea, sic enim Xaraguae, occidentalis partis quam supra
memoravimus, rex vocabatur ad Adelantatum nuncios mittit,
qui gossampium caeteraque vectigalia, quae sibi suisque incolis
5 imperaverat, parata esse significarent. Ad iter se accingit Adelantatus, pergit, honorifice a rege recipitur et eius sorore, quae,
quondam Caunaboae regis Cibavi uxor, non minoris erat in
fraterni regni gubernatione momenti et consilii quam frater.
Aiunt enim eam esse urbanam, facetam ac prudentissimam
10 fratrique ut Christianis assentetur, blandiatur, obtemperet,
exemplo mariti eius edoctus, persuaserat. Haec foemina *Anacaona* nuncupatur. Duos et triginta ibi regulos in Beechii Anacaucheae regia congregatos, cum tributis expectantes reperit;
qui omnes, praeter imperata vectigalia ad benivolentiam cum
15 nostris captandam, munera tulerunt ingentia ex utroque pane,
radicali scilicet ac paniceo, *utias*, id est cuniculos insulares,
innumeros piscesque, sed ne putrescerent aut corrumperentur,
assos tulerunt et de serpentibus, quos inter edulia principatum
obtinere crocodillisque simillimos esse supra descripsimus.
20 *Iuannas* serpentes vocant. Has in insula nasci sero didicerunt
neque ex eis nostri ob foeditatem, quae horrorem non modo
nauseam inducere videbantur, gustare hactenus ausi fuerant.
Praemordere paulatim Adelantatus iuannam, regis sororis pellectus facetiis, statuit, sed ubi demulcere carnium earum sapor
25 palatum et guttur coepit, plenis deinde faucibus eas expetere
videbatur. Non mordicus deinde neque vix uncto labello illas
delibabant, sed helluones omnes effecti, de re nulla iam praeterquam de serpentium suavitate sermocinabantur lautioresque
esse dapes illarum quam aut pavonis aut phasiani vel perdicis
30 apud nos. Sed, si aliter quam uno condiantur modo uti pavones et phasiani, nisi lardo involuti, verubus assentur, saporem
perdunt. Evisceratas a iugulo ad inguina, lotasque ac detersas
diligenter et in gyrum postea in modum anguis dormientis,
in se recepti, insinuatas in ollam sui tantum capacem, paulisper
35 aquae, cum pipere insulari super iniecto, comprimunt tenuiter,
igne ex quodam ligno odorato, minime fumoso supposito. Ex
abdomine sic stiilato ius efficitur, ut aiunt, nectareum, nullum-
que esse epularum genus ovis ipsarum serpentium par ferunt,
quae per se et lenius coquuntur. Si coctae et recentes suavis-
40 simae et servatae per aliquot dies iucundissimae sunt. De edu-
liis satis, ad alia veniamus. Quum vectigali gossipio insularem

province of *Xaragua*, as we have mentioned earlier) sent messengers to the *Adelantado* to inform him that the cotton and other tributes, which had been asked of him and his subjects, had been readied. The *Adelantado* prepared for the trip, set out and was received with honor by the chief and his sister who, once wife of the *Cibao* chief Caonabó, did not have any less decision-making power than her brother in the government of his kingdom. Indeed, they say that she was courteous, elegant and very prudent, and that she had persuaded her brother to please, soothe and obey the Christians, having learned from the example of her husband. The name of this woman was *Anacaona*. The *Adelantado* found there 32 chieftains gathered at the house of Beechio Anacauchea, all waiting with their tribute. In order to ingratiate our men, all of them brought numerous presents, in addition to required tributes, both types of bread, one from roots and one from wheat, many *utia*, that is, their rabbits, and fish; but, so that the fish would not rot or spoil, they brought them roasted, and along with them some of those snakes which, as we said earlier, constitute delicacy for them but look very much like crocodiles. They call them iguanas and later learned that these are native to the island; our men did not dare taste them until now, because their disgusting look seemed to provoke not only nausea but horror. Slowly, the *Adelantado* decided to put his teeth in an iguana, charmed by the humor of the chief's sister; but, once that tasty meat began to reach his palate and throat, he seemed to go after it with gluttony. Then, not only did the Spaniards taste them in small bites or with the touch of their lips, but, having all turned gluttons, they would not speak of anything but of such delicacy, claiming that the banquets prepared with them were more sumptuous than ours based on peacocks, pheasants and partridges. If iguanas are prepared in any but one method, they lose their flavor, just as do peacocks and pheasants, if they are not roasted wrapped in lard on spits. Once completely gutted, washed and cleaned with care, iguanas are pressed gently into a container of sufficient capacity coiled up like a sleeping snake, covered with water, and sprinkled with island pepper; underneath it a small fire is built of odorous wood that does not produce much smoke. The meat marinated in this fashion produces, a very savory juice they say, reporting also that no food is as good as the eggs of these animals when

301

20

quandam casam Adelantatus implevisset, panis sui quantum-
cunque vellet se libenter impartituros reguli pollicentur. Is,
oblata eorum acceptans, gratias agit. Interea igitur dum per
regiones panis conficeretur ad regiamque Beechii Anacaucheae,
5 Xaraguensis regis, portaretur, ad Isabellam nuncios mittit, qui
adduci peractam caravelam de duabus quas inceptas reliquerat
suo nomine imperent. Pane namque se onustam ad eos illam
remissurum renunciavit. Laeti nautae, navim ad Xaraguense
littus, insulam circumeuntes, plenis velis, tendunt; Beechii
10 Anacaucheae regis soror illa faceta, prudens et magni ingenii
mulier Anacaona, uxor quondam Caunaboae, ubi navim nostram ad patrium littus suum applicatam cognovit, fratri persuadet ut ambo ad illam videndam proficiscantur; sex tantum
passuum millia littus a regia distabat. Itinere autem medio in
15 vico, quod est ipsius regiae sororis gazophylacium, pernocta-
tum est; illius vero thesauri non aurum, non argentum, non
gemmae, sed utensilia tantum resque ad humanum usum attinentia, ut puta, sedilia, paropsides, lances, pelves, patellae ex
ligno nigerrimo, lubrico, lucido, quod hebenum[31] eximius ar-
20 tium et medicinae doctor tuus Ioannis Baptista Elisius esse
contendit confectae et arte mira laboratae. In his enim quidquid est incolis ingenii a natura tributum exercent. Sed haec
illi foeminae in insula sua *Guanabba* quam in faucibus occidentalibus Hispaniolae insulae, si pictam videris, iacere con-
25 spicies, fabrefiunt. In eis lemurum, quos noctu videre se praedicant, serpentum, hominum et aliarum rerum quascunque semel intuentur, vivos vultus caelant. Quid facturos illos,
illustrissime Princeps putares, si ferrum et chalybem assseque-
rentur? Illa enim omnia, igni prius interius mollefacta, lapillis
30 postmodum fluvialibus quibusdam cavant et diducunt. De sedilibus Adelantato quattuordecim, de utensilibus autem men-
sariis et coquinariis fictilibus sexaginta dono dedit; quattuor
praeterea neti gossampi glomos ponderis immensi tribuit. Ad
littus igitur postero die cum pervenissent ubi pagus erat alter
35 regius, servitoriam iussit Adelantatus cymbam instructam ad-
vehi. Rex autem canoas suo more depictas duas, unam qua
ipse cum familiaribus suis, alteram qua soror Anacaona et eius

---

[31] Ebony plants were known since antiquity. Virgil reported them growing only in
India (*georg.* II 116: *Sola India nigrum fert hebenum*), whereas Herodotus says Africa (Her. III
114) yet in India and Ethiopia (XVII 7, 36) for Isidore [of Seville] *nat. hist.* XII 17.

cooked slowly by themselves. If you cook and eat them fresh, they are delicious, and if kept for a few days, very flavorful. Enough about foods; let us proceed to other matters. After the *Adelantado* had filled one of the huts of the natives with cotton tributes, the chieftains promised they would give him as much of their bread as he wanted. Thanking them, he accepted their offerings. In the meantime, as bread was being collected through the regions and taken to the house of Beechio Anacauchea, ruler of the *Xaragua* territory, the *Adelantado* sent messengers to La Isabela so that in his name be sent the completed caravel of the two unfinished ones at the time he left and did announce he would send it back to them full of bread. The delighted sailors, tacking around the island, directed the ship at full sail to the shore of *Xaragua*; Anacaona, sister of king Beechio Anacauchea, an elegant woman, wise and with great intelligence, former wife of Caonabó, when she learned that our ship had approached the shore of *Xaragua*, persuaded her brother that they both should set out to see it; the shore was only six miles from the house of the king. Halfway through the trip they spent the night at a village, one she used as her treasures storage; what made up that treasure was not gold, silver or precious stones, but only utensils and objects pertinent to human use, such as chairs, fruit platters, dishes, basins, trays manufactured and wrought with remarkable art, made of very black wood, smooth and shiny, which Giovanni Battista Elisio, your famous doctor of arts and medicine, claims is ebony. These objects truly reveal whatever ability has been given by nature to the inhabitants. They, however, are made for her in her island of *Guanabba*, which, if you look at the map, you will see located at the west end of the island of Hispaniola. Chiseled and embossed are lively images of phantoms, which they claim to see at night, of animals, people or anything else they see, even once. O most illustrious Prince, imagine what they would do if they had iron and steel? Indeed, all those crafted objects, are first softened by fire, then carved out and worked with some river stones. She gave fourteen of those chairs to the *Adelantado*, besides sixty table utensils and kitchenware; in addition, she gave him four bales of spun cotton of exceptional weight. The following day, they reached the shore where there was another royal village where the *Adelantado* ordered that a service ship be outfitted and brought

ancillae veherentur, apparat. Sed in servitoriam cymbam voluit
Anacaona cum Adelantato vehi. Cum navi iam appropinqua-
rent, ex composito, ignem tormentis suffigunt, mare tonitruis,
aer pulvereo fumo implentur. Tremunt, terrentur, mundi ma-
5 chinam [32] laborare ea concussione arbitrati sunt. Verum enim
ubi Adelantatum ridere in faciem eorum versum vident, sedant
animos; cum autem propius irent, fistulae, tibiae timpanaque,
instructis choreis, pulsantur. Illi sonitus dulcore allecti stupent,
admirantur. Ingressi navim ubi proram, puppim, castella, ta-
10 bulata, carinam, cubicula diligenter percurrerunt, frater in sororem, soror in fratrem oculos vertentes obmutescebant, neque
quid, prae nimia admiratione invicem loquerentur, inveniebant.
Dum his intenti per navim vagarentur elevari anchoras, ex
temporeque, vela ex antennis devolvi et protendi in altumque
15 dirigi iubet. Tum vero stupidiores cum sine remis, sine hominum robore, molem ita grandem adeo celeriter per aequor
volitare conspicerent (flabat enim e terra optatus ad id ventus),
sed tunc multo magis, cum eodem vento duce, ire modo, modo redire, modo in dextram in laevam modo, uti libebat, ver-
20 tere navim cernerent admirabantur. His ita peractis, navi pane
radicali caeterisque muneribus repleta nostris etiam muneribus
donatis, non modo Beechium Anacaucheam regem sororemque
eius, sed ministros ancillasque utriusque alacres stuporeque
plenos dimisit. Ipse vero terrestre iter aggressus cum militibus,
25 ad Isabellam concessit. Ibi Roldanum quendam Ximenum facinorosum, quem fossorum et calonum ductorem ex famulo
suo, deinde iusticiae praesidem, Praefectus erexerat malo vivere
in Adelantatum animo, significatum est. Comperit insuper
Guarionexium regem huius Roldani et aliorum relictorum in-
30 solentias et rapinas pati ulterius nequivisse, cum familiaribu-
sque suis et ditionariis pluribus, desperato animo, ad montes
quosdam qui ab Isabella decem tantum lequas occidentem versus, in littore septentrionali distant, secessisse. Montes mon-
tiumque incolas uno nomine *Ciguavos* vocant; regem regulo-
35 rum monticolarum principem *Maiobanexium* appellant, eius regia *Capronus* dicitur. Montes asperi, alti, inaccessi, in arcum
a natura dispositi ad mare cornua porrigunt. Inter utrunque
montis eius cornu pulchra planities, per quam in mare plura

[32] See Lucr. V 96.

out. The king, for his part, prepared two canoes, painted according to his rank, one for himself and his family members, and the other one for his sister Anacaona and her maids. But Anacaona wanted to go aboard the service ship with the *Adelantado*. When they got near the ship, the crew, fired the mortars as planned: the sea filled with thunders and the air with powdery smoke. The natives were shaken and frightened; they thought the entire universe was damaged by that quaking. But when they saw the *Adelantado* turn toward them and smile, they were reassured and, as they got closer, dances and songs started and reed pipes, fifes and drums were played. Amazement and astonishment followed the attractive and sweet music. Having climbed aboard ship, where they walked carefully around the prow, stern, hold, bridge, keel, and the place reserved as a dormitory, brother and sister, looking at each other, became mute and, astonished beyond measure, found no words to exchange with each other. While they toured the ship, busy looking at these things, the *Adelantado* ordered that the anchors be raised and that, right there and then, the sails be unfolded and set for going out on the high sea. They were quickly dumbfounded, indeed seeing that such a large thing could move so swiftly on the sea without oars, without human force (the needed wind was blowing from land to the sea), but even greater was their astonishment when they saw the ship go forward and backward, now turning right or left, as desired, in the same wind. After all this, the ship was filled with bread roots and other gifts, and we presented our gifts as well. The *Adelantado* then let off not only king Beechio Anacauchea and his sister, but also their advisors and maids, all excited and full of astonishment. He himself, then, marching on land with the soldiers, returned to La Isabela. Here he found out that a certain Roldán Jiménez, an evil man, whom the Admiral had raised from his personal staff to the position of chief of the miners and carriers, and later to chief justice, had ill-will feelings toward the *Adelantado*. In addition, he learned that chieftain Guarionex could no longer tolerate the arrogance and robberies of this Roldán and others who had been left there, and so had left in desperation with his family members and several subjects for some mountains which are only ten leagues West of La Isabela on the northern coast. They call the mountains and the people by the same name, *Ciguavi*; and they call

flumina a montibus ipsis delabuntur. Gens fera, bellicosa, quae
a Canibalibus originem traxisse creditur: cum enim e montibus
ad planitiem, bellum finitimis illaturi, descendunt, si quos pe-
rimant comedunt. Guarionexius igitur ad hunc regem monti-
5 colam confugiens, dona illi regia multa, suo more, quibus
monticolae carent impartitus est; rettulitque sese nefarie, foede,
violenter a nostris tractatum, nec humilitatem nec superbiam
quicquam sibi apud nostros profuisse conqueritur; propterea
se supplicem ad eum venire ut illum tutetur defendatque ab
10 iniuriis facinorosorum hominum precatur. Maiobanexius autem
omnem illi opem, tutelam, praesidium contra Christianos pollicetur. Ad Conceptionem igitur Adelantatus proficiscitur; Roldanum Ximenum qui in insularium pagis ad milliare duodecimum, cum iis qui eum sequebantur, hospitabatur, accersiri
15 facit. Quid sibi vellent hi motus interrogat. Ille, perfricata
fronte, respondet: "Almirantum fratrem tuum interisse Regi-
busque nostris parvae curae res nostras esse videmus; fame,
dum te sequimur, perimus, cogimur infoelicem victum per
insulam quaeritare; praeterea me una tecum insulae guberna-
20 torem Praefectus reliquit. Quare mens nobis est nolle ulterius
tuo imperio parere". Haec et alia Roldanus. Adelantatus autem
manum in eum iniicere, cupiens, nequivit. Evasit enim secutique illum sunt septuaginta homines; quibus comitatus ad occidentem in Xaraguam regionem se contulit; ibique, uti Al-
25 mirantus nunc et frater eius testantur, solutis habenis, stuprari,
praedari, trucidare coeperunt. Interea dum haec fierent in insula, a Regibus tandem navigia Almiranto obsignantur octo;
de quibus primum duo ex Gadibus Herculeis recta cum alimentis mittit ad Adelantatum fratrem. Haec duo navigia ad
30 eam insulae partem occidentalem, in qua Roldanus Ximenez
cum consortibus agebat, casu, primum appulsa sunt. Seducit
illos Roldanus, pro ligone puellarum papillas tractandas, pro
labore voluptatem, pro fame affluentiam, pro lassitudine et
vigiliis quietem promittens. Guarionexius interea, comparata
35 manu amicorum, ad plana saepenumero descendens, insulares
nostrorum amicos Christianosque, quoscunque assequebatur,
trucidabat, agros hostiliter vastabat, sementes diripiebat, pagos
depopulabatur. Roldanus comitesque, quamvis Almirantum
propediem venturum sensissent, quandoquidem novos homines
40 cum duobus navigiis praemissis vectos subornaverant, minime
perterrebantur. Dum inter hos fluctus miser Adelantatus fra-

the most important of the chieftains living in the mountains *Maiobanex* and his residence *Caprone*. The mountains, rugged, tall, and inaccessible, are disposed by nature in a semicircle extending to the sea. Between the peaks of each mountain there is a beautiful plain, through which several rivers flow from the mountains into the sea. The fierce and bellicose people, are believed to have drawn their origin from the cannibals: in fact, when they come down from the mountains to the plain to fight with the bordering people, if they kill someone, they eat him. And so, Guarionex, taking refuge with this mountain chief, gave him many presents as was customary, things that the people of the mountains lack; he related that he had been treated shamefully, wickedly and violently by our men and complained that neither humility nor pride were of any use to him in dealing with our men; therefore, he was coming to him to beg him for assistance and ask for his protection from the attacks of violent men. Maiobanex promised all the help, protection and defense he could offer against the Christians. The *Adelantado*, then, left for Concepción; he summoned Roldán Jiménez, who was living as a guest twelve miles away in the villages of the islanders, together with his followers. He asked him what those revolts meant to him. And Roldán, with a frown on his face, answered, "Your brother, the Admiral, is dead. We realize that our concerns matter very little to our Sovereigns; as long as we follow you, we die of hunger, we are forced to look for meager sustenance throughout the island; besides, the Admiral has placed us both in charge of the island. Therefore, we have no intention of obeying you any longer." Roldán said these and other things. The *Adelantado*, however, could not lay his hands on him, although he wished to. Roldán actually fled and 70 men followed him; with them, he took refuge in the western region of *Xaragua* and there, as now the Admiral and his brother testify, without any restraint they began to commit rapes, robberies and murders. In the meantime, while these things were taking place on the island, eight vessels were finally given by the Sovereigns to the Admiral, who first sent two of them to his brother the *Adelantado*, with food and supplies, directly from Cádiz Hercules. These two vessels by chance arrived first in that western part of the island in which Roldán Jiménez lived with his companions. Roldán lured them by promising breasts of young girls to touch instead

trem, in dies expectans, versaretur, Praefectus frater ex Hispanis littoribus, cum reliquis navigiis, discedit, sed non itinere
recto ad Hispaniolam: vertit enim se ad meridiem. Qua navigatione quid sit operatus, quas maris ac terrarum oras pera-
graverit, quid, novos tractus detegens, invenerit, prius enarremus. Harum enim seditionum et tumultuum eventum in se-
quentis libri calce late referemus. Vale!

of hoes, pleasure instead of toil, plenty instead of famine, rest instead of weariness and watches. Meanwhile, Guarionex, after assembling a band of friends, came down repeatedly to the plain, slew several natives who were friends of our men and whatever Christians they found, ravaging fields, ripping out plantings and destroying villages. Roldán and his followers, although knowing now the Admiral would come soon, were not at all afraid since they had won over the new men sent ahead with the two vessels. While the poor *Adelantado*, floundering amid these waves, was waiting for his brother day by day, the Admiral left with the remaining vessels from the coast of Spain, but not directly for Hispaniola, really heading South. First, let us tell what he accomplished during this voyage, what shores and land he explored, and what he found when he discovered new lands. At the end of the next book we will certainly report fully on the outcome of these rebellions and tumults. Fare well!

I 6: ad cardinalem Ludovicum, nostri Regis nepotem

Ex oppido Barrameda, Baetis ostio, a Gadibus parum
distanti, cum octo navibus onustis tertio Kalendas Iunii anni
octavi et nonagesimi, Colonus dat vela assuetumque iter suum
per Fortunatas, ob piratas quosdam Gallos, qui ut illum adori-
5 rentur in itinere recto operiebantur, detorsit. Ad Fortunatas
ituris, ad milliare vigesimum et septingentesimum laevorsum,
Madera occurrit insula, quae australior Hispali est quattuor
gradibus. Elevatur enim Hispali polus arcticus gradus sex et
triginta, huic autem insulae, uti nautae referunt, duo et triginta.
10 Maderam igitur primum adnavigavit. Inde, missis ad Hispaniolam, itinere recto, navibus reliquis commeatus vehentibus,
cum una navi caveata et duabus mercatoriis caravelis australis
plagae iter aggressus est, lineam petiturus aequinoctialem, deinde ut eius, occidentem sequens, locorum quae reperiret natu-
15 ram, Hispaniola ad septentrionem dextrorsum relicta, vestigaret.
Iacent in eo discursu mediae Hesperides, Portugalensium insulae terdecim, praeter unam inhabitatae, quae *Caput Viride* ap-
pellantur. Hae sunt interiori Aethiopiae e regione ad occidentem duorum, tantum dierum navigatione vicinae. Ex his vocant
20 Portugalenses unam *Bonavistam*: cuius testudinibus multi, quotannis, leprosi sua labe mundantur. Inde cum esset ibi aer
contagiosus, subito discedens ad Africum, qui medius est inter
austrum et favonium, millia passuum quadrigenta et triginta
navigavit. Ibi malachiis et ardoribus (nam erat is Iunius mensis)
25 adeo, ut ait, oppressus fuit ut fere navigia ihi incenderentur;
cadorum circuli crepebant et rumpebantur, aqua dispergebatur,
homines eos aestus sufferre nequibant: elevabatur enim eis, ut
ipse rettulit, ab horizonte polus gradus quinque tantum. Octo
dierum, quibus ea perpessus est, primus fuit serenus, reliqui
30 nubili ac pluviosi, nec eo minus fervidi; quare saepius adisse
non mediocriter poenituit. Actis in eo discrimine et angustia
his octo diebus, Vulturnus ihis flatu secundo exoritur; quem
ventum secutus recta ad occidentem eius paralleli, aliam stella-
rum faciem aliamque aeris gratiam ait Praefectus se reperisse:
35 nam in tertium inde diem temperiem se amoenissimam sensisse
inquiunt omnes. Asseverat enim Praefectus se a malachiis et
ardoribus semper ascendisse per maris dorsum, veluti per altum

I 6: To Cardinal Ludovico, Nephew of our King

From the city of Barrameda, located at the mouth of the Guadalquivir, not too distant from Cádiz, Columbus left with eight loaded ships on May 30, 1498 and deviated from his Fortunate Isles usual route because of some French pirates who were coming directly at him to attack. Those heading for the Fortunate Isles, 720 miles to the left, they will find the island of Madeira, 4° S of Seville. Seville is actually 36° from the pole star whereas Madeira as sailors report, is at 32°. From here, he sent directly to Hispaniola the provision-carrying ships but he, with a square-rigged ship and two merchant caravels, chose the southern route up to the equinoctial line, to then proceed West and investigate along that route the nature of the places he would find after leaving Hispaniola to the North, on the right side. Half way along that route lie the *Hesperides*, thirteen Portuguese islands, which are called *Cape Verde*, all of them inhabited except one. They are hardly two days' sail from the interior of Ethiopia and the region to the west. The Portuguese call one of them 'Bonavista:' every year many lepers are cured there of their sores by its turtles. Because the air was contagious, Columbus, left right away, sailed south-west for 430 miles with the *Africo* wind which is between the South [Austro] and West [Favonius] winds. Here, as he says, he was so overwhelmed by the calms and the heat (for it was precisely the month of June) that the ships almost caught fire; the staves of the barrels were cracking and breaking, the water lost and the men could no longer bear that heat: as a matter of fact, we are given to understand from him that the pole star was above them only 5° over the horizon. The first of those eight days, during which he had to tolerate this, it was clear; the other days were cloudy and rainy, but not any less hot; therefore, he often much regretted having travelled through those places. When these eight days, spent in such hardships and difficulties, were over, the South-West wind rose, blowing favorably for them; following this wind due West of the parallel, the Admiral said that he had found a new arrangement of the stars and a much milder climate, consequently they all agree that, due to this, in two days they came to enjoy the

montem coelum versus ascenditur; nec tamen adhuc in omni prospectu terram ullam viderat. E cavea tandem grandioris navis, pridie Kalendas Iuhi, nauta quidam speculator tres montes altissimos, sublatis prae laeticia ad coelum vocibus, se conspicere proclamat; ne frangantur animo [33] hortatur: moesti enim erant, tum adusti solis ardoribus, tum quoniam aqua illis deficiebat, cum cadi, qui prae nimio calore concrepuerant, aquam per scissuras evomuissent. Laeti ergo adeunt. Attamen, ubi primum terram attigerunt, eo quod ibi esset mare vadosum, quamvis portum a longe viderint alias satis commodum, non potuerunt terram capere. Habitatam esse regionem et bene cultam perpenderunt e navibus: namque cultissimos hortos et amoena viridaria vident, ex quorum herbis et arboribus matutini rores ad eos suaves efflabant odores. Ad vigesimum inde lapidem in portum incidit recipiendis navibus satis aptum, sed nullus in eum amnis decurrebat. Procedens igitur, reperit tandem portum reparandis navibus aptum et aqua et lignis sumendis accomodatum, *Arenalis Puntam* hanc terram vocat. Vicina portui domicilia nulla reperere, sed innumera quorundam animalium vestigia, veluti caprina, invenerunt; de quorum genere unum videre mortuum, ut aiunt, quasi capreae simile. Altero die canoam a longe venientem prospiciunt, qua viginti quattuor homines vehebantur, iuvenes omnes elegantes et procerae staturae, scutis praeter arcus et sagittas, ultra morem aliorum, armati, capillis oblongis, planis et, quasi more Hispano, scissis in fronte; pudibunda vitta gossampina variis coloribus intexta [34] tegebant, caeterum nudi. Tunc vero terram illam reliquis eius paralleli regionibus coelo proximiorem esse et a crassis convallium ac paludum vaporibus remotiorem credidit, quanto altorum montium a profundis vallibus suprema culmina recedunt. Quoniam se ab Aethiopiae parallelis nunquam exiisse in tota ea navigatione pertinaciter Almirantus affirmat tantaque sit in utriusque terrae incolis, continentis, scilicet Aethiopiae et insularum, naturae varietas (Aethiopes enim nigri, crispi, lanati, non autem capillati; hi vero albi capillis oblongis, protentis, flavis), unde discrimen hoc tantum oriri possit, alias non video. Terrae igitur dispositio, non coelorum flatus eam causantur

---

[33] See Cic. *Phil.* II 15.
[34] See *rhet. ad Her.* IV 60.

most beautiful weather. The Admiral claims to have overcome the calms and torrid heat on the sea surface, in much the same way one climbs up to heaven through a lofty mountain; however, he had not yet sighted land anywhere. Finally, on 30 June, from atop the crow's nest of the larger ship a sailor on watch cryed out with joy he had sighted three very lofty mountains: the Admiral then exhorted them not to lose courage; they were readly sad, being exhausted by the burning heat of the sun and because they had no water: it had leaked after the barrels cracked due to the excessive heat. And so they were happy on approach. Just as soon as they got near the shore, they realized there was no landing place because of shallows; yet from far away they could see in another place a rather convenient port. From the ship they saw an inhabited land, well-cultivated; indeed, they saw very well-tended gardens and delightful orchards: everything was covered by morning dew and pleasant perfumes exhaled toward them. Twenty miles from there, they ran into a port wide enough to take in the ships, but no water course flowed into it. So, continuing his voyage, he finally found a port suitable for sheltering the ships and obtaining water and wood: he called this *Punta del Arenal*. He could not find any dwellings near the harbor, only innumerable tracks of unidentified animals, perhaps goats; they saw a dead one, they say, which looked like a goat. The following day they saw a canoe with twentyfour rowers coming from far away. They were all young and well-kept, tall, armed differently than the other islanders with shields in addition to bows and arrows, and they wore their hair long, smooth and parted on their forehead, almost in a Spanish fashion. Their loins were covered with a multicolored cotton cloth, with the rest of the body naked. Columbus really thought, at the time, that this land was closer to the sky than all other regions on that parallel and much farther removed from the dense steam rising from valleys and swamps than loftiest mountains are from deep valleys because the Admiral firmly claims that he never deviated from the parallels of Ethiopia during that crossing, and yet, the natural difference between the inhabitants of one land and the other — that is, of the continent of Ethiopia and these islands — was so great (Ethiopians are black, hairy, with curly hair but not long whereas these are white, with long, smooth, blond hair), that he could not fathom where

varietatem. Scimus in torridae zonae montibus nives cadere durareque; scimus et in valde distantibus ab ea, ad septentrionem, urgeri magno calore habitatores. Iuvenes obvios ut alliceret, Praefectus specula, vasa aenea, tersa, lucida, tintinnabula aliaque eiuscemodi, ignota illis, ostendi iussit. Illi autem, quo magis vocabantur, tanto magis fraudem inesse et strui timentes retrocedebant, cum summa tamen admiratione nostros et eorum res ac navigia, fixis oculis, intuentes, remis semper innixi. Videns Praefectus muneribus illos adduci non posse, iussit e cavea grandioris navis tympana tibiasque pulsari cantarique inferius ac instrui choreas, cantus et insoliti sonitus dulcedine illos posse vinci existimans. Iuvenes autem ad certamen canere nostros e caveis arbitrati, citius ictu oculi, relictis remis, sagittas arcubus scuta brachiis aptarunt cuspidibusque in nostros directis, quid sibi vellent hi sonitus parati operiebantur. Nostri e converso, paratis sagittis, ad illos paulatim movent; illi vero a navi praetoria discedentes, dexteritate remorum freti, unam ex minoribus adeunt adeoque illi adhaeserunt ut navis gubernatori sagulum cuidam primario pileumque alteri e puppi porrigere licuerit. Per signa ut eius navis gubernator in littus descendat, ibi invicem collocuturi, ut aptius poterunt, data fide conveniunt. Sed cum ipsum navis gubernatorem ad praetoriam navim, veniam colloquii petitum, accedere conspexerunt, insidias veriti, statim in canoam prosiliunt auraque velocius advolarunt. Non longo ab ea insula spacio, semper ad occidentem, Praefectus se fluxum aquae rabidum ab oriente in occidentem atque adeo impetuosum reperisse ait ut nihilo torrenti vasto, ex altis montibus decidenti, cederet. Ibi se, ex quo navigare a teneris[35] coepit, nusquam tantum formidasse fatetur. Ulterius aliquantulum per id discrimen procedens, fauces reperit quasdam octo mihiarum, veluti alicuius maximi portus introitum, ad quas aquarum ille defluxus ruebat; *Os draconis* fauces appellavit et insulam ori oppositam *Margaritam*. Ex faucibus autem non minor impetus aquarum dulcium, venientibus salsis occurrens, egredi conabatur ita quod ibi esset inter utrasque undas non leve certamen. Sinum ipsum ingressus tandem, potabiles ac suaves aquas esse cognoscit, atque aliud maius ipse Praefectus et reliqui navigationis eius comites fide digni mihi diligentius omnia, percun-

[35] See *ep*. 812 C, p. 188.

such a difference did originate. The location of the earth, then, not the climate, causes this difference. We know that on the mountains of the torrid zone the snows fall and stay a long time; we also know that in regions very distant from it, to the North, the inhabitants are overcome by great heat. In order to lure the young men who were approaching, the Admiral ordered that mirrors, clear and shiny bronze vases, bells and similar objects unknown to them be exhibited. But the greater the calling, the farther these people would pull back, fearing trick or some kind of plot, staring intently at our men, their things and the ships with the greatest admiration, but always ready at the oars. Seeing that with the gifts we could not get them to come near, the Admiral ordered that from the crow's nest of the larger ship the kettle drums and fifes be played and, below, the men should sing and dance, hoping thus that the young men might be attracted by the sweetness of songs and music never heard before. But the young men, thinking that our men were playing before battle, dropping the oars, fitted arrows to the bows more rapidly than a twinkling of an eye and, shields in their arms, were pointing to our men, ready in wait to see what those sounds meant. Our men, conversely, moved slowly toward them and readied their lances; but they, backed away from the flagship and trusting the agility of their oars, approached one of the smaller ships and came so close that the pilot of the ship from the stern was able to hand a cloak to one and to another a cap. By means of signs they agreed the pilot of that ship would go down onto the beach and they would negotiate there with fairness, as best they could. But as they saw the same pilot of the ship approach the flagship to ask for the favor of a consultation they quickly regained the canoe fearing some trick and vanished faster than the wind. The Admiral says that he found, not far away from the island, to the north, a forceful east-west current, so impetuous to resemble a large torrent falling from high mountains. He admits that since he began to sail as a child, in no place had he been more afraid than here. Proceeding a little farther, in the midst of such danger, he found a strait eight miles long, with a mouth of a very wide port, toward which the current rushed; he named this *Boca del Dragon* and the island opposite to it *Margarita*. Now, from the strait a fresh water current just as large was flowing out against the rushing salt

ctanti rettulerunt se videlicet lequas sex et viginti, hoc est millia
passuum quattuor supra centum, per semper dulces aquas ad-
navigasse; quantoque ulterius ad occidentem praecipue procederet tanto asseverat dulciores. Occurrit deinde monti altissimo
5 quem cercopithecorum, [36] ab ea parte orientali, multitudo tantum incolebat. Id latus asperum, propterea hominibus inhabi-
tatum; apud littus tamen in terram exploratum missi cultos
plaerosque satosque agros reperisse rettulerunt, gentem autem
aut casas nullas, ut ruricolae nostri saepius etiam a villis aut
10 stationibus, quas incolunt, seminatum longius forte proficiscun-
tur. In montis eius occidentali latere latam agnoscunt iacere
planitiem, hanc laeti adeunt, iaciunt anchoras in lato flumine.
Cum primum indigenae gentem ad eorum littora novam appulsam esse cognoscent, certatim visendi studio, sine ullo metu,
15 ad nostros festinant; a quibus per signa *Pariam* vocari terram
illam, quam maxima esset et quanto ulterius ad occidentem
tanto populosiorem collegerunt. Quattuor igitur hominibus ex
eius terrae incolis in navem suam sumptis, occidentale latus
prosequitur. Ex aeris temperie, ex amoenitate terrae, ex popu-
20 lorum amplitudine quibus in dies magis ac magis inter navigandum occurrebant quod regio illa magni aliquid portenderet
omnes recensent neque illos sua fefellit opinio, uti suo loco
videbimus. Sole nondum exorto, surgere tamen iam volente,
quodam die locorum suavitate allecti (sentiebant enim ex terrae
25 viretis gratissimos odores afflari), terram captant. Ibi numero-
siorem, quam alibi usquam, incolarum multitudinem esse perpenderunt. Statimque nostris propius se applicantibus, eius
terrae cacichi nomine, nuncii ad Praefectum mittuntur: se suaque omnia, hilari fronte, per signa et nutus, offerendo, a Prae-
30 fecto ut in terram descenderet nec quicquam vereretur petunt.
Renuente Praefecto, ecce visendi studio, cum eorum cymbis,
innumeri ad naves confluunt, colla lacertosque maiori ex parte
auro et unionibus Indicis torquati armillatique atque id adeo
populariter gestabant ut ex vitro non maiora calculorum serta
35 foeminae nostrates ferant. Ubinam illa quae gerebant legerentur
interrogati, proprium littus digito monstrabant, manuumque
ac labiorum torsione et motu uniones apud se non magnifieri
signifcare videbantur, immo et, canistris manu captis, posse

---

[36] See Plin. *nat. hist.* VIII 72; Varro *ap.* Non. 296, 26 L.; Mart. XIV 128, 202;
Iuv. XV 4.

water, making for a great clash of the two currents. Finally, once he entered the bay, he realized that the water was potable and palatable. The Admiral himself and his traveling companions told me, when I was diligently collecting information on everything, another more important detail, that is, that he sailed for 26 leagues, or 104 miles, always in fresh waters; he claims that the farther west he proceeded, the fresher was the water. Then he found a very lofty mountain where, on its eastern part, lived only a multitude of long-tailed *monkeys*. That slope was rugged, therefore not inhabited; however, those who had been sent ashore to explore reported finding several cultivated fields, clearly sown but no people or huts, just as our farmers rather frequently leave their homes, where they live, to go and sow elsewhere. On the western slope of that mountain they saw a large plain; they happily approached and dropped anchor in a large river. When the natives realized that new people had landed, they fearlessly raced one another and came to observe our men; from the gesturing natives they found out that this quite vast land was called *Paria* and that the farther West it extended the more populated it was. So, having taken on board his ship four men from among the inhabitants of that land, he proceeded along the western side. From the climate, the charm of the land and the large population they found during the voyage, each day greater, they all concluded that the region portended great surprises, and their opinion did not deceive them, as we will see at the right time. One day, just before dawn, with the sunrise minutes away, they landed, enticed by the pleasantness of the place sensing the presence of most agreeable perfumes (coming from the verdant meadows of that region). They felt that larger crowds of people than at other places liked them. As our men approached, messengers were sent in no time to the Admiral on behalf of the cacique of that land, cheerfully requesting the Admiral, through signs and gestures, while offering themselves along with all they had, to come ashore and not to fear anything. When the Admiral refused, they crowded our ships with their boats, wishing to see the Spaniards. These natives wore necklaces and bracelets on their arms and necks, mostly made of gold and Indian pearls, and more used to wearing these than our women with glass beads. Indeed, asked where they had found the things they wore, they pointed to their beach and, with movements

317

21

ibi, si apud eos versari vellent, canistratim colligi insinuare
videbantur. Sed, quoniam frumenta quae vehebat ad Hispaniolam fere iam sale corrumperentur, differre id commercium in
accomodatius tempus statuit. Duas tamen ex servitoriis cymbis
ad terram hominibus onustas misit, qui de unionibus aliqua
serta, per rerum nostrarum permutationem referrent et de locorum ac hominum natura quaecunque possent scrutarentur.
Illi nostros adeuntes hilares et animo laeto suscipiunt; mirus
ad nostros tanquam ad portentum aliquod erat numerus con-
fluentium. Duoque viri graves nostris primum obvii, quos
reliqua turba sequebatur, prodeunt grandaevus alter, alter iunior. Patrem et filium successurum autumant fuisse. Salutatio-
nibus utrinque peractis, in domum quandam sphaericam, cui
magna platea adiacet, nostros adducunt. Ex ligno nigerrimo
arte mira laborato, sedilia feruntur multa. Postquam nostri et
eorum primates assederunt, ecce veniunt ministri, dapibus alii,
alii vino onusti; sed eorum cibi fructus tantum, varii tamen
generis, nostris penitus ignoti. Vina vero, tam alba quam ru-
bentia, non ex uvis, sed ex diversis fructibus compressa, non
iniucunda tamen. Sumptis apud seniorem cibis, iunior illos
ducit in tabernaculum suum. Viri foeminaeque astabant plures,
sed ubique viri semper a foeminis separati. Utriusque sexus
indigenae, albi veluti nostrates, praeter eos qui sub sole ver-
santur, mites, hospitales, pudenda gossampino velamine variis
coloribus intexto contegunt, caetera nudi. Nemo aderat qui non
esset unionibus et auro aut torquatus aut armillatus; multi
utrunque, sed uti vitreos nostri rurales calculos, ferunt. Interrogati ubinam aurum illud quod gestabant gigneretur, digito
signabant e regione in quibusdam montibus, sed nostris, tanquam minitantes, accessum dissuadere videbantur. Comedi enim
illis homines gestu manibusque innuebant, sed an a Canibalibus
dicerent an a feris silvestribus non bene perceperunt. Quod
nostros intelligere a nostrisque intelligi nequirent ingenti molestia afficiebantur. His, qui missi fuerant, hora tertia post
meridiem, cum quibusdam unionum sertis ad naves redeunti-
bus, anchoras elevant; neque propter frumenta, uti ipse ait,
quae vehebat diutius moratus est animo, tamen, compositis
rebus Hispaniolae, intra paucos dies redeundi; sed tanti prae-
mium inventi surripuit alter. Institit et eius pelagi profunditas
modica aquarumve cursus praecipites qui, assiduis conflictibus
grandiorem navem, si vis ventorum aliqua surgebat, conquas-

and gestures of the hands and lips, seemed to want to say that the pearls were not valued very much by them, and, more than that, after taking some baskets in their hands, seemed to let the Spaniards know that, if they wanted to stay with them, they could pick pearls by the bucket. But, since the wheat, which he was taking to Hispaniola, was about to spoil from the salt water, he decided to postpone that business to a more opportune time. Nevertheless, he sent ashore two life boats loaded with men that might bring back some pearl necklaces in exchange for some of our objects and also investigate as much as possible the surroundings and their inhabitants. Cheerfully and all excited these natives welcomed our approaching men; extraordinary was the number of those who came near our men, as if to witness some wonder. Two majestic-looking men approached first, one older than the other, and the rest of the people behind. Our men thought they might be the father and the son destined to succeed him. Once some greetings had been exchanged from both sides, they accompanied our men inside a round house near a large square. They brought many seats made with very black wood, remarkably decorated. After our leaders and their chiefs were seated, the servants came, either loaded with food or with wine; but such food consisted only of fruits, although of different kinds, completely unknown to us. In truth, the wines, both white and red, made not from grapes but from various fruits, were not bad tasting. After the food was consumed at the house of the older chief, the younger one took them into his tent. There were several men and women there, but everywhere the men were always separated from the women. The natives of both sexes were white like us, except those constantly exposed to the sun; they are mild, hospitable and nude but for their loins covered with a multicolor cotton cloth. Not a single person stood there without a necklace or a pearl bracelet or some kind of gold ornament; many wear both, just as our peasants do with glass beads. Asked where that gold they were wearing had come from, they pointed out a region in the middle of some mountains, but they seemed to discourage our men in an almost threatening manner from going there. In fact, with hand gestures they made our people understand that men there had been eaten, but they could not understand well if they said by cannibals or by wild beasts. Their disappointment for not being able to

sabant. Ad evitanda vadorum discrimina, leviorem ex caravelis,
quae brevi fundo contenta erat, tanquam exploratricem, plum-
batis fundi altitudinem tentantem semper permittebat; sequebantur aliae. *Cumana* et *Manacapana* in vasta Pariae provincia,
dicebantur ab incolis illae regiunculae, in spacio milliarium
ducentorum triginta; quibus altera regio distat lequas sexaginta,
nomine *Curiana*. Cum autem longum ita maris tractum percur-
risset, putans assidue insulam esse dubitansque posse per occidentem se ad septentrionem, ut ad Hispaniolam iter caperet,
exolvere, in fluvium incidit profunditatis triginta cubitorum,
latitudinis vero inaudita: ait enim octo et viginti lequarum
fuisse. Paulo autem ulterius, ad occidentem tamen semper, sed
meridionalius aliquantisper, cum ita littorum se flectentium
ratio exigeret, mare herbidum ingressus est: supernatans herbarum semen lentisci bactras aemulabatur; quare herbarum
densitas ne bene fluerent navigia impediebant. Ibi Praefectus
refert diem esse nullum toto anno multo longiorem aut bre-
viorem altero; arcticum polum in ea regione quinque tantum
gradus, sicuti Pariae, disputat elevari, in cuius tractu haec omnia
littora iacent; de poli etiam varietate quaedam refert: quae
quoniam contra omnium astronomorum sententiam prolata
mihi videntur, sicco pertingam pede. Compertum est, illustrissime Princeps, polarem illam stellam, quam nautae nostri *Tra-*
montanam vocant, non esse arctici poli punctum, super quo
coelorum axis vertatur; quod facile dignoscitur si, stellis primum apparentibus, per angustum aliquod foramen stellam
ipsam conspexeris eandemque si, ultima vigilia aurora illas
fugante, per idem foramen conspicies, locum mutasse compe-
ries. Sed quomodo fieri possit ut, primo noctis crepusculo, in
ea regione quinque tantum gradus, tempore Iunii, elevetur,
stellis autem discedentibus, obvenientes solares radios, sumpto
eodem quadrante, quindecim non intelligo; nec rationes quas
ipse adducit mihi plane nec ulla ex parte satisfaciunt. Inquit
enim se orbem terrarum non esse sphaericum coniectasse, sed
in sui rotunditate tumulum quendam eductum, quum crearetur,
fuisse: ita quod non pilae aut pomi, ut alii sentiunt, sed piri,
arbori appensi, formam sumpserit, Pariamque esse regionem
quae super eminentiam illam coelo viciniorem possideat; unde
in trium illorum culmine montium, quos e cavea speculatorem
nautam a longe vidisse memoravimus, paradisum esse terre-
strem asseveranter contendit rabiemque illam aquarum dulcium

understand our men or be understood was evident. Since those who had landed had returned to the ships with some necklaces, the anchors were lifted at three o' clock in the afternoon. The Admiral did not delay any longer because of the provisions he carried, as he says, intending, however, to return in a few days after taking care of the problems at Hispaniola. But someone else (P. Alonso Niño) took from him the prize of such a great discovery. The shallows were a great threat to him, as well as the impetuous watercourses, which, combined with a strong wind, would repeatedly affect the larger ship. In order to avoid the dangers of shallow waters, he kept sending ahead the lighter of the caravels, which had little draught, so as to sound and explore the depth of the bottom; the others followed. Those small regions in the vast province of *Paria* were called by the inhabitants *Cumaná* and *Manacapana*, 230 miles away; the other region, named *Curiana*, is 60 more leagues beyond them. But, after having traveled across so much sea, continually thinking that the land was an island and doubting they would be able to reach North by going West in order to head toward Hispaniola, he encountered a river 30 cubits deep and of un-heard-of width: they indeed claim it was 28 leagues wide. However, a little farther on, still going West, but a little more to the South, since the bending coast line required that they curve, the Admiral entered into a sea of weeds. The floating seed of this weed looked like the berries of the lentisc, with its thickness preventing the swift progress of the vessels. The Admiral reports that here throughout the whole year there is not one day much longer or shorter than another; he claims that in this region, where all these shores are, the pole star rises only by five degrees, as in *Paria*. He ados as well some details on the nature of the pole: since his reasoning seems to go against the opinion of all the astronomers, I will relate it without compromising myself. It is well known, illustrious Prince, that the pole star, which our sailors call *Tramontana*, is not the pole's rotating point of the axis of the heavens. That is easily realized if one looked at the same star through a small opening at its first rising and then again later, through the same opening but in the last part of the night, when dawn puts the stars to flight; at that point one realizes that the star has moved. Yet, I cannot understand why, at twilight in that region, the star rises only by five degrees in the month of

de sinu et faucibus praedictis exire obviam maris fluxui venienti conantem, esse aquarum ex ipsis montium culminibus in praeceps descendentium. De his satis, quum fabulosa mihi videantur. Ad historiam a qua digressi sumus, revertamur! Cum se, praeter optatum, tam vasto sinu implicitum cerneret nec iam reperiendi ad septentrionem exitum, quo ad Hispaniolam vertere proras posset, spem ullam haberet, eadem qua profectus fuerat regreditur iterque suum, per septentrionem eius terrae, ab oriente ad Hispaniolam capit. Hanc qui postmodum accuratius, utilitatis causa, investigarunt continentem esse Indicum volunt, non autem Cubam, uti Praefectus; neque enim desunt qui se circuisse Cubam audeant dicere. An haec ita sint an invidia tanti inventi occasiones quaerant in hunc virum, non diiudico, tempus loquetur in quo verus iudex invigilat. Sed quod Paria sit vel non sit continens, Praefectus non contendit: continentem ipse arbitratur; Pariam, autem, esse Hispaniola octingentis octoginta duobus millibus passuum australiorem Praefectus refert. Ad Hispaniolam tandem, visendorum militum, quos ibi cum frattibus reliquerat tertio Kalendas Septembris octavi et nonagesimi cupidissimus, tetendit. Sed, uti pleraque mortalium solent, inter tot secunda, dulcia, laeta absinthii semen fortuna in medium proiecit, zizaniaque omnia eius suavia commaculavit.

June, but when the stars set at sunrise, it rises by fifteen degrees, always in the same quadrant. The reasons he gives do not satisfy me fully or in all respects. Actually his conjecture implies as he says, that the world is not evenly rounded but a sphere with a protrusion since creation time which gives it the shape not of a ball or of an apple, as others believe, but that of a pear hanging on a tree, and that the *Paria* region is located on that protrusion closer to the heavens. Hence his firm claim that, at the top of those three mountains which, as we have mentioned, the watch sailor sighted from afar, the earthly paradise is found, and that the raging fresh waters from the inlet and narrow straits we talked of previously, struggling against the waves of the sea, are the ones descending from these mountaintops. We have talked enough about these things; they seem so incredible to me. Let us go back to the narrative from which we strayed. Realizing that he was enclosed by a gulf bigger than he anticipated and by now without hope of finding a way out to the North where he could direct his prow to Hispaniola, Columbus went back to the same place from which he had taken off and began his Northbound voyage going East toward Hispaniola. Those who later explored that land with greater care for purposes of exploitation claim that it is the Indian continent, not Cuba, as the Admiral claims. Indeed, there are those who dare say that they have sailed around Cuba. I do not judge if these things are true or if these men are looking for pretexts against this man out of jealousy of such a great discovery; time will speak as the only true judge. The Admiral, however, does not argue whether *Paria* is a continent or not: he believes it is a continent, and, on the other hand, reports that *Paria* is 882 miles farther South than Hispaniola. Finally, wishing very much to see the soldiers whom he had left there with his brothers, on 30 August 1498 he headed for Hispaniola. As it often occurs in human endeavors, however, in the midst of so many favorable, pleasant, happy events, fortune threw in the seed of absinth, and darnel spoiled all his satisfactions.

I 7

Veniens ad insillam Praefectus, ultra spem omnem, per-
turbata omnia in praecepsque iam labentia cuncta invenit.
Roldanus enim, qui, eo absente, a fratre discesserat, multitudine quae eum sequebatur fretus, ad Praefectum quondam
5 dominum, qui eum evexerat, non modo non venire instituit,
sed conviciis illum lacerare scribereque ad Reges de utroque
fratre nefanda incoepit. Praefectus autem ad Reges nuncios
mittit, qui de eorum defectione certiores faciat instatque simul ut militares homines ad se mittantur quibus vires eorum
10 infringere punireque pro commissis quemque valeat. Illi, de
utroque fratre graviter conquesti, iniustos, impios, Hispani
sanguinis hostes et profusores vocabant, quod levibus de
causis torquere, iugulare, obtruncare, quoquo modo perimere
delectarentur; ambitiosos, superbos, invidos, intolerabiles ty-
15 rannos esse proclamabant: propterea se ab eis tanquam a feris
sanguine gaudentibus et Regum inimicis discessisse. Perspe-
xisse enim se aiebant nil aliud ipsos moliri aut animo versare
quam de usurpando insularum imperio idque mille coniectu-
ris perpendisse argumentabantur, sed praecipue quod adire
20 aurifodinas, aurum collectum neminem, praeter familiares
suos patiebantur. Praefectus autem, e contrario, quum a Regibus auxilia, quibus debitis illos poenis posset afficere, po-
scebat homines eos esse, qui talia in se commentarentur,
omnes flagitiosos, facinorosos, lenones, fures, stupratores,
25 raptores, vagos, quibus nihil pensi, nulla ratio inesset, pe-
riuros, falsos, convictos in praetorus aut pro commissis minas
iudicum timentes, sese de medio sustulisse. Ibique violando,
rapiendo, ocio, ventri, somno, libidinibus deditos, nemini
parcere et qui ut foderent officioque calonum fungerentur
30 adducti fuerant, nunc neque stadium domo egrediuntur pedibus: ab insularibus namque miseris pensiles per totam insulam, tanquam aediles curules, feruntur. Ioci etiam gratia,
ne manus ab effundendo sanguine desuescat, ut lacertorum
vires experiantur, eductis ensibus, inter se certant super ob-
35 truncandis innocentum capitibus uno ictu et qui agilius ictu
suo caput miseri deiiciebat in terram, ille fortior honoratior-
que inter ipsos censebatur. Illi in Praefectum ea, Praefectus

I 7

The Admiral, as he came to the island, most unexpectedly found everything in disorder, actually near disaster. During his absence, Roldán, relying on those who followed him, had turned against the Admiral's brother. Now he not only decided not to follow the Admiral, who, as his previous master, had brought him there, but he also began to malign him with accusations and to write slanderously to their Majesties about both Columbus brothers. The Admiral, then, sent messengers to the Sovereigns to inform them of the rebellion and at the same time insist that soldiers be sent to break their strength and punish each of the rebels for his crimes. The rebels, complaining seriously about both brothers, called them unjust, impious, enemies of the Spanish blood, and squanderers, because they took delight in torturing over trifles, hanging, slaughtering, and killing in all kinds of ways; they depicted them as ambitious, arrogant, envious, unbearable tyrants: so they deserted them being just wild animals thirsty for blood and enemies of the Sovereigns. In addition, they claimed they had seen the brothers plot or meditate nothing but taking over the rule of the islands, as could be seen from a thousand instances, but especially from the fact that they would allow no one but their own men to reach the gold mines or gather it. On the other hand, the Admiral, when requesting help from the Sovereigns to punish the rebels for their crimes, stated that those men who wrote such accusations against him were all wicked and quarrelsome, pimps, thieves, rapists, kidnappers, outlaws, men deprived of any value or good sense, brainless perjurers, liars either with previous criminal record or escapees fearing being sentenced by judges for crimes committed; that was the reason of their desertion. And given over to violence, robberies, laziness, carousing, inactivity and pleasures, they did not spare anybody there: those originally brought to dig and provide services, now did not even walk out of the house for a stadium: as a matter of fact, they have the poor natives carry them throughout the whole island, like high-ranking magistrates. And for fun, so as not to loose their blood-shedding habit and test their strength, they draw the swords and compete

in eos haec et alia multa. Dum haec ita geruntur, ut Ciguavis populis, de quibus supra, Guarionexio duce, multa damna inferentibus obviaretur, Adelantatum fratrem cum nonaginta tantum peditibus, equitibus vero paucis mittit, tribus tamen
5 millibus insularium, qui a Ciguavis, alias acriter stimulati, inimicitias cum eis capitales exercebant, sequentibus illum. Cum igitur Adelantatus, ad cuiusdam magni fluminis ripam per eam planitiem quam supra inter Ciguavorum montium cornua et mare iacere memoravimus defluentis, exercitum
10 duxisset, exploratores hostium, in dumis quibusdam latentes comperit duos. Quorum alter in mare se praecipitans, per fluminis fauces trans fluvium ad suos evasit; alter autem, captus in nemore trans fluvium delitescere dicebat sex Ciguavorum armatorum millia, ut nostros transeuntes incautos ado-
15 riantur. Quam ob rem Adelantatus adversa ripa, vadum quo traiiceret quaeritans, ascendit. Vado tandem reperto, in lata planitie intraiicere volentes nostros, emissis uno spiritu horrendis clamoribus, e silvis Ciguavi, facto agmine, aspectu foedo ac formidoloso prosiliunt. Prodeunt ita Maroniani
20 Agathyrsi[37], picti omnes et aspersi maculis. Nigro enim coccineoque, coloribus quos ex quibusdam fructibus piro similibus ex hortis ad id summo studio enutritis legunt, sese a fronte ad genua usque depingunt, crinibus mille modis compactis quos nigros longosque arte, si natura negat, nu-
25 triunt. Lemures[38] e Tartareis speluncis prosilire videbantur, nostris fluvium superare adnitentibus sagittarum ac missilium, sudium, iactu transitum prohibentes obviam prodeunt. Tanta erat telorum multitudo quae solem fere illi demeret, et, nisi scutati in se ictus recepissent, male actum fuisset. Adelanta-
30 tus, vulneratis utrinque in eo certamine non paucis, traiecit

---

[37] A Thracian tribe living in Banat [Hungary] and Transylvania. The peculiarity of their costumes (flashy tattoos on their body) was described by Herodotus (Her. IV 48, 78, 100, 102, 104, 125). See also Virg. *Aen.* IV 146; Mela II 10 (*ora artusque pingunt*). According to other sources (Plin. *nat. hist.* IV 88; Solin. 15, 3), the term *picti* often used to identify them, would be a reference to their tinted hair.

[38] In supersticious Ancient Rome lemures were the ghosts of the dead of a family, floating specters. Lemuralia was the annual city festival observed in May to placate them.

with each other in cutting off the heads of those innocent people with one blow; the man who would more swiftly decapitate an unfortunate native in a single blow was declared the strongest and more worthy of honor among them. They formulate accusations against the Admiral, and the Admiral makes these and many others against them. While these events took place, in order to oppose the people of Ciguava, of whom we spoke earlier, and who, under the command of Guarionex, caused many problems, the Admiral sent his brother, the *Adelantado*, with only 900 foot-soldiers and few cavalrymen, accompanied, however, by 3,000 natives who, having been violently provoked by the Ciguani before, had a deep hatred for them. Therefore, the *Adelantado*, after leading the army to the banks of a large river that flowed through the plain and, as we mentioned earlier, located between the mountaintops of the Ciguani and the sea, found out that two enemy scouts were hiding in the bushes. One of them, diving into the sea and crossing the stream through the mouth of the river, was able to escape to his people; the other one, instead, once captured, said that in the woods across the river 6,000 armed Ciguani were hiding ready to attack our men when they crossed with little caution. Therefore, the *Adelantado* climbed on the opposite bank looking for a ford they could take. Finally, when a passage was found and our men wanted to cross in the vast plain, the Ciguani yelling in unison terrifying screams, jumped from the woods in tight formation, with a disgusting and terrifying look reminiscent of Virgil's Agathyrsi, all made up and covered with blobs of color. Indeed, the Ciguani paint themselves from head to knees in black and scarlet dies, which they extract from certain fruits, similar to our pears, cultivated in orchards with the greatest care for this purpose; they also fix their hair in a thousand ways if it is not so naturally, since they like it long and black. They resembled ghosts out of some hellish caves; they resisted our men, who were trying to cross the river, impeding their passage with the throwing of arrows, darts and sticks. The number of arrows was so great that it almost obscured the sun: and had they not shielded themselves they would have ended up badly. The *Adelantado*, after scores of men had been wounded on both sides in that battle, finally made it through; the enemies fled with our men in pursuit, but killing few, for they have greater strength in their feet.

tandem; fugiunt hostes, insequuntur nostri, perimunt, paucos tamen: valent enim pedibus maiorem in modum. Ad silvas se illico recipiunt ex quibus tuto nostros accedentes arcubus conficiebant: ipsi enim nudi per vepres et dumos et arbusta,
5 uti apri, sine ullo obiice, silvis assueti, prolabuntur; nostris autem scuta, vestes, longae hastae, locorum imperitia, intra dumos officiunt. Quare, quum frustra ibi pernoctasset, posteroque die neminem in silvis moveri sentiret, insularium qui Ciguavos veteri odio prosequebantur consilio et ductu,
10 ad montes, in quibus Maiobanexius rex Capronum vicum regiam habebat proficiscitur; ad milliareque duodecimum in alterius reguli vico incolis omnibus prae metu vicum deserentibus castra metatus [39] est. Duos assequuntur a quibus esse apud Maiobanexium decem regulos in Caprono eius regia
15 cum octo millibus Ciguavorum congregatos cognoverunt. Levibus incursionibus sese invicem duabus lacessunt nec procedere Adelantatus ausus est, donec regionem diligentius exploraret. Nocte sequenti intempesta, exploratores mittuntur, ductu insularium qui terram noverant. Ciguavi e montibus
20 nostros senserunt, ad pugnam se, uti solent, sublatis clamoribus accingunt neque tamen e silvis egredi audent, Adelantatum cum omni exercitu adesse existimantes. Altero die, Adelantato exercitum ad eos ducente, bis fortunam belli, e silvis pugnando prosilientes, tentarunt. Impetu maximo in
25 nostros ruunt, vulnerant plerosque priusquam scutis se tegere licuerit. Profligant illos, insequuntur, perimunt, capiunt multos. Ad silvas non ulterius egressuri revertuntur. Ex captis unum cum altero insulari ex amicis ad Maiobanexium cum mandatis huiuscemodi mittit: "Non ut tibi, o Maiobanexi,
30 aut incolis tuis bellum inferret, exercitum duxit Adelantatus; amicitiam enim tuam exoptat, sed efflagitat ut Guarionexius, qui ad te confugit tibique ut arma in maximum tuorum incommodum sumeres persuasit, commissorum poenas, deprehensus, luat; propterea hortatur monetque ut Guarionexium
35 tradas. Id si feceris, te Praefectus marinus, frater eius, in

[39] See Iord. *Get.* 277.

They took refuge in the woods and thus sheltered, would kill with their bows our men as they approached. Naked, they slipped among the bushes, thickets and shrubs, like wild boars used to underbrush, without hindrance; whereas our men's shields, clothes, long spears, and lack of knowledge of the place were obstacles in the thickets. Therefore, the *Adelantado*, spent the night there invain for the following day, realizing that nobody was moving in the woods, with the advice and guidance of the natives with him who pursued the Ciguani because of an ancient hatred, set out toward the mountains for a village called *Capronus* where king Maiobanex resided; he marched 12 miles and camped in the village of another chieftain, whose inhabitants fled the village out of fear. They captured two of them, from whom they learned that with Maiobanex at his residence in *Capronus* ten chieftains had gathered with 8,000 Ciguani. In two light raids the forces provoked each other without much consequence, with the *Adelantado* not daring advance before he had explored the region with greater care. During the next, gloomy night, explorers were sent out guided by natives who knew the territory. The Ciguani, who in the mountains became aware of our men, got ready to fight and shouting, as is their custom, but did not dare leave the woods, thinking the *Adelantado* was present with a full army. The following day, while the *Adelantado* was leading the army against them, they twice tried their luck in battle by coming out of the woods to fight. With the greatest vehemence they rushed against our men and wounded several before those men could protect themselves with shields. Yet, our men defeated them: they pursued, killed and captured many. The Ciguani went back to the woods resolved not to come out. The *Adelantado* sent a native friend of his with one of the prisoners to Maiobanex carrying this message: "Maiobanex, the *Adelantado* did not lead an army in order to make war with you or your subjects; indeed, he desires your friendship, but he asks that Guarionex, who has taken refuge with you and has persuaded you to take up arms with very great harm to your men, be apprehended and pay for the crimes he has committed; therefore, he exhorts and warns you to turn Guarionex in. If you do so, the Admiral, his brother, will accept you as a friend and will respect and defend your vast territory. If, however, you refuse, he will toil to make sure you regret your action.

amicitiam admittet et tuorum regnorum amplitudinem integram servabit ac tutabitur. Sin facere recusaveris, dabitur opera ut te facti poeniteat. Regni enim quicquid tibi est ferro ignique vastabitur, omnia diripientur". Maiobanexius autem,
5 propositione intellecta, illis respondit: "Guarionexium virum bonum esse omnique virtute praeditum neminem latet, propterea auxilio praesidioque dignum illum esse iudico". Ipsos autem violentos et malos homines, qui aliena tanto opere expetant, qui sanguinem innocentum semper exoptent; nolle
10 se cum sceleratis hominibus commercia aut amicitiam inire. His auditis, Adelantatus vicum, ubi castra metabatur, aliosque vicinos complures cremari iussit. Maiobanexioque propior factus, iterum nuncios mittit qui cum eo agant ut ex familiaribus intimis aliquem ad se venire iubeat, quocum possit
15 de pace tractare. Charissimum quendam ex primoribus, duobus aliis illum comitantibus, rex ire imperat. Huic Adelantatus proponit suadetque ac monet ne floridum eius regnum Maiobanexius diripi pro Guarionexio patiatur. Ut tradat illum hortatur, nisi perditum iri se suaque omnia simul et incolas
20 in praedam abduci mallet. Nuncio redeunte, populum Maiobanexius convocat, quae acta sint praeponit. Populus autem tradi debere Guarionexium proclamat detestarique et execrari diem, quo Guarionexius turbatum eorum quietem venerat, incipiunt. Maiobanexius autem Guarionexium virum esse bo-
25 num et de se benemeritum, quod regia illi dona, cum ad eum veniret, multa praebuisset uxoremque suam et ipsum chorizare[40] tribudiareque docuisse, quod non parvi faciebat, sibique curae esse respondit; propterea se, nullo pacto, eum, quandoquidem ad se configerat et ipse tutandi fidem dederat
30 deserturum. Malleque se extrema omnia cum eo perpeti quam obloquendi causam, quod hospitem tradiderit detractoribus praebere. Ita, populo suspiriis anhelante dimisso, Guarionexium ad se vocat, omnem opem denuo pollicetur: velle se fortunam omnem, quoat vixerit, cum eo expectare neque ad
35 Adelantatum quicquam referendum censet, immo et eum qui

---

[40] See p. 290 n. 29.

Whatever territory you have will be devastated with arms and fire; everything will be destroyed." Maiobanex, once he understood the message, replied this way: "Everyone knows that Guarionex is a good man, endowed with every virtue and so I deem him worthy of help and protection." They, on the other hand are violent and wicked men, avidly seeking what belongs to others always going after the blood of innocent people, and so he does not seek business connections or friendship with wicked people. After hearing those words, the *Adelantado* ordered the village, where he was camped, and many others nearby to be burned. And as he got closer to Maiobanex, sent messengers again to request that he would order one of his close staff to come to him and negotiate peace. The king bid one of his more important people, a dear friend, to go, accompanied by two others. The *Adelantado* presented his proposal to them advising and warning Maiobanex not to let his prosperous kingdom be destroyed for the sake of Guarionex. He urged him to turn him in, unless he preferred to be killed and to have all his goods and inhabitants taken as booty. When his messengers returned, Maiobanex assembled the people so they may hear the proposed conditions. The people proclaimed that Guarionex ought to be turned in, and they began to hate and curse the day when Guarionex had come to disturb their peace. Maiobanex, however, answered that Guarionex was a good man and deserving of his gratitude because, when he came to him, he had offered him many gifts worthy of a king and he had taught him and his wife how to dance and sing, things which he did not deem of little importance and which were dear to his heart; therefore, in no way would he abandon him, since he had taken refuge with him and he had promised to defend him. He preferred to suffer with him every extreme rather than to give slanderers a reason to rebuke him for turning in his guest. And so, after dismissing the people sighing and moaning, he called in Guarionex and once more pledged him all his help: as long as he could, he wanted to share with him the events of fate and decided to ignore the *Adelantado*; moreover, he placed under trusted guard the man first sent by him and had returned with the messengers of the *Adelantado* giving orders as traditionally done to kill anyone who came and not to accept proposals from anybody. Two men sent next by the *Adelantado*, one chosen from the

primus ab eo missus fuerat in itinere, quo Adelantati nuncii
venire ad se soliti erant, cum fida custodia locat, imperans
ut venientes interimat nec cuiusquam sermones admittat. Mittuntur ab Adelantato duo, unus ex captivis Ciguavensibus,
5 ex amicis insularibus alter: obtruncantur ambo. Sequitur illos
Adelantatus cum decem tantum peditibus, equitibus quattuor,
mortuos reperit in itinere nuncios; quare iratus saevire acrius
in Maiobanexium constituit. Vadit, instructo exercitu, ad Capronum regiam. Fugiunt reguli per diversa. Imperatorem
10 Maiobanexium deserunt. Ad montes asperos Maiobanexius
cum omni familia profugit, alia vero Guarionexium, quod
tanti mali causa fuisset Ciguavi, ut eum perimerent, quaesie-
runt. Sed pedibus vitam servavit intra rupesque desertorum
montium fere solus delituit. Cum iam longo bello, vigiliisque
15 ac laboribus et fame Adelantati milites fatigarentur (agebatur enim iam tertius mensis quo inceptum fuerat), veniam
multi Petunt et ut redire ad Conceptionem liceat ubi plurimi
ex eis praedia, insulari more, habebant cultissima. Datur
commeatus, recedunt multi; triginta tantum cum Adelantato
20 comites permanent. Id trimestre bellum satis aerumnose egerunt: neque enim trimestri toto cibos ullos sunt assecuti
praeter *cazabi*, id est radicalem eorum panem (atque ex eo
raro ad saturitatem) et de utiis, id est eorum cuniculis, si
quos ipsimet cum suis canibus venando capiebant; potusque
25 eorum suaves interdum, interdum coenosae et palustres
aquae. Inter has delicias sub dio fere semper ac in perpetuo
motu: sic enim belli natura exigebat. Cum his igitur paucis
Adelantatus montana scrutari et latibula quaeritare, si qua
Maiobanexi aut Guarionexi vestigia reperiat, constituit. For-
30 te fortuna venatores quidam ipsius Adelantati, quos fames,
ubinam utias venando captare possent indagare coegerat,
cum caetera deessent, in duos Maiobanexii familiares inci-
dunt qui, ad pagos quosdam ipsius missi, panem ferebant
ab incolis datum. Hi ubinam dominus delitesceret propalare
35 coguntur. Quibus ducibus, Ciguavo more duodecim ex nostris depictis, per dolum Maiobanexius cum uxore et filiis
capitur; ad Conceptionem ad Praefectum ducuntur. Paucos
post dies Guarionexium de speluncis exire fames compulit,
quem insulares, Praefectum veriti, venatoribus quibusdam
40 prodiderunt. Praefectus ubinam versetur certior fit, peditum
turmam mittit qui ex insidiis, de plano ad montana redire

prisoners of the Ciguani, the other from his native friends: both were slain. The *Adelantado*, following them with only ten foot soldiers and four cavalrymen, found the messengers dead on the road; enraged, he decided to fight Maiobanex with greater ruthlessness. After preparing an army, he heads for *Caprone*. The chieftains fled in different directions abandoning the commander Maiobanex. Maiobanex with all his family took refuge in the rugged mountains, while the people of Ciguani went another way looking for Guarionex in order to kill him because he had been the cause of such a great evil. But he saved his life on account of his swiftness and hid himself almost alone among the cliffs of isolated mountains. Now, exhausted by the long war, the watches, hardships and hunger (now in the third month of battle) the soldiers of the *Adelantado* begged for mercy in great numbers and asked that they be allowed to go back to Concepción, where many of them, as was the custom of the natives, had plots of well-cultivated land. They were given permission to leave and many went back; only 30 companions remained with him. They had spent three months at war in rather rough circumstances: during those three months they did not have any food other than *cazabi*, that is, the bread made from cassava roots (and even so, rarely in sufficient amounts) and *utia*, that is their rabbits, when they caught them hunting with dogs; the water they drank was sometimes tasty and sometimes muddy and swampy. Among these "delights," they were almost never under cover and constantly marching, for the nature of the war so demanded. With his few men then, the *Adelantado* decided to explore the mountains and look for hiding places to see if he could find any traces of Maiobanex or Guarionex. Some of the *Adelantado's* hunters whom hunger had pushed to track down *utia* where they could, in absence of other foods, by chance ran across two of Maiobanex followers, who, having been sent to some of his villages, were carrying bread given them by the natives. These two were forced to reveal where their chief was hiding. With them as guides, after twelve of our men had tattooed themselves according to the custom of the Ciguani, Maiobanex was captured with his wife and children through trickery; they were taken to the Admiral in *Concepción*. Few days later, hunger forced Guarionex out of the caves, and the islanders, afraid of the Admiral, turned him in to some hunters.

333

22

volentem, adoriantur. Eunt, capiunt, ducunt. Ita illius regionis convicina pacata sedataque sunt omnia. Maiobanexium cognata quaedam alterius reguli, cuius regnum intactum adhuc erat, uxor in his adversis comitabatur. Eam foe-
5 minarum omnium quas natura in ea insula creavit formosissimam omnes praedicant. Hanc, quom vir ipsius ut eius forma merebatur, arderet, insanus et mentis inops, uxore capta, per deserta, quid consilii caperet ignarus, vagabatur. Ad Praefectum tandem se suaque omnia dicioni eius
10 sine ullo obiice subditurum, si uxorem redderet, promittens, venit. Uxor redditur et ex incolis primarii plures iureiurando astringuntur se imperata facturos. Sponte sua regulus hic idem incolarum quinque millia inermium cum agricultoriis instrumentis solum ducens adiit maximamque Praefecto se-
15 mentem in convallis eius amplissimae[41] fundis sua impensa cultam reliquit. A Praefecto donatus, laetus revertitur; haec fama ad Ciguavos delata regulorum animos ad clementiae spem movit. Ultro igitur veniunt, se deinceps imperata facturos fidem praestant pro rege suo et omni familia supplicant. Uxor et tota
20 domus eius regulorum rogatu liberantur, rex vinctus detinetur. Haec in insula a Praefecto, quid contra se apud Reges adversari molirentur inscio, gerebantur. Cum Reges tot querelis undique conflictati, et maxime quod ex tanta auri et aliarum rerum amplitudine parum, ob eorum discordias et seditiones afferretur,
25 gubernatorem instituunt novum qui diligenter inquirat haec omnia, sontesque deprehensos corrigat aut ad se mittat. Quid in Praefectum et eius fratrem, quidve in illos qui eis adversati sunt fuerit perquisitum non bene percipio; hoc unum scio: capitur uterque frater, in vincula omnibus bonis spoliatus,
30 coniectus ducitur, uti vides, illustrissime Princeps. Cum primum tamen Reges Gades vinctos adductos esse didicerunt utrunque, statim, per celeres tabellarios, solvi iubent utque liberi adeant permittunt, moleste se tulisse eam ipsorum iniuriam ostendentes. Novus ille gubernator ad Reges Praefecti dextera exaratas
35 ignotis characteribus scriptas litteras misisse dicitur, quibus,

---

[41] See Liv. XXVI 50; Frontin. II 11, 5.

The Admiral, informed where he was, sent a squadron of foot soldiers to ambush him, as he wanted to return from the plain to the mountains. They went, captured him and took him to the Admiral. And so all the neighboring territories of that region were returned to peace and calm. A relative of Maiobanex, the wife of another chieftain whose kingdom had remained intact up to then, accompanied him throughout these adversities. Everybody said that she was the most beautiful woman that nature had created in that island. Her husband, who loved her most passionately, as her beauty deserved, crazy and out of his own senses because his wife had been captured, was wandering through deserted places without knowing what to do. He finally came to the Admiral, promising to hand over himself and all his possessions, without any resistance, if he would give him back his wife. The wife was given back and several native chiefs took an oath to follow orders. This same chieftain came of his own will, leading 5,000 unarmed natives who carried only agricultural tools and left to the Admiral a crop planted through his own effort in the fields of his very large valley. Showered with gifts by the Admiral, he went back happy; this news, taken back to the Ciguani people, raised hope for clemency in the hearts of the chieftains. They therefore came voluntarily pledging to follow his orders from then on and begged for their king and his whole family. The wife and his whole household were freed upon the request of the chieftains, but the king was kept tied in chains. These actions were taking place on the island by authority of the Admiral, who was not aware of what his enemies were plotting against him to the Sovereigns. The Sovereigns, troubled by so many complaints from every direction and especially because so small a quantity of gold and other products was obtained regardless of availability, on account of the dissensions and rebellions appointed a new governor who would diligently investigate all these matters and enforce new orders or send back to them those guilty who were caught. I do not know precisely what was found out against the Admiral and his brother, or against those who were his enemies; I only know this: both brothers were caught, stripped of all their possessions, and taken away in chains, as you see, most Illustrious Prince. However, as soon as the Sovereigns learned of their having been taken to Cádiz in chains, they at once ordered, by means of speedy messengers,

Adelantatum, fratrem absentem, armata manu ut se, si vim gubernator inferre pararet, ab eius iniuria tutaretur venire propere hortabatur monebatque. Propterea, quum Adelantatus praecessisset armatos, incautos ambos, priusquam multitudo conveniret, gubernator apprehendit. Quid futurum sit, tempus, rerum omnium iudex prudentissimus, aperiet. Vale!

that they be unchained, freed and given permission to come to them as free men, showing they did not appreciate but took personal offense at that. We are given to understand that the new governor had sent to the Sovereigns letters written by the Admiral, in an unknown language, in which he urged and warned his brother the *Adelantado*, who was then absent, to come immediately with armed troops and defend him from such insult should the governor use force. And so, having *the Adelantado* gone ahead of his armed troops, the governor caught both brothers unprepared, before an army could be assembled. Time, a very wise judge of all events, shall reveal what is in store. Fare well!

III 4

Hic sistere Pater Beatissime, statueram, sed igniculus quidam, tortor animi, producere parumper sermonem hortatur. Beraguam dixi primo repertam a Colono. Defraudare virum et admittere scelus mihi viderer inexpiabile, si labores
5 toleratos, si curas eius perpessas, si denique discrimina, quae subivit, ea navigatione, silentio praeterirem. Is, a salute nostra .M.D.II. sexto Idus Maii, cum classicula navium quattuor, cuparum in singulas quinquaginta et sexaginta cumque hominibus centum septuaginta solvit e Gadibus et, felici
10 cursu, Canarias praehendit in diem quintum. Inde appulsus est ad insulam Dominicam, quae Caribium est patria, die sexto decimo captavit, e Dominica Hispaniolam die quinto. Sexto igitur et vigesimo die, ventis lapsuque oceani ab oriente in occidentem fluentis adiuvantibus, ab Hispania
15 navigavit ad Hispaniolam, qui cursus mille ac ducentarum lequarum a nautis esse perhibetur. In Hispaniola, sive libens, sive monente prorege, parum moratur. Occidentem rectam secutus, Cuba Iamaicaque insulis a septentrione in dextram relictis, in insulam se incidisse meridionaliorem Ia-
20 maica scribit, nomine incolarum *Guanassa*, virentem universam uberemque, supra quam credibile cuiquam sit. Eius insulae littora percurrens, duobus occurrit provincialibus monoxylis, de quibus satis late diximus in superioribus. Restibus iugata mancipia nuda trahebant uti, adversis flumini-
25 bus, solet fieri. Monoxylis primarius insularis vehebatur cum uxore ac liberis nudis omnibus. Nostris, qui descenderant in terram, superbe mancipia innuebant, ex heri mandato, ut cederent venientibus, minabantur recusantibus; tanta est eorum simplicitas quod nec veriti sint neque admirati
30 nostrorum vel navigia vel potentiam aut multitudinem. Putabant nostros, ea qua ipsi reverentia colebant herum, assurecturos. Ab alienis terris mercatorem esse redeuntem intellexerunt (nundinas exercent): nundinarias merces ille ferebat, aurichalcea tintinnabula, novaculas cultellosque ac

338

O Most Holy Father, I had decided to stop here, but a little flame which tortures me urges me to continue the narrative a little longer. I said earlier that *Veragua* was discovered by Columbus. It would seem that I cheat the man or commit an unforgivable sin if I passed over in silence the hardships endured, the griefs suffered, and, finally, the dangers faced during that voyage. He left from Cádiz on 10 May of the year 1502 with a small fleet of four ships weighing between 50 and 60 tons each, and with 170 men; after a successful navigation of four days he reached the Canaries. From there, on the sixteenth day, he landed on the island of *Dominica*, which is the country of the Caribs; from there it took him five days to land at Hispaniola. Therefore, in 26 days, with the help of the winds and with the push of the ocean currents from East to West, he sailed from Spain to Hispaniola, a voyage which is reported by the sailors to be 1200 leagues long. He stayed a short time in Hispaniola, either of his own volition or on the advice of the governor. After following the course West, he left on the right, to the North, the islands of Cuba and Jamaica; then he writes that he found an island farther South of Jamaica, called by the natives *Guanassa*, all green and fertile beyond anyone's belief. While traveling the shores of that island he ran into two single-oar local boats as described quite extensively earlier. Nude slaves tied with ropes dragged them, as is usual when they go against the current. The chief of the island, with his wife and children all naked, was carried in the boats dug out of a single tree. When our men went ashore, the slaves gestured haughtily, by order of their master, so that our men would yield to them, and they advanced, threatening them if refused; such was their simplicity that they did not show any fear or astonishment at our ships or at the power or number of our men. They thought our men would respect their master with the same reverence they did. Our men thought he was a merchant coming back from other lands (indeed they do hold markets): he was carrying merchandise bought at the market, such as zinc-rich brass [oricalchum] bells, razors, knives and hatchets made of a yellow stone, transparent

secures e lapide flavo, diaphono lucido genere quodam ligni
tenaci manubriato, utensilia etiam coquinariaque vasa et fictilia arte mira e ligno partim, partim ex eodem marmore
laborata, sed lodices praecipue supellectiliaque gossampina
5 variis intexta coloribus vehebat. Dominum et universam
eius familiam remque omnem praehenderunt. Solvi tamen
mox Praefectus illos iussit et rerum partem maiorem resti-
tui, quo benivolos redderet, imperavit. De natura terrae
ulterioris ad occidentem didicit. Recta carpit iter ad occi-
10 dentem. Ad milliaria decem paulo amplius tellurem reperit
vastam, nomine incolarum *Quiriquetanam*, ipse vero *Ciambam*
nuncupavit. Rem divinam in littore iussit celebrari; habitatoribus nudis plenam reperit. Hi mites et simplices, posito
timore, ad nostros, ut ad rem mirandam, provincialibus ci-
15 bis et aqua recenti onusti confluebant. Oblato munere, ver-
sis vestigiis, capite obstipo, reverenter retrocedebant. Pen-
savit munera illorum muneribus rerum nostrarum: calculorum, puta, vitreorum sertis et speculis quibusdam
acubusque ac spinteribus et huiuscemodi mercibus illis pe-
20 regrinis. In magno illo tractu regiones sunt duae, *Taia* haec,
Maia illa appellatae; universam scribit terram illam esse salubrem, amoenam, clementia coeli fortunatam optime, nulli
terrarum ubertate agrorum postferendam, temperie mira
praeditam, et montanam refert partim, partim, lata planitie
25 nobilem arboriferam ubique herbidamque ac perpetuo vere
autumnoque gaudentem, arboribus toto anno frondentibus
et pomiferis. Ilicetis pinetisque ait esse refertam ac palmarum generibus septem, quarum aliae dactiliferae steriles aliae
sunt; pelgoras uvis pendentibus maturis, sed labruschis, ter-
30 ra gignit suapte natura inter arbores. Tantam refert esse
apud hos suavium, utiliumque fructuum nativorum copiam
aliorum, quod de uvis colendis nulla sit cura. Ex palmarum
quodam genere *machanas*, id est enses ligneos latos et iacu-
lares hastas construunt. Gossampinas arbores nutrit ea tellus
35 vulgo mirabolanos[42] etiam diversarum specierum, *emblicos*

---

[42] See Plin. *nat. hist.* XII 100 ff.: Diosc. I 109.

and clear, with handles made of strong wood, and also kitchen utensils and vases, pottery, crafted with remarkable artistry, partly wood and partly of the same stone; but he was mostly carrying blankets and multicolored, woven cotton swaths. Our men captured the master with his whole family and all his goods. However, the Admiral ordered that they be freed right away and insisted that most of the things be given back so as to make them well disposed toward us. He gathered information on the nature of the region which was located farther West. He took a direct route West. A little more than ten miles farther he discovered a vast land, called by the natives *Quiriquetana*, but which he renamed *Ciamba*. He ordered that a religious service be held on the beach which he found full of naked inhabitants: kind and simple people that fearlessly ran toward our men as to a miraculous sight, bringing loads of native foods and fresh water. After giving their gifts, they turned and departed respectfully, their heads bowed. Columbus reciprocated with some of our own things: necklaces of glass beads and some mirrors, needles, bracelets and goods of this type, new to them. In that vast land there are two regions, one called *Taya*, the other *Maya*; he writes that the whole land is wholesome, pleasant, very fortunate for the mild climate, with first rate fields of unmatched fertility, endowed with wonderfully moderate temperatures; he reports that it is partly mountainous and partly beautified by a vast plain, everywhere full of trees and grass, and blessed by an eternal spring and fall, so that the trees are covered with leaves and fruits throughout the whole year. He states that it has abundant oak and pine trees, and seven kinds of palm trees, of which some produce dates and some are sterile; the land spontaneously produces among the trees hanging vines of ripe wild grapes. He relates that with them there is such an abundance of other native fruits, deliciously edible, that there is no need to grow grapes. From a certain type of palm they build *macanas*, i.e. large wooden swords and javelins. The land produces cotton trees everywhere, and also myrabolans of different kinds, such as *emblicos* and *checubos*, according to the name given by physicians. This land also yields maize and yuca, *ages* and sweet potatoes, just as other regions there do; the same land also nourishes lions and tigers, deer and wild goats and similar animals, also diverse species of birds, including fowl similar to

puta et *checubos*, medicorum appellatione. Maizium et haec
terra generat ac iuccam, ages et batatas, uti caeterae regiones illae; eadem et leones nutrit ac tigres, cervos capreolo-
sque et huiuscemodi animalia, volucres etiam diversas, inter
quas pro altilibus habent eas quas, pavonibus foeminis colore ac magnitudine similes, esse gustu etiam et sapore diximus aliquando. Proceros esse aiunt ac pulchre formatos
incolas utriusque sexus; quos ait pudenda tegere gossampinis velaminibus, intextis diversis coloribus. Ad elegantiam
seipsos depingunt quorundam pomorum succo, ad id in
hortis nutritorum (nigris ac rubentibus uti Agathyrsos legimus). Totum inficiunt alii corpus, partes alii, plerique
autem tractim flores aut rosas effigiant aut implicitos laqueos, prout cuique sedet appetitu. Idiomata sunt penitus
alia ab insularibus convicinis. More torrentis, aquae defluebant ad occidentem; statuit tamen orientem eius terrae
quaerere animo, vertens Pariam Osque Draconis et alias
quas iam descripsimus, ab oriente repertas oras, contiguas
esse, uti erant, existimans. Ex ampla igitur Quiriquetana
decimo tertio Kalendas Septembris solvit. Ad lequas triginta fluvium reperit extra cuius ostium dulces haustus
sumpsit in mari. Littus erat scopulis et rupibus purgatum,
fundo ad iacendas anchoras ubique apto. Tantam scribit
fuisse vim oppositi torrentis oceani quod diebus quadraginta lequas vix potuerit septuaginta percurrere. Claudican-
do semper et gyris per altum agendo classiculam, procedebat. Interdumque se repulsum et retro raptum reperiebat
impetu aquarum, terram captare volens, ad vesperum, ne
per noctis tenebras in ignotis littoribus naufragarentur.
Intercapedine lequarum octo, tria se ingentia flumina niti-
darum aquarum scribit reperisse, in quorum marginibus
cannae crassiores humano femore gignebantur pisciumque
ac magnarum testudinum copiam ingentem et plerisque in
locis crocodillorum multitudinem, in arena vasto hiatu solem captantium; varia etiam animalia, quibus nomen non

female peacocks in color and size and, as we have said earlier, similar in taste and flavor. They say that the inhabitants of both sexes are tall and well-formed; he reports that they cover their loins with woven, multicolored cotton bands. For beauty they paint themselves with the juice of some fruits grown in gardens for this purpose (black and red colors just as we read about the Agathyrsi). Some paint their whole body, others only parts, but most draw flowers or roses or interlaced knots designs, as each wishes. Their language is profoundly different from that of the inhabitants of the nearby islands. The streams, flowing like torrents, run toward the West; he decided, however, to explore the eastern part of the land, heading toward *Paria* and *Boca del Dragon* and other shores earlier described found to the East, thinking that they were near, as indeed they were. So, on 20 August, he set sail from the vast *Quiriquetana*. After 30 leagues, he discovered a river and, beyond its outlet he drew fresh water from the ocean. The shore was clear of rocks and cliffs, with sufficient fathom everywhere for dropping anchor. He writes that the strength of the opposing ocean current was so great that he could hardly travel 70 leagues in 40 days. He advanced the fleet by constant rolling at sea and tacking. At times he found himself repulsed and held back by the force of the water, when toward evening he recalls, trying to make land, so as not to be shipwrecked on unknown shores during the dark of night. He writes that he has found, in the space of eight leagues, three large rivers with clear waters, on whose banks were growing canes thicker than human thigh-bones. He reports an enormous quantity of fish and huge turtles and in many places a large quantity of crocodiles taking in the sun on the sand with big yawns; there were also other animals that he did not name. He relates that the appearance of that land is diverse: in some places rocky, held in by barren promontories and rugged cliffs, and in others, not inferior to any other land for the fertility of the soil. Varied also are the names of the kings and chiefs on the different coasts. They call the chieftain *cacique*, as we said on another occasion, elsewhere *quebí*, in some places also *tibá*; a person with authority is called *saccus* in some places, elsewhere *jurá*. They call *cupra* and consider a hero someone who has acted bravely in battle against the enemy and shows a face marred by scars. They call people *chiuys* and a man, in some places,

dedit. Variamque referti eius telluris faciem esse: saxeam
alicubi et promontoriis fultam squalidis ac rupibus ambe-
sis, alibi, benignitate soli, nulli terrae cedentem. Varia
etiam, in variis oris, regum et primariorum nomina. Vocant regulum *cacicum*, ut alias diximus, alibi *quebi, tiba* vero
alicubi; primarium autem, alicubi *saccus*, alibi *iura*. Eum,
qui strenue se gessit in pugna hostili et signatam cicatri-
cibus faciem ostentat, *cupram* appellant, habentque pro he-
roe. Vulgum nuncupant *chiuys*, hominem alicubi dicunt *ho-
mem*. Accipe homo si quis dicere voluerit, *hoppa home* dicet.
Alius deinde fluvius grandibus navigiis aptus occurrit, ante
cuius fauces quattuor insulae parvae floridae atque arbori-
ferae iacebant, quae portum efficiebant. Has *Quattuor Tempora* vocitavit; ab his ad lequas terdecim ad orientem, semper contra vim aquarum tendens, duodecim parvas praehendit insulas: has quia praeditas novo genere fructuum,
limones nostros aemulantium, *Limonares* appellavit. Eadem
via pererrans ad lequas duodecim, magnum reperit portum
lequarum trium spacio sese in terram insinuantem pauloque minus latum, in quem fluvius ingens cadebat. Ibi
amissus est postmodum Nicuesa, Beraguam quaeritans,
uti supra diximus, unde *Perditorum fluvium* recentiores
nuncuparunt. Continuo cursu tendens contra pelagi furo-
rem, Almirantus Colonus varios reperiebat montes, valles
varias fluminaque ac portus; spiritus rerum omnium suaves fuisse atque recreantes naturam refert neque incidisse
in adversam valitudinem e sociis quemquam ad regionem
usque incolarum appellatione *Quicuri*, ultima acuta, in qua
ponus est *Cariai*, ab ipso Almiranto *Mirabolanus* appellatus, quia nativa sit ibi arbor illa. In hoc portu Cariai sese
obiiciunt circiter ducentum incolae manu, gestantes terna
quaternaque iacula, mites tamen et hospitales, sed quid
sibi gens haec nova quaereret, parati expectantes. Colloquia petunt, dato signo pacis; natando nostros adeunt,
commercia ineunt: permutationem rerum postulant. Dari

home. If one wishes to say "take, o man," one says, *hoppa home*. Then, there appeared another river, suited for large vessels and in front its outlet are four little islands, rich in flowers and trees, which formed a port. He called them *Cuatro Estaciones*; from them, sailing East thirteen leagues always against the current, he reached twelve little islands: he called them *Limonares*, because they have a new kind of fruit similar to our lemons. Sailing along the same way for another twelve leagues he found a large port which extended into the land for a distance of three leagues and was a little less wide: in it flowed a great river. Later on, here, they lost Nicuesa, searching for *Veragua*, as we have already said, and for that reason the explorers that followed called it *Río de los Perdidos*. Continuing to sail against the current, Admiral Columbus found various mountains, valleys, rivers and ports; he reported that the air of all those places was suave and rejuvenated the bodies and that none of the companions had become sick until the region called by the inhabitant *Quicurí*, with the stress on the last syllable, in which there is the port of *Cariai*, named by the Admiral himself *Myrabolano*, because there grows that tree. In that port of *Cariai*, about 200 inhabitants came to meet him, carrying in their hands three or four javelins, but nevertheless kind and hospitable, although ready, waiting to know what those foreigners wanted from them. They asked to speak, after exhibiting signs of peace; swimming, they reached our men and began trading: they asked for an exchange of goods. The Admiral ordered that objects from our country be given to them freely, to gain their good will; they refused the favor, trough gestures, and in fact, not a word of their language could be understood. Having suspected some deception in our gifts because our men refused to accept their offerings, they left on the beach whatever had been given them. The inhabitants of *Cariai* are so courteous and generous that they would rather give than receive. They sent to our men two beautiful young girls and made these men understand that they could take them away. These, as all the other women, wore a cotton band over their pubis. This is indeed the custom of the Cariai women; the men, however, go naked. The women also part the hair on their heads; the men, on the contrary, let theirs grow on the back of the head, but shave it from the forehead and, they tie it with white bands twisting it around the head, just as we

e nostratibus rebus ad eorum benivolentiam captandam, Almirantus, sed gratuito imperat; per signa gratiam recusant neque enim ullum ex horum idiomate vocabulum perceperunt. Fraudem aliquam inesse nostris donis suspicati, quod ipsorum oblata nostri recipere renuissent, quicquid fuerat impartitum in littore liquerunt. Tanta pollent Cariairenses urbanitate atque animi benignitate ut magis dare quam accipere studerent. Puellas ad nostros virgines formae elegantis misere duas, quas ut abducere liceret insinuabant. Hae, ut caeterae foeminae, pube tenus fascia tegebantur gossampina. Is enim est foeminarum Cariairensium mos; virorum autem nude agere. Scindunt et crines foeminae; viri nutriunt occipite, a fronte radunt, colligunt quos vittis candentibus et in orbem circunducunt capiti, uti nostrates videmus puellas. Almirantus indutas ac bene donatas, cum rubro laneo pileolo genitori earum praebendo, remisit. Sed cuncta iterum in littore locata sunt, quia ipsorum dona recusassent nostri; duos tamen viros et eos non invitos secum advexit, quo vel illi nostram vel nostri Cariairensem perdiscerent linguam. Maris aestu parum quati tractus illos cognovit, quod haud secus littori ac fluviorum ripis, arbores inhaererent. Idem aiunt et caeteri oras illas tractantes, exiguo fluxu ac refluxu omnium illarum terrarum insularum etiam littora madefieri. In huius terrae prospectu, inquit, in mari ipso gigni arbores quae ramos incurvent, postquam altius emerserint, ad profundum quo applicatae cuspides, uti propagines vitium solo demersae, radices creant et in sui generis arbores perpetuo virentes prodeunt. De huiuscemodi arboribus Plinius[43] in duodecimo *Naturalis historiae*, sed in arido solo, non autem in mari. Animalia nutriri in ora Cariai eadem, quae alibi diximus, sed unum reperere naturae longe dissonae. Id

[43] These trees remind Peter Martyr of those similarly described by Pliny (*nat. hist.* XII 22), namely, the *ficus religiosa* and *ficus Indica* (see Theophr. *hist plant.* IV 4, 4-5; Curt. IX 1, 10; Solin. 52, 47).

see our girls do. The Admiral sent them back dressed and with beautiful gifts, with a cap of red wool to give to their fathers. But again, all the gifts were placed on the beach, because our men had refused theirs; he did take with him two men who followed him voluntarily, so that either they would learn ours or our men would learn the Cariai language. He observed that those shores were little beaten by breakers, because on them no less than on the banks of rivers trees were also growing. Others sailing along those coasts say the same thing, that is, that the shores of all those lands and islands are lapped by a rather weak ebb and flow. He says that within view this land's trees grow right onto the sea and from a certain height bend their branches into the deep water, their tips sticking like shoots of vines embedded in the ground, form roots and grow into evergreen trees of their own species. Pliny talks of trees of this kind in the XII book of the *Naturalis Historia*, but he says that they grow in the barren land and not in the sea. On the shores of *Cariai* live the same animals of which we have spoken elsewhere, but there is found one of a totally different kind. This is similar to a huge monkey as it hangs by a rather long and thick tail; rolling three or four times in order to gain strength, it jumps from branch to branch and throws itself from tree to tree, as if it were flying. An archer of ours hit one of them with an arrow; wounded, the monkey threw itself down and furiously attacked the enemy which struck him. The hunter, drawing his sword, fought the animal, cut off an arm of the monkey and captured it maimed but fiercely resisting. Taken on board, it became somewhat tame among the men; while they were keeping it tied with iron chains, other hunters dragged from the swamps of the coasts a wild boar (the desire for meat pushed them to explore the woods). The boar was shown in his ferocity to the monkey. Both bristled; the monkey, in a fury, flung itself against the boar and wound its tail around it; with the surviving arm, it grabbed the boar by the throat; the monkey choked the boar as it struggled to resist. That land nourishes these and other such monsters. Moreover, the inhabitants of *Cariai* preserve the bodies of their chiefs and relatives on bed-trellises wrapped in tree leaves; for the common people, woods and forests serve as burial places. Advancing from *Cariai* for about twenty leagues, they found a gulf so ample that they think it measured

est grandi cercopitheco par, cauda longiore procerioreque cauda suspensus et vim terque quaterque sese devolvens capiendo ex ramo transilit in ramum et ex arbore sese proiicit in arborem ac si volitaret. Arcuarius e nostris unum sagitta confixit;
5 vulneratus se deiicit cercopithecus, hostem vulneratorem, rabidus adoritur. Stricto ense agit in pecus venator, lacertum cercopitheco abscidit cepitque mancum ferociter renitentem. Ad classem perductus, mansuevit inter homines parumper; dum sic ferreis vinctum catenis servarent, e littoribus trahunt
10 paludibus aprum venatores alii (cogebat namque carnium desiderium nemora perlustrare). Cercopitheco aper et ipse ferox ostenditur. Setas excutit uterque, in aprum cercopithecus furibundus salit, cauda circunligat aprum; cum servato a venatore victore suo lacerto guttur apro praehendit: reluctantem aprum
15 suffocavit cercopithecus. Haec et huiuscemodi monstra nutrit alia tellus illa. Servent et Cariairenses desiccata cratibus procerum et parentum cadavera, foliis arborum involuta; populo nemora silvaeque sunt addicta sepulchris. Procedentes ex Cariai ad lequas viginti circiter, sinum reperere amplum adeo ut in
20 gyrum putent lequas continere decem. Quattuor insulae parvae feraces, exiguo discretae intervallo, sinus faucibus obiectae, tutum efficiunt portum. Is est portus, quem alias diximus appellari ab incolis *Cerabaro*, ultima acuta, sed unum eius littoris latus tantum ita vocitatum nunc didicere atque id dextrum
25 ingrediendo, laevum autem *Aburema* nuncupatur. Insulis inquiunt universum feracibus et frequentibus celebrem esse atque arboriferis, fundo ad anchoras iaciendas ubique apto nitidoque, ac mira piscium copia pollentem. Utraque terra adiacens, ubertate soli, nulli terrarum eorum iudicio cedit. Duos incolas ad
30 manus habuere: colla incolae monilibus, quae appellant *guanines* aureis, in aquilas aut leones vel animalia huiuscemodi affabre effigiatis ornant, sed aurum id minime purum esse cognoverunt. A duobus illis Cariairensibus, quos abductos diximus, nostri didicerunt Cerabaroam et Aburemam regiones auro dites
35 esse Cariairensesque rerum suarum permutatione, universum aurum, quo ornantur, ab his adeptos fuisse. Quinque pagos,

ten leagues around. Four small, fertile islands, separated by a brief distance, opposite the mouth of the gulf, make a safe port. This is the port which elsewhere we said was called by the inhabitants *Cerabaró*, with the stress on the last vowel; but now they learned that only one side of that coast is thus called, the right side, when entering, with the left side called instead *Aburema*. They claim the entire bay is full of numerous islands, fertile and rich in trees, with clear bottom everywhere, suitable for anchoring and remarkably abundant fish. It is their opinion that both adjacent territories are not less fertile in soil than any of the others. They held two natives: they adorn their necks with golden jewels, which they call *guanines*, wrought with mastery in the shape of eagles or lions or other similar animals, but our men realized the gold was not at all pure. From those two natives of *Cariai*, whom we said had been taken, our men learned that the regions of *Carabaro* and *Aburema* are rich in gold and that the natives of Cariai, by bartering some of their own goods, had obtained from these regions all the gold with which they adorned themselves. The inhabitants of Cariai explained to our men that in the regions of *Carabaro* and *Aburema*, not very far from the shore, toward the interior, there were five villages famous for the gathering of gold; as a matter of fact, both populations always had done business with each other since the time of their forefathers. They reported these names for the villages: *Chirará, Purén, Chitazá, Iureche, Atamea*. All the men of the province of *Cerabaro* are completely naked, but they paint their bodies in different ways, and take delight in garlands of flowers and crowns intertwined with claws of lions and tigers. The women cover only their groin area with a narrow band of cotton. When they finally left this place, sailing along the same coast for eighteen leagues on the bank of the river just discovered, 300 nude men, yelling and shouting, came to meet them, menacing our men and spitting at them either water (which they had put in their mouths), or herbs of the shore. Throwing javelins and brandishing lances and *macanas* (identified earlier as wooden swords), they attempted to keep our men away from shore. They were painted in various degree: some their faces, others their entire body or parts of it. They made clear they did not want peace or any business with our men. He ordered that some shells be fired against them, but from on

auro legendo egregios, inesse Cerabarois et Aburemanis regionibus a littore in internis distantibus non longo tractu Cariairenses nostris aperuerunt; commercia namque a maioribus eorum utraeque nationes frequentarunt semper. Pagorum nomina
5 haec esse perhibentur: *Chirara, Puren, Chitaza, Iureche, Atamea.* Viri omnes Cerabaroae provinciae nudi sunt penitus, sed variis depicti modis sertis floridis et coronis ex leonum et tigrium unguibus contextis oblectantur. Foeminae, angusta gossampina vitta, pudenda tantum contegunt. Hinc iam tandem egressi,
10 per idem littus ad lequas octodecim in fluminis reperti ripa occurrunt viri nudi tercentum, sublatis clamoribus, minitabundi, expuentes in nostros, aqua sumpta in os aut littoralibus herbis. Iaculando missilia vibrandoque hastas et machanas (enses diximus esse ligneos) a littore arcere nostros conabantur.
15 Depicti variis modis erant: alii, praeter faciem, corpus universum, tractim alii. Pacem nolle se aut commercium ullum cum nostris insinuabant. Solui tormenta quaedam in illos, sed ab alto, ne perimerent quemquam imperat: hoc enim semper sedit Coloni animo ut pacato ageret cum novis gentibus. Fragore
20 discussae ballistae bombardae perterriti, sternuntur omnes, pacem optant, commerciantur invicem, guaninorum aureorum ex adverso calculorum vitreorum atque huiuscemodi rerum permutatione. Tympana hi habent et marina conchilia, quibus ad excitandos animos pugnae tempore utuntur in bellis. In eo
25 tractu flumina sunt *Acateba, Quareba, Zobroba, Aiaguitin, Urida, Durubba, Beragua*: in omnibus aurum colligere licebat. Foliis arborum latis ab aestu pluviaque, penularum loco, se tuentur. Oras inde perlustravit *Ebetere* et *Embigar*: in his flumina labuntur dulcium aquarum et piscium copia egregia, *Zahoram* et
30 *Cubigar*; hic sistit auri ubertas, quinquaginta circiter lequarum tractu. Distat inde lequas tantum tres ea rupes quam in infausto Nicuesae discursu diximus appellari *Pegnonem*, a nostris, incolarum autem appellatione, regio dicitur *Vibba*; in quo etiam tractu est portus, ad lequas tantum sex, quem *Bellum*
35 diximus a Colono vocitatum: cuius regio *Xaguaguara* dicitur

350

high, in order not to kill anyone; this was always Columbus' true intention, to deal with new peoples peacefully. Frightened by the crash of the mortar shells that exploded in the air, they all prostrated themselves, asked for peace and engaged in trade, exchanging the golden *guanines* for glass beads and things of that sort. These people have drums and sea shells which they use in war to arouse their hearts at the time of battle. In that region there are the following rivers: *Acateba, Quareba, Zobroba, Ayaguitín, Uridá, Durubbá, Veragua*; in all of them one could gather gold. With big tree leaves worn as a cloak, these people protect themselves, from heat and rain. Then he explored the coasts of *Ebeteré* and *Embigar*: where *Zahorán* and *Cubigar*, rivers flow distinguished for an abundance of fresh water and fish; here one can find plenty of gold along a stretch of 50 leagues. Only three leagues from there is the cliff which we said, was called by our men *Peñón*, during the unfortunate voyage to *Nicuesa*, but in the words of the inhabitants the region is called *Vibbá*; in this stretch at the sixth league there is also a port which we said was named *Bello* by Columbus, and its territory is called *Xaguaguará* by the natives; that whole land is very populous, and everyone goes nude. In *Xaguaguará* the inhabitants paint themselves with colors, the chieftain with black, the people with red. The king and seven notables had gold leaves hanging from their nostrils down to their lips. They believe that in this ornament there is the greatest dignity. The men cover their genitals with a sea shell, but the women cover theirs with a cotton band. In gardens these natives grow a fruit similar to a pine nut, which elsewhere we said comes from a shrub like a cardoon, but a delicacy, food worthy of a king; they also grow gourds which they use to carry water. Of these I have spoken extensively elsewhere. They call this plant *hibuero*. In some places our men ran into crocodiles which, when they ran away or dove, left behind a smell sweeter than musk or castoreum. The people of the Nile have told me the same thing about the female crocodile, especially her abdomen, because her smell recalls Arabic perfumes. From here the Admiral turned back with his small fleet, both because he could no longer hold out against the force of the currents and because the ships were rotting more and more every day and consumed by worms, which are born in the heat of the waters in all those lands situated near the equator. Venetian merchants call

ab incolis; populis est ea tellus universa frequens sed nudis. In Xaguaguara regulus nigro, populus rubro, coloribus fucantur. Regi et primariis septem e naribus pendebant aurea lamina labiorum tenus. In hoc ornatu summum putant esse decorem.
5 Testa marina viri pudenda includunt, foeminae gossampina tegunt vitta. In hortis hi pineae nuci fructum similem nutriunt quem diximus alias e frutice nasci veluti carduo, sed mollem et regia dignum esca; cucurbiteas quoque arbores ad potus ferendi usum. De his late alias. Vocant arborem *hibuero.* Cro-
10 codillis alicubi occurrebant qui, quum aufugerent aut mergerentur, odorem a tergo musco vel castoreo suaviorem relinquebant. Nili accolae de crocodillo foemina idem mihi rettulerunt, de abdomine praesertim, quod arabicos aequet odores quosque. Regressus hinc est Almirantus cum sua classicula,
15 tum quia nequibat adversum aquarum cursum sustinere, tum etiam quia magis ac magis, in dies, navigia putrescebant atque terebrabantur vermium aculeis, qui, ex aquarum tepore, in universis tractibus illis aequinoctio fere suppositis gignuntur. *Bissas* vermes illos mercator Venetus appellat; hos et Alexan-
20 drini duo portus Aegypti generant navesque labefactant si diu in anchoris morentur: cubitales sunt et interdum longiores, digitulo nunquam crassiores. Hispanus nauta pestem hanc *bromam* vocat. Bromam igitur veritus Colonus Almirantus et renitente pelago vexatus, secundo oceano ad occidentem regre-
25 ditur. *Hiebram* fluvium, a Beragua fluvio duas distantem lequas, quia sit maioribus navigiis suscipiendis aptior, captat. A Beragua minore regio nomen tenet quia utriusque fluminis possessor regulus Beraguam inhabitat; quid dextrum quidve sinistrum hic acciderit dicamus. Stans in Hiebra Colonus fra-
30 trem suum Bartholomaeum Colonum, Hispaniolae Adelantatum, cum cymbis servitoriis et hominibus octo et sexaginta mittit ad fluvium Beraguam. Obvius fit Adelantato cum patriis monoxylis, secundo flumine, regionis regulus, more patrio depictus, nudus cum ingenti comitatu, sed inermis. Quum pri-
35 mum ad colloquium deventum est, reguli familiares quidam,

those worms *bisse*; the two ports of Alexandria in Egypt also have these worms and ships are ruined if they remain anchored there for a long time: they are a cubit long, sometimes longer but never thicker than a small finger. Spanish sailors call this pest *broma*. Therefore, Admiral Columbus, fearing the *broma* and vexed by an adverse sea, headed back toward the West with a favorable current. Two leagues from the river Veragua he reached the river *Hiebra*, which is better suited to take in larger ships. The region takes its name from Veragua, which is smaller, because the chieftain who rules over both rivers lives on the Veragua; let us describe the good or bad events that happened here. While on the Hiebra, Columbus sent to the Veragua river his brother Bartholomew, the *Adelantado* of Hispaniola, with service cutters and 68 men. The chieftain of the region, painted according to the native custom, and naked, accompanied by a large number of men, but unarmed, went to meet the *Adelantado* in their native one-piece vessels, helped by a favorable current. As soon as he began to talk, some relatives of the chieftain, anxious for the tranquillity of their master and mindful of the royal dignity, so that the chieftain would not conduct business standing up, took a stone from nearby and, washing it on the bank and polishing it carefully, they carried it with reverence and placed it under the chieftain. The latter, sitting, seemed to communicate by signs that he would let our men sail on the rivers under his rule. On 8 February, the *Adelantado*, after leaving the cutters, went by foot along the opposite bank of the Veragua river; he came to the *Durabá* river and said that this river is richer in gold than the Hiebra and the Veragua. In all the rivers of that land there certainly is some gold. In between the roots of the trees clinging to the bank and among the stones and pebbles deposited by the torrents and wherever they would dig holes of about a palm and a half, they could find gold mixed with the dug-out dirt; for that reason they decided to stop there, but the natives prevented it, suspecting future misfortunes. In compact formation, with terrible shouts, they hurled themselves against our men who had begun to build huts. Our men could barely resist the first attacks; initially, the naked barbarians fought with several javelins from far off; then, furiously, fought hand to hand with wooden swords that we said are called *macanas*. Then — amazing to report it — so great was their rage that they

de quiete sui heri anxii et maiestatis regiae memores ne stans regulus negocietur, saxum e proximo sumptum in ripa lavant confricantque decenter et reverenter allatum regulo supponunt. Sedens regulus, per signa, visus est annuere ut nostris liceat dicionis eius flumina percurrere. Sexto Idus Februarii pedes Adelantatus adversa tendit Beraguae fluvii ripa, cymbis relictis. In *Durabam* fluvium incidit: hunc Hiebra, et Beragua inquit esse ditiorem auro. In omnibus quippe terrae illius fluminibus aurum gignitur. Inter arborum radices ripis inhaerentes interque saxa et lapillos a torrentibus relictos et ubicunque scrobes ad sexquipalmum effodiebant, egestam reperiebant terram, auro mixtam; propterea figere ibi pedem fuit consilium, sed incolae, futuram perniciem olfacientes, vetuerunt. Facto agmine, cum horrendo clamore ruunt in nostros, qui domos aedificare iam coeperant. Primos impetus vix sustinuere nostri; certarunt eminus crebris missilibus primo barbari nudi, mox cominus, strictis ensibus ligneis, quos diximus nuncupari *machanas*, rabidi pugnare cogitarunt. Dictu mirandum, tanta erat concepta in eis iam ira ut neque arcubus aut scorpionibus et, quod maius est, neque bombardarum e navibus iactarum fragore terrerentur. Cesserunt loco semel; iterato maiore numero comparato redeunt ferociores: satius emori fore iudicant quam perpeti patriam occupatum iri a peregrinis. Hospites benigne susceperant, habitatores recusant. Quo magis instabant nostri, eo maior finitimorum multitudo confluebant. Nocte dieque a fronte modo, modo a lateribus, urgebantur nostri. A tergo, stans in littore classis, tutos reddebat. Deseruere igitur terram hanc et qua venerant regrediuntur. Iamaicam insulam, Hispaniolae Cubaeque collateralem a meridie, navigiis, in cribrorum modum pertusatis a *broma*, ut Hispano utar vocabulo, vix praehendere potuerunt; fere ex itinere perierunt. Viribus lacertorum exhaurientium maris aquas, per amplas rimas, ingredientes, vitae discrimen evaserunt tandem et ad Iamaicam semianimes appulsi sunt; obrutis ibi navigiis omnibus intercepti, vitam egere mensibus decem Vergiliani Achemenidis[44] vita, in

---

[44] Achaemenes, companion of Ulysses, was abandoned on the Cyclopes' island and saved by Aeneas (see Virg. *Aen.* III 588 ff.). Peter Martyr mentions his misfortunes also in *Dec.* II 10.

were not frightened by bows and crossbows nor, what is more, by the crash of mortars fired from the ships. Once, they retreated from that place, but, gathered in bigger numbers, they returned again more ferociously: they believe it is better to die than see their country occupied by foreigners. They had received the Spaniards kindly as guests, but refused to have them as permanent inhabitants. The more our men pressed, the more the number of nearby peoples crowded together. Day and night our men were attacked, now on the front, now on the flanks. The fleet anchored at shore protected thus from behind; therefore, they abandoned that land and returned the same way they had come. They were just able to reach the island of Jamaica, next to Hispaniola and Cuba, to the South, with the ships pierced like sieves by *broma*, to use a Spanish term; they almost perished in this voyage. With the strength of their arms, empting the sea water that kept coming in through the ample cracks, they finally were able to avoid the danger which hung over their life and, exhausted, they landed in Jamaica where they were stranded and the ships wrecked. They lived for ten months a life more calamitous than that of the Virgilian Achaemenes, at the mercy of naked barbarians, satisfied with foods of that land, when sometimes it pleased the barbarians to give them any. An advantage for our men was the mortal hatred native chieftains had for each other: to keep our people as their allies when they would wage war on neighboring enemies, they occasionally fed our hunger with local bread. But, O Holy Father, may Your Holiness consider how wretched and painful it is to live on begged bread, especially when everything else is lacking, such as wine and meat, or any kind of dairy products which the stomachs of the Europeans are accustomed to from the cradle. Necessity forced them to try their luck. Columbus resolved to find out what plans God reserved for him through his steward Diego Méndez who climbed into a canoe after taking with him, however, two natives of Jamaica as guides, who were experts of those coasts. In an already choppy sea, they went from reef to reef, promontory to promontory, tossed by the waves given the small size and shape of the canoe, before Diego Méndez finally landed at the extreme corner of Hispaniola, 40 leagues off Jamaica. With the hope of receiving the gifts promised by Admiral Columbus, the two natives of Jamaica felt again

nudorum barbarorum potestate, calamitosiorem eius, terrae cibis, contenti si quando barbaris placebat impartiri. Profuit nostris odium capitale, quo sese invicem barbari reguli prosequuntur; ut enim nostros fautores haberent, si quando cum
5 finitimis hostibus bella ingruerent, pane aliquando patrio famelicos recreabant. Sed quam miserum et aerumnosum, Pater Beatissime, sit, mendicato pane, adipisci coniectetur Tua Sanctitas, ubi praesertim caetera desint vinum, puta carnesque vel omne pressi lactis genus, quibus Europeorum hominum sto-
10 machi a cuna solent enutriri. Fortunam tentare necessitas coegit. Per oeconomum suum Diecum Mendem, ducibus tamen Iamaicensibus duobus eorum littorum peritis, quid de se Deus cogitet, statuit experiri. Canoam conscendunt mare iam undosum. E scopulo in scopulum, e rupe in rupem, quassatus un-
15 dis, ob navigioli brevitatem et formam, appulsus est iam tandem Diecus Mendez ad ultimum Hispaniolae angulum, e Iamaica distantem lequas quadraginta. Spe munerum ab Almiranto Colono promissorum, Iamaicenses laeti revertuntur. Ipse pedes ad Sanctum Dominicum, urbem primariam metro-
20 politanam, proficiscitur, duo nostratia comparat navigia, dominum adit. Invalidi omnes et egestate rerum extenuati veniunt ad Hispaniolam. Quid inde illis successerit non intellexi. Ad generalia redeamus. Universos tractus illos, quos percurrisse Colonum diximus, (ipse scribit, idemque fatentur omnes
25 laborum socii), toto anno esse frondosos, virentes, amoenos et, quod maius est, salubres, in quibus ex universo comitatu nullus unquam aegrotaverit; neque horrenti frigore unquam aut aestu fervido, quinquaginta lequarum intercapedine a Cerabaroo magno portu ad usque Hiebram et Beraguam, vexa-
30 tum se fuisse iactat. Cerabaroi populi quique iacent medii, ad Hiebram usque Beraguam, non, nisi certis anni temporibus, auro intendunt quaeritando. Suntque negociationis eius opifices exerciti, uti apud nos argenti ferrique fodinatores. Quae loca magis auro fortunentur a specie defluxi torrentis, a terrae co-
35 lore aut huiuscemodi argumentis, longo hi callent experimento.

happy. Diego set out on foot for Santo Domingo, the main city, got two of our ships, and returned to his master. Thus all of them returned to Hispaniola sick and exhausted from lack of food. I do not know what happened to them after that. But now let us go back to the general news. All those coasts which we said Columbus has traveled (he himself writes about it and all his companions confirm such hardships) are leafy throughout the whole year, verdant, pleasant and, what is more important, wholesome: not one man of his crew ever became ill; he boasts of having never suffered any horrible cold or stifling heat for the whole span of 50 leagues, from the great port of Cerabaro to that of Hiebra and Veragua. The natives of Cerabaro and those who live in the middle, between the Hiebra and the Veragua, busy themselves looking for gold, but only at certain set times of the year. They are also workers experienced at their trade, just as miners of silver and iron are among us. Their long experience points them to where there is more gold using the look of the current, the color of the earth and such similar clues. They believe there is a divinity in gold because, according to ancestral customs, they do not look for it without rituals of purification: for instance, they abstain from sexual relations and other pleasures, making very moderate use of food and drink for the whole time during which they prospect for gold. They think men, and all animals, have been given permission to live and to die, and therefore do not worship anything else; but the sun which they greet with reverence as it rises on the horizon. Let us now talk about the mountains and the nature of the land. From all the coasts of those regions one views tall mountains rising to the South but extending without interruption from East to West. That is why we think that those two large seas, which elsewhere we have extensively talked about, are separated by these embankments, so that the seas do not touch each other, just as Italy divides the Tyrrhenian from the Adriatic Sea. As a matter of fact, regardless of wherever one sails from *Point San Augustín*, which belongs to the Portuguese and faces Atlas, to Uraba or to the port of *Cerabaró* and other lands to the West discovered up to now, mountains are ever present to the sailors without interruption: near and far, now tall, now low, now rugged and rocky, now full of trees and grassy and suitable for tilling, just as it is the case on the Taurus and various slopes of our

Credunt inesse auro numen, quandoquidem ad id negocii minime tendunt inexpiati, ex priscorum religione, puta qui a coitu et omni oblectamento abstinent cibisque ac potu parcissime utantur, universo legendi auri tempore. Vivere tantum ac mori
5 datum hominibus, ut caeteris animantibus, arbitrantur, propterea nil colunt aliud, solem tamen venerantur et surgentem ab orizonte reverenter excipiunt. De montibus et terrae situ sermo trahatur. Ex universis illarum regionum littoribus vastos attolli montes a meridie, sed protentos ab oriente in occiden-
10 tem, continuo tractu prospicitur. Quare ita disterminari duo illa magna maria, de quibus alias late fecimus mentionem, his aggeribus, ne invicem collidantur, existimamus, veluti Tyrrhenum Italia dirimit ab Adriatico. Quacunque enim proficiscantur, ab ea cuspide Sancti Augustini, quae ad Portugalenses
15 attinet, ad Atlantem spectante, Urabam usque ac Cerabaroum portum atque ultimas ad occidentem terras, alias ad hunc usque diem repertas, perpetuo tractu, eminus cominusque sese montes navigantibus offerunt, nunc lenes, elati nunc modo asperi et petrosi; arboriferi herbidique atque apti culturae mo-
20 do, uti accidere solet in Tauro nostrique Apennini costis variis, reliquis etiam huiuscemodi vastis montibus. Vallibus quoque egregiis horum, uti aliorum, montium intersecantur iuga; ea pars montium, quae Beraguae fines recipit, superare suis verticibus nubes creditur raroque cerni eius culmina dicunt,
25 ob nubium et nebularum fere continuam densitatem. Quinquaginta amplius attolli milliaria Beraguensia cacumina contendit Almirantus ipse; qui ea primus exploravit, in eadem praeterea regione inquit, ad montium radices, iter esse apertum ad australe pelagus et Venetias comparat cum Genua, sive mavis
30 Ianua, uti eius cives iactitant, qui a Iano conditam fabulantur; protendique vult terram ad occidentem et capere hinc initium lati corporis, uti ab Alpibus nostris, ex angusto Italiae femore, videmus amplas eas Galliarum terras Germaniarumque ac Pannoniarum distendi ad Sarmatas Scythasque varios, ad usque
35 Riphaeas[45] rupes et glaciale pelagus; complecti etiam, nexu

---

[45] Oby mountains, in Tatary.

Apennines or on all other mountain chains. The slopes of these mountain ranges, and others, are intersected by beautiful valleys. The peaks of the mountains within the Veragua borders are believed to rise above the clouds, and they say that the summits are rarely seen because of the constant thickness of clouds and fog. The Admiral himself asserts that the peaks of the mountains of the Veragua region extend more than 50 miles; he, who first explored those lands, also says that in the same region, at the base of the mountains, there is a road open to the southern sea, as at Venice and Genoa (or, if you prefer, *Ianua*, as its citizens call it, boasting that it was founded by Janus); he believes that the land extends to the West and from here begins a great body, just as beyond our Alps we see stretch out from the narrow leg of Italy those vast countries of Gaul, Germanies and Pannonia up to the Sarmats and the various Scythians, as far as the Riphe Mountains and the glacial sea; included in one link are the Thracians and the whole of Greece, and whatever is enclosed to the South by Cape Malea and the Hellespont, but to the North by Euxine Sea and the Palus Maeotidus. The Admiral, then, thinks that this land includes the Ganges' India to the left of those traveling West, but on the North it extends up to the glacial sea, beyond the Hyperboreans and the arctic pole, so that both seas, that is the south ocean and our ocean, reach the corners of that land; the waters, however, do not surround that land in the way that Europe is washed all around by the Hellespont, the Tanais, the glacial and Atlantic oceans and the Mediterranean sea; on the contrary, the strength of the ocean current to the West, in my opinion, prevents that land from being enclosed and joined on the northern coasts, as we have said earlier. Most Holy Father, we have dealt long enough with the topic of longitude; let us try to understand what is thought about latitude. We said at one time that the south ocean and our ocean are separated by a narrow territory and this was demonstrated by the journey of Vasco Núñez and his companions. But, as our Alps in Europe become narrow in one place and wider in another, this land, by analogous natural arrangement, now stretches out and extends widely, now is constrained by narrow valleys by both seas and thus enclosed in short spaces. Where we have said that the regions of *Urabá* and *Veragua* lie, the seas are separated by a narrow margin; however, we have to believe

continuo, Thraces et Graeciam omnem et quicquid Malea promontorio et Hellesponto, a meridie, a septentrione vero Eu-
xino et Meotide concluditur. Vult ergo Almirantus iste a laeva
tendentibus ad occidentem, terram hanc India recipi Gangeti-
5 de, a septentrione vero in dextram ad glacialem oceanum ultra
Hyperboreos et arcticum polum distendi, ita ut utrunque mare,
australe illud scilicet et nostrum oceanum, in eius telluris an-
gulis sese insinuet; non autem sepiant aquae terram ipsam,
veluti Europa Hellesponto Tanaique et oceano, tum glaciali,
10 tum Hispano ac Nostro mari circum ambitur; sed furor dela-
bentis oceani ad occidentem vetat, meo iudicio, clausam esse
coniungique septentrionalibus oris terram illam, uti supra di-
sputavimus. Sit satis de longitudine tractatum, Beatissime Pater, quid de latitudine sentiatur, intellegamus. Diximus aliquan-
15 do angustis limitibus dirimi australe pelagus et hunc nostrum
oceanum atque ita constitit experimento, quandoquidem Va-
scho Nunez et commilitonibus eius iter patuit; sed quod varie
nostrae Alpes in Europa exangustantur hic, alibique late pate-
scunt, eodem naturae consilio, tellus haec modo protenditur
20 et vagatur late, modo ab utroque mari repertis vallium aditibus perstringitur et brevibus contenta est intervallis. Ubi Urabam et Beraguam diximus iacere regiones, parva discluduntur
intercapedine maria; eam autem, quam Maragnonus amnis in-
terluit, late patere regione, credere oportet, si flumen, non
25 mare Maragnonum esse fatebimur; fateamur vero, suadent
aquarum eius dulces haustus! Nequeunt enim in angustis terrae
specubus voragines adeo vastae considere, quae aquarum eam
amplitudinem queant enutrire, idem de flumine magno *Dabaibae*, quem diximus ex angulo sinus Urabae ulnarum quadra-
30 ginta quinquagintaque alibi profunditate, latitudine autem milliarium trium in mare defluere. Latam ibi terram dare necesse
est, quae ab altis Dabaibae montibus non ab austro, sed ab
oriente fluvium demittit. Hunc aiunt constare fluminibus quattuor a Dabaibae montibus collabentibus, *(Sancti Ioannis* flumen
35 nostri appellant); inde in sinum, uti Nilum, per septem cadere
ostia ferunt. In eadem regione Urabae angustias esse alicubi
miras, quae vix lequas colligunt quindecim, at invias ob per-
petuas paludes medias frequentesque lamas aiunt, quas Hispani
tremedales appellant, alias *trampales, cenagales* etiam et *fumideros*
40 ac *zahondaderos*. Priusquam ultra progrediamur opere, precium
etit unde illi montes nuncupentur enarrare. *Dabaibam* ferunt

that the region which the river Marañón washes is very vast, if we admit that the Marañón is a river, not a sea; let us admit it: the sweet draughts of its waters convince us. Indeed, in narrow channels there cannot be chasms wide enough to feed that mass of water; the same can be said of the great river Dabaiba, which we said flows into the sea from an angle of the gulf of Urabá, with a depth of 40 ells and elsewhere of 50, but with a width of three miles. We must concede that the land from which the river flows down from the high mountains of Dabaiba, not going South but East, is wide. They say that this river is formed by four streams which come down from the mountains of Dabaiba (our men call it the river of *San Juan*); from here they say that it flows into the gulf through seven mouths like the Nile. They also claim that in the same region of *Urabá* there are some exceedingly narrow zones which measure only fifteen leagues, but are impassable because of the perpetual swamps in the middle and the frequent quagmires, which the Spaniards call *tremedales* or *trampales* and also *cenagales* and *fumideros* and *zahondaderos*. Before we proceed with our work, we may find it useful to tell from where those mountains take their name. They say that, according to their ancestors, Dabaiba was a woman of great courage and wisdom whom the men of the past respected when she was alive; they add that, when she was dead, all the people of those regions venerated her with reverence. They say that the region has been named after her and that, if ever she becomes angry, lightning and thunder come and crops destroyed; as a matter of fact, they suppose that Dabaiba becomes angry if they neglect her ceremonies. Some deceitful people have instilled in those unfortunate natives such a superstition under the name of religion, so that they may bring to the ceremonies of Dabaiba numerous gifts which the former themselves can enjoy. We have said enough about this subject. They say that the swamps of this narrow land nourish crocodiles, dragons, bats and poisonous mosquitoes. And so, if one plans to march South, one must take to the mountains and avoid being near those quagmires. There are some who believe that a valley, through which flows the river named by our men *Rio de los Perdidos* (for the terrible accident to Nicuesa and his companions), not far away from Cerabaro, separates those mountains on the south side. But, since its waters are drinkable, they think that those believing

fuisse foeminam apud maiores eorum magni animi et providentiae, quam viventem antiquitas observabat; mortuam, inquiunt reverenter coli ab universis regionum illarum incolis. Ab ea regiones nomen sumpsisse aiunt et mitti fulgura tonitruaque ac segetum stragem, si quando irascatur; irasci namque balbutiunt Dabaibam, si negligenter sacris eius intendatur. Eam miseris inbibere superstitionem genus hominum fallax, sub nomine religionis, quo frequentia dona portent ad Dabaibae sacra, quibus ipsi fruantur. De hoc satis. Paludes illas angustae telluris crocodillorum draconumque ac vespertilionum et culicum valde noxiorum altrices esse dicunt. Ad montes propterea divertitur, quando ad austrum carpere iter consilium est, et paludum illarum vicina fugiuntur. Sunt qui putent vallem unam, qua fluvius labitur *Perditorum* a nostris dictus, ob Nicuesae sociorumque infortunium, a Cerabaroo non multum distantem, findere montes illos ad austrum. Sed, cum potabiles sint eius aquae, fabulatos esse eos putant, qui talibus argumentis innituntur. Hoc perpendiculo perficiamus opus. A dextra laevaque Darienis praedicant viginti flumina decurrere auro feracia: quae dant accipimus, nemo est, qui non id ferat. Sed, interrogati cur parvam auri copiam inde asportent, fossoribus opus esse inquiunt; qui autem eas adiere terras, minime sunt assueti laboribus. Propterea dicunt minorem auri copiam inde vehi quam tellus ipsa sua benignitate, polliceatur. Videtur et nitidas promittere gemmas. In cuius rei argumentum est quod, praeter ea, quae dixi in Cariai et Sanctae Marthae vicinia reperta. Andreas quidam Morales nauclerus [46] per ea maria, Ioannis Cossae amicus et socius, dum Cossa viveret, ad manus habuit adamantem a iuvene Pariensi in Cumana nudo, mire preciosum, longum, uti signant, duos infamis digiti [47] articulos, magni autem pollicis primum articulum aequantem crassitudine, acutum utrobique et costis octo pulchre formatis constantem; eo inquiunt infixisse incudibus vibices vectesque ac limas corrosisse, adamante illaeso. Collo gestabat pendulum adaman-

[46] In classical times it appears to have meant "owner of the ship" (see Plaut. *mil.* 1110; Isid. XIX 3; Firm. *Math.* 8, 20; Tert. *adv. Marc.* 5, 2) whereas Peter Martyr rather implies "pilot."

[47] It is the middle finger. Peter Martyr uses such an expression without the obscene meaning attached to it occasionally in antiquity. See Ov. *ars. am.* II 707; *Priap.* 56, 2; Pers. II 33; Mart. I 92, 2; II 28, 2; VI 70, 5; *schol.* Iuv. X 52.

so are telling stories. Let us complete the book with this appendix. They say that to the right and left of Darién there flow twenty gold-laden rivers we simply accept the news they give us, but there is no one who would not believe it. However, asked why they took only a small quantity of gold, they blame the lack of miners; yet many who went there were not used to hard work. This is their explanation for the small quantity exported when gold is so abundant in that land, which seem to promise also precious stones. Beside those precious stones which I said had been found in the vicinity of *Cariai* and *Santa Marta*, here is some further evidence. A certain Andrés de Morales, a helmsman of those seas, friend and companion of Juan de La Cosa, while La Cosa was still alive, had in his hands a diamond given him by a naked young man of *Paria*, in the region of *Cumaná*; the diamond was very precious: its length was two joints of the middle finger, as they say, but with a thickness of the first joint of the thumb; it was pointed at both ends and had eight beautifully cut facets; the claim is that it scratched lines onto anvils and left notches in iron bars and on files, and it remained unscratched. That young man from *Cumaná* used to wear this diamond around his neck but sold it to Andrés de Morales for five of our green and blue glass beads, captivated as he was by its vivid colors. On the beach they also found topaz; but since they have only gold on their minds, they do not care about these precious stones. They Pay attention only to gold, prospectiong for it. In addition, most Spaniards mock those who wear rings or precious stones and consider it shameful to wear jewels, especially common people; but the nobles, during wedding feasts or, on other occasions, such as the numerous festivities at court, like to wear gold necklaces mounted with jewels, and they weave into their garments pearls mixed with precious stones, but on other occasions they do not. They consider it effeminate to wear ornaments of this kind as well as to smell of perfumes of Arabia and of constant aromatic sprayings; if they run into someone who smells of castoreum or musk, they think he is stained with a sinful passion. In the same way from a single fruit picked from a tree, one infers that there is a fruit tree; or that from a fish caught in a river, people realize that fish live in rivers so, it is that — in like fashion — from a little gold and one precious stone, we ought to conclude that this land

tem iuvenis ille Cumananus et Andreae ipsi Morali, precio quinque calculorum vitreorum nostratium veridium et glaucorum, varietate colorum delectatus, vendidit. Offenderunt et topazios in littore; sed, cum auri faciem animo gestent, nulla est his de gemmis cura. Auro tantum invigilant, aurum sectantur. Maior praeterea Hispanorum pars annulatos aut gemmatos derident et probro ascribunt gemmarum gestamina, populares praecipue; nobiles autem, si quando nuptiales vel alias regiae parentur pompae celebres, torquibus aureis gemmis consutis gaudent et vestibus margaritas gemmis admixtas intertexunt, alias minime. Effoeminatorum esse huiuscemodi ornatus atque arabicorum odorum spiritus et suffumigationes continuas diiudicant; obscoena venere obvolutum putant, si cui castoreum vel muscum olenti occurrant. Ab uno pomo ab arbore decerpto, pomiferam intelligemus eam esse arborem; ab uno pisce in fluvio capto piscium esse nutritorem fluvium dignoscemus. A modico igitur auro et ab uno lapillo auri et lapillorum esse genitricem terram hanc assentiamur oportet. Quid etiam in portu Sanctae Marthae, in regione Cariai, repererint transeunte classe integra, duce Petro Aria, commilitones eius et e regiis magistratibus plerique, loco suo diximus. Pullulant, germinantur, coalescunt, maturescunt legunturque cotidie opimiora praeteritis. Vilescit quicquid manu Saturni, Herculis et aliorum huiuscemodi heroum patefecit antiquitas; si quid indefessus labor Hispanorum detegat, animadvertemus. Valeat Tua Sanctitas et crebro quid sentiat de his suae sedis apostolicae culturis mihi significet, quo animum sublevet ad laborem futurorum subeundum.

yields gold and precious stones. We reported at its specific time what the companions of Pedro Arias and many royal officials found in the port of Santa Marta, in the region of *Cariai*, while the whole fleet was going through under Arias' command. With each passing day new treasures — greater than those in the past — are acquired and produced, collected, processed and accumulated. Whatever was discovered in ancient times by Saturn, Hercules and other similar heroes is now of very little value; should Spain's unfailing efforts unveil yet new things, everyone shall heed. May Your Holiness fare well, and convey to me what the Apostolic See thinks of these new cultures that my intellect be induced to withstand the labor of future undertakings.

INDEX OF CORRESPONDING PASSAGES

We list the concordances between some passages of the Decades de Orbe Novo presented here and those of other parts of the work in which Peter Martyr, by his own admission at times even unintentionally (see Dec. VII 6, p. 226; VIII 8, p. 257), deals with clearly related topical analogies. His frequently identical espressions, however, typical of his writing style, have not been included in this list.

(The numerical refences are from the Graz anastatic reprint).

Decades de Orbe Novo	Topic	*Decades de Orbe Novo*
I 1, p. 39	Canaries	III 5, p. 122; III 7, p. 129
1, p. 40	*Juana* = Cuba	I 3, p. 50; I 10, p. 76; II 7, p. 97; III 9, p. 138: III 10, p.143, IV 1, p. 146; VII 1, p. 215; VII 8, p.232; VIII 1, p. 241
1, p. 40	Hispaniola	I 3, p. 48; I 10, p. 76; III 7, pp. 129-131; V 9, p. 198; VIII 1, pp. 215-216; VII 8, p. 232
1, p. 40	Single-oar canoes	I 8, p. 67; II 4, p. 89; II 7, p.98; III 1, p. 105; III 4, p. 116; III 7, p. 129; III 10, p. 140, V 2, p. 168; VII 4, p. 224; VIII 6, p. 251
1, p. 40	Cannibals	I 2, pp. 43, 45-47; I 8, p. 68; I 10, p. 75; II 1, pp. 79-80; II 3, p. 87; II 4, p. 90; II 6, p. 93; II 8, p.99; III 3, p. 115; III 5, pp. 122-123; III 9, p. 138; III 10, pp. 141-142; VII 4, pp. 223-224; VIII 6, p. 251
1, p. 41	Food	I 3, p. 53; II 1, p. 81; I 7, p. 66; II 4, p.88; III 2, P. 111; III 4, p. 116; III 5, p. 124; III 8, p. 136; III 9, pp. 136-137; III 7, p. 131; V 9, p. 198; VII 2, p. 219; VIII 3, p. 245
I 1, p. 41	Gold	I 4, p. 56; I 10, p. 76; II 3, p. 87; III 2, p. 112; III 3, pp. 114, 115; III 4, pp. 118, 119; III 5, p. 125; III 6, p. 127; IV 4, p. 150; IV 10, p. 158; V 5, p. 174; V 9, p. 198; VII 6, p. 227; VII 8, p. 232; VIII 6, p. 251
1, p. 41	*utía*	I 7, p. 66; III 7, p. 130; VII 9, p. 235
1, p. 41	Snakes and crocodiles	I 3, pp. 50, 51; I 10, p. 75; II 1, p. 82; II 9, p. 101; III 4, pp. 117, 119, 121; V 9, p. 198; VIII 7, pp. 252, 254

NOTES

by
ERNESTO LUNARDI

I. – PETER MARTYR OF ANGHIERA: A MAN IN THE WINGS OF HISTORY.

The autobiographical data are scarce, the documents refer almost exclusively to his titles and stipends, the pages of his letters do not yield many revelations: what would seem a life of no consequence — is instead one of the most remarkable testimonies in history of the last years of the XV century and first decades of the XVI.

According to one of his statements, Peter Martyr was born on February 2, 1457 in Arona — where the family had homes and land — to Giovanni d'Anghiera, called de Boldo, Milanese, who was perhaps in the service of the Borromeo family.

We accept such a date because it is clearly specified: the references that can suggest other years from 1455 to 1459 are vague and inaccurate. In 1488 Peter Martyr told Talavera he was twenty-nine years old in order to convince Talavera to support his request to the Queen to serve as a soldier; Lucio Marineo Siculo speaks of Peter Martyr as a twenty-four year-old teacher in Rieti in 1480, but from official documents his appointment appears dated 1482. Really Peter Martyr speaks of his family history only once, in a letter of 1502 when he visited his native Arona on his return leg from his embassy to the Sultan of Egypt. In this letter he refers to a text in three "notebooks" concerning the family history which had been sent to him by his relatives when he was serving at the court as tutor of the aristocracy.

The timing of the letter and that of the "notebooks" are particularly significant in helping us understand one and maybe the greatest of his aspirations, that of obtaining from the Spanish sovereigns an honorary title with which he could deck himself in his homeland, as a revenge against those who, in a past perhaps not too remote, had caused his illustrious family to decline. After achieving almost unexpected success in Egypt, a difficult and risky mission, Martyr again dreams of obtaining a noble title, a fantasy which perhaps he had begun to pursue while participating in the war for Granada.

Throughout all of the fifteenth century, D'Anghiera appears as "last name" or "family name" of several persons of rank of the Milanese and Verbano area, judges, administrators, public servants, men of letters associated with the ducal power or the powerful Borromeo family. "D'Anghiera" is never used in reference to a locality of Lake Maggiore called today Angera, and the title of "Count of Anghiera" is attributed beginning with the XIV century to the heir of the Visconti, lords of Milan, while the jurisdiction on Anghiera is granted in the second half of the 1400's to the Borromeos, counts of Arona and the Verbano.

While one must exclude any ties with the legendary lineage of the sovereigns of Anghiera, whose power might have extended from the Verbano to the Gotthard, it is plausible that the D'Anghiera belonged to the minor nobility incorporated in the Milanese territory at the ascent to power of the Visconti by whom they were deprived of the title and jurisdiction because they had clashed with them. But, perhaps in contrast to the Visconti, they obtained the protection of the Borromeos from whom they also gained trust and friendship. Being related to the Trivulzios and the Marlianos, a certain cultural tradition and, the familiarity with the Borromeos, upon whom in a sense they were dependent, might have assured a dignified life but deprived of great expectations.

Most likely what the D'Anghieras suffer from at the time in which Peter Martyr appears is the loss of a previously more elevated rank due to causes that cannot be determined from local history. This can be demonstrated from the certain fact that two of the three brothers, given their character, try, to again become influential outside of their own land. Peter Martyr follows the path of humanistic studies whose necessary premises are deep commitment and intellectual brilliance; Giovanni Battista chooses an army career, more aleatory and risky but perhaps, with luck, quicker and brighter.

The two did not get along with the third brother, Giorgio, the shrewd administrator of the family estate, who expected some recognition because of his constant respect for power.

And up to the first years in the 1500s it seems as if all aspirations were being realized: Giorgio becomes governor of Monza; Giovanni Battista, who serves under the Venetian flag, becomes captain of the fortress of Brescia. But the power of the Sforzas declines and Giorgio returns into obscurity; the fortunes of war move against Venice, and Giovanni Battista withdraws from Brescia, taking refuge in Mantua, where he dies in 1514. Only Peter Martyr in fact, obtains, in addition to his fame as a great humanist, prestigious appointments; but because of his ecclesiastical status, his "fortune" can be extended only indirectly to the rest of the family.

We have an interesting letter of recommendation from Queen Isabella to Ludovico il Moro, with whom she certainly was not on the best of terms, on behalf of the D'Anghiera family and in particular Giorgio. The letter was undoubtedly solicited by Peter Martyr, who is highly praised in it.

As for the humanist, when Giorgio is nominated governor of Monza, Peter sends him advice and suggestions, useful for absolving his duties. He remembers him again in his will, entrusting to him the care of his niece Laura, with the obligation that she attend to him.

Peter Martyr is much closer to his younger brother, Giovanni Battista, who is also eager to better his own condition, not through studies but by pursuing a military career: he enlists in the service of Nicolò Orsini, count of Pitigliano, who was employed by the Republic of Venice, and he achieves a certain prestige. Queen Isabella writes on his behalf to the Senate of the *Serenissima* [the Republic] while Peter Martyr sends him suggestions and advice.

Peter Martyr probably spends his infancy in Arona, and returns there from time to time during his adolescence, which he spends in Milan, where under the protection of the Borromeos he begins his humanistic studies at the school of Filelfo, in the court of the Sforzas. A remarkable disposition, an always-sharp curiosity and the belief that perhaps education was the only path by which he could better his condition, motivate him to a constant and profitable engagement, so much that he soon stands out among all the young people who take courses from Filelfo the humanist. Even the Visconti-Sforzas wanted to be equal to the other Italian Princes and thus protected men of letters and artists.

Peter Martyr will keep some friends among Milanese society, favored perhaps by his relationship with illustrious families, but a certain uneasiness about these ties which surfaces in the correspondence of later years is evident; he will leave for Rome when he is not yet twenty years old, with letters of recommendation from the Borromeos and Archbishop Arcimboldi.

In 1477 he is in Rome, where he tries to find employment: he has a good humanistic preparation, but he must also find an occupation which will assure him a living. So he accepts the offer to teach in Rieti in a narrow-minded and spiteful provincial milieu, becoming a colleague of another man of letters, the envious Cantalicio, with whom he clashes in lively polemic compositions.

In 1483, Cantalicio obtains the teaching position in Rieti and Peter Martyr is nominated secretary to Antonio Negro, who was appointed governor of Perugia. Is it a promotion or a dismissal? Whatever the case, his stay in Perugia lasts a year and subsequently, still serving as secretary to the same Antonio Negro, now governor of Rome, he returns to the capital of Christianity and has the opportunity to come in contact with Roman humanists.

He spends a few years among these scholars and high dignitaries of the Holy See: among others we mention the great humanist Pomponius Letus, Alonso Carrillo, bishop of Pamplona, and Diego de Sousa, archbishop of Braga (who consider themselves his "pupils" in that they come to him to enrich their own knowledge of humane letters), Ascanio Visconti Sforza, brother of Ludovico il Moro, and Cardinal Arcimboldi, archbishop of Milan. In spite of the recognition that he receives in this cultured ambience, there are conflicts with governor Negro, brought about by the latter's severity, and a few mishaps, such as the episode involving the beautiful Francesca — a lovely girl, perhaps involuntarily a central figure in a public scandal and who ends up in prison — whom he loves and personally defends, even composing some verses on her behalf.

Nonetheless he enriched his culture, learned to know men better, value the causes and effects of political action, determine the favorable moment for making a choice or a decision: in other words, he prepared himself for what would later be his role at the Spanish court. Literature and poetry remained almost peripheral for lack of time, or, better, lack of inspiration in a day to day environment that was mediocre and often mortifying.

Suddenly his destiny changes because of an unexpected circumstance that exhaults his mind. In Rome people are living daily with worry; hunger already oppresses them, and everywhere there is rumor of war — the army of the King of Naples is near, and the French threaten to intervene. Then one night a knight arrives in Rome who manages to be received by the pontiff and convinces him to negotiate an agreement with him, and the city is saved.

This mysterious knight is Don Iñigo López de Mendoza, Count of Tendilla, chief of the mission sent by Queen Isabella of Castile and King Ferdinand of Aragon to make a gesture of homage to the pontiff Innocent VIII. Don Iñigo, whose deeds in the war of Granada were already famous in Italy, arriving in Florence and, realizing that the situation was by now almost irreparable (the task of settling the disagreement between the pontiff and the King of Naples was, however, in the secret instructions given to him), decides to act as circumstances dictate: he leaves his followers in the city of the Medici and rushes alone to Rome. The action is certainly unusual, even if such audacity is characteristic of him. The outcome is unexpectedly resounding: when Don Iñigo, a month later, officially enters the Eternal City as the head of the Spanish delegation, the people applaud him as a conqueror, as their liberator from the spectre of war.

Peter Martyr, impressed by the knight and his bold gesture, feels his poetic inspiration awakening and composes for him the *Inachus*, a short poem in Latin, in which he praises past deeds and the recent triumph. The valiant knight Don Iñigo, Alonso Carrillo's cousin, probably met Peter the poet at Carrillo's house. The Count of Tendilla [Iñigo] is not only a representative of the highest Spanish nobility and a brave soldier, but is also by family tradition well-versed in literature, indeed, a recognized poet: Don Iñigo Lopez de Mendoza, marquis of Santillana, a representative Castilian writer of the XV century.

The meeting marks a turning point for Peter Martyr: the noble Spaniard is particularly sensitive to the poetic homage of the Italian humanist, and in his mind resurface the worries of the Queen, who would like to offer young Spanish noblemen that humanistic formation without which, she thinks, even military conquests fail to bring about progress in the country.

Born in this climate is the invitation by Tendilla to Peter Martyr to follow him to Spain, where he will be introduced to the Queen: his learning and poetry will be able to find in Iberia full recognition. At the base of this invitation and its quick acceptance there is, undoubtedly, an understanding, a spiritual affinity, a reciprocal trust which allow them to overcome their socially notable differences. We have dwelled upon this decisive moment in the life of the writer precisely because it gives us the key to better understand his later behavior: the image of a calm courtier who observes and records events because he is a man of letters and also of confidant to the Sovereigns—an image which could also be derived from his work, with the exception, however, of his epistolary — is a totally wrong perception.

The meeting with Tendilla gives him a surge of energy which he will never lose, a flair for bold deeds, for the always tense climate that one breathes where the destiny of peoples is decided, the conviction that the writer must perform the role of witness of life in all its facets, the vision of culture as a constant search for the new. We will see him as warrior, priest, teacher, advisor to the Sovereigns, ambassador *extraordinaire*, mediator between two kings—Ferdinand and Philip the Fair, father-in-law and son-in-law—a man charged with assisting Queen Juana the Mad, referee between two ferociously opposed factions, and, in this capacity, forger of documents, commissioner of "Indian affairs," defender of the oppressed.

Tendilla's invitation arrived at an appropriate time: in the first letter from Spain to Ascanio Sforza the reasons which prompted the Lombard humanist to leave are made quite clear. Even if, as it is held by most, the letter is written afterwards, the reasons stated in it are fully in harmony with the psychological conditions of Peter Martyr, above all with his belief that he will never be able to distinguish himself in a Rome where political intrigues, material interests, and noble rank dominate everything, in an Italy where the dissension among the powerful anticipates the imminent storm.

On the other hand, there was proof of the possibility of quick advancement in Spain, through Antonio Geraldini, who had accompanied Don Iñigo on his mission and had delivered for him the official oration in Latin to the pontiff and who was, with his brother Alessandro, tutor of the monarchs' children at court, and Lucio Marineo Siculo, brought to Spain by the "Almirante de Castilla," Don Fadrique, who was a professor at the famous University of Salamanca. Peter Martyr leaves in the summer of 1487 with his protector after a stop in the Florence of Lorenzo il Magnifico, where Italian culture seems to lay down the law for the rest of Europe, and he arrives at the Court of Isabella and Ferdinand, who are moving from Saragossa to Alcalá de Henares, where the Mendozas live.

The meeting of Peter Martyr with Queen Isabella proves to be decisive: there is an immediate understanding, a spiritual affinity, an absolute trust which seems to erase any class distinction. The Italian humanist represents, for the Castilian Queen, culture at its highest expression, and she recognizes immediately also his communicative gifts, indispensable for his mission as guide on the road to culture, his honesty and uprightness, his religiosity, energy, and diligence.

On the other hand, Peter Martyr cannot avoid being fascinated by the Queen. Not beautiful, perhaps too rigid in her religious zeal, energetic and unyielding, she has nonetheless an exceptional sensitivity which helps her understand the intimate dramas of the protagonists whom she singles out among the multiform crowd of courtiers that surrounds her, and she always knows how to find the most opportune formula to help, without too much clamor, and to give timely rewards.

With the most eulogistic words, Tendilla presents the humanist to the Queen, who congratulates him and declares that his presence at the court will be of great usefulness to the Spanish people.

For the moment, however, the problems of culture are secondary: the war of Granada has been going on for six years and its outcome is still uncertain and remote. Yet Isabella wants neither to humiliate Don Iñigo, who had made so many promises, nor to disappoint Peter Martyr for fear that he might go back to Rome, so for the time being she employs him on the staff of her retinue, which enjoys greater remuneration than that of the King's. Peter Martyr perhaps struggles to find his way: he has left the luxurious dwellings of Renaissance Rome and finds himself in a court which does not even have its own seat. Welcomed with much respect, he enjoys a stipend but lacks a definite assignment, and around him he feels the fighting spirit of the last war of the Re-Conquest which has been going on for eight centuries.

He found at the court also a certain cultural milieu, represented by, among others, the Italian Geraldinis, Tendilla, Fray Hernando de Talavera, bishop of Avila, confessor of Isabella and member of the royal council, a man of profound learning, former professor at the University of Salamanca, with whom he quickly develops a spiritual affinity, just as he had done with Tendilla.

Still, it seems to him he is not being "employed," and Isabella, who has understood his state of mind, has Talavera ask him which assignment he would like to have at the court. Surprising everyone, he asks to serve as a soldier in the war against the Moorish kingdom of Granada. Certainly no one could have expected that Peter Martyr, brought to Spain as a representative of the Italian culture, would ask to bear arms.

The request could surprise us, too, but in reality, aside from his religious spirit and the influence that Queen Isabella exerted on everyone, there were many valid reasons for that choice. Peter Martyr knew well that the court would soon be transferred to the war front where he, armed only with his culture, would have been really like a fish out of water, the object of contempt and scorn, especially since Spanish nobility traditionally appreciated military virtues above all else. Even the mission that the Queen had led him to envisage after the war, that of teacher of liberal arts to the nobles of the court, would be anything but easy if he did not manage first to gain a clear prestigious reputation.

So that his request be accepted, he even tells a little lie to Don Hernando, saying that he is twenty-nine years old, and he writes a letter to the Queen using most persuasive and flattering language. Isabella accepts the request and has him admitted to the royal guard (the *cohors pretoria*, writes the humanist), which receives orders directly from the Count of Tendilla, head of the Castilian forces: the royal guard is deployed for the defense of the Sovereigns, and is made up of select elements, but it must earn this privilege by proving itself through swift and violent actions of the greatest risk.

At the school of his protector and friend, the humanist learns well the art of war and he conducts himself so well that the Sovereigns allow

him to add an oak crown to his coat of arms; the memory of his partici-
pation in the campaign will be recorded among the many titles on his
tombstone.

We must add that Peter Martyr was anything but an individual with
a strong physique. Probably short in height and frail, his strength is all
in his strong will. From the letters sent from the front, we learn that
often he returns to camp extremely tired, too tired to be able to write;
that he suffers for insufficient food, the hard bed, the weight of the
armor, and the long rides. But he does not give up: his involvement in
the fighting can also be deduced by the more dramatic tone, or the more
precise details, by the use of "we" (in place of "our soldiers," which he
employs instead when he is not taking part in the fighting). Yet Peter
Martyr does not reap the first real victory in Spain on the battlefield, but
in his specific capacity as a humanist: from the University of Salamanca
he receives an invitation to deliver a lecture on a topic of his choice, an
invitation perhaps intended as mild provocation toward this Italian, who
has just arrived and already has been so successfully accepted by the
Court and who pretends also to be a soldier.

At first he tries to fend off the invitation, then he accepts it and, in
a moment when the various battle fronts are calm, he starts a venturesome
trip that seems of bad auspice; introduced by Lucio Marineo Siculo, he
teaches his lesson on Juvenal's second satire before an audience made up
of professors, students and guests, scoring great success. According to
his lively report to the Count of Tendilla, because of the large crowd,
some people were bruised, first while trying to enter the hall then in
trying to congratulate him, so that they had to use clubs to let him
through. The success of Salamanca is a confirmation of his learning and
increases his prestige, so that besides serving as a soldier (the Queen
sometimes invites him not to go when the operations take place too far
away because she does not want him to get too fatigued) he becomes the
drafter of Latin letters for the Sovereigns and counselor and confidant
on political problems as well as family matters.

But the war continues, with its ups and downs, and the most concrete consequences, for the moment, are only sacrifice, pain, and physical
and moral sufferings of the army and, above all, of the civilian population,
all for a cause whose most legitimate motives are perhaps on the side of
the Muslims, who are defending both the soil on which they have been
living for eight centuries and their faith and traditions.

What makes him weary is not physical exhaustion, but the belief
that wars are always unjust and inhuman. One can anticipate from his
experiences as a soldier what his future attitude will be, especially when

the echo of the horrors of the wars in Italy and the slaughters in the New World finally reach him. During the moments in which the fighting stagnates, the man of culture emerges in him again on the battle field. Perhaps simply in reaction to the harshness of war he converses with his Roman friends, and in military tents the great problems of philosophy, history, poetry and science are passionately discussed. During these moments Peter Martyr is a teacher, and around him gather Tendilla and Talavera, the young people from the high nobility, perhaps sometimes the Queen herself, who was much interested in cultural problems, and her ladies-in-waiting, so numerous in that military camp where even Moorish poetry did abound.

In the encampment below Granada, which after the terrible fire of August 1491 was transformed into a fortified city with all white buildings and the significant name of Santa Fe, from time to time there would make an appearance a singular character, all caught up in his dream of opening a new route through the "Dark Sea," the Genoese Christopher Columbus, strong in his indomitable will, supported more or less openly, but always firmly, by the great Queen.

In the context of the above-mentioned learned discussions, to which frequent reference is made in the correspondence of the following years, the great friendship between Peter Martyr and Christopher Columbus is born and grows. Perhaps the support of the humanist and his learning, combined with the Crown's political motivations, was important in overcoming the last oppositions of the Court and making the great voyage possible.

The war ends: the Catholic Sovereigns enter Granada on January 2, 1492, and in their retinue are present the Genoese Columbus and the Milanese Peter Martyr.

Here another change of life occurs: the humanist-soldier sheds his armor and puts on the cassock, joining the clergy of the Cathedral of Granada. Peter Martyr vaguely speaks of being tired of court life, speaks of his love for solitude, but these are reasons that we consider neither determining nor very plausible, especially since barely a few months later he is busy petitioning all the friends that he believes he has at the Court that they have him called back.

Possibly he had too many illusions, especially in his hope that his conduct during the war would have brought him some recognition. If that had been the cherished dream for which he had not spared risks or sacrifices, one must admit that this time he was completely wrong: Isabella and Ferdinand tended rather to diminish the importance and number of nobles, and they would not have been easily able to elevate a foreigner to nobility without causing great discontent.

One can imagine an irreconcilable conflict with a very powerful figure of the Court; joining the clergy was, in those times, a device often adopted to solve very difficult situations.

One could also suppose there was some disappointment in love. We have mentioned the presence in the camp of many women in the Queen's retinue of high nobility, daughters, sisters, wives of soldiers, about whom much is said in the chronicles of the time. Peter Martyr remembers the Marquise of Moya wounded by a criminal who thought she was the Queen, and Navagero talks of a "gentle war" in which the warriors would accomplish brave deeds in order to please their lady loves.

In the letters of those years feminine figures do not appear, but in later years and in poems are remembered the sisters of the heroic Pedro Fajardo, his student and friend, and particularly the oldest sister, Eleanora, beautiful, virtuous, and learned.

The climate of war is suited to create dreams and illusions, perhaps as a necessary compensation for the cruelty and suffering; the humanist was for four years in close contact with the Sovereigns, their closest advisers, and their retinue. In other words, he lived fully the atmosphere of the Court and, still young and admired for his learning and courage, he might have attributed in his heart a much more ample significance to the affection and the kindnesses of a young noble lady.

We do not have certain proof at all, but the change of state took place quite quickly and, what is most important, the "renunciation of the world" was of very short duration.

Whatever the occasion might have been, we must exclude a sudden spiritual crisis that would have made him shun earthly possessions to lock himself up in one of the strictest religious orders: the secular clergy in fact provides one with a privileged "status," especially in the Spain of the Catholic Monarchs, but does not prevent one from living a busy but comfortable life similar to that of all the others, which is, as Peter Martyr acknowledges, one of his unrepressible needs. He may not have noble or academic titles, but belonging to the clergy can mean that he has already reached a stable, albeit for the time being modest, condition, which in some way complements the personal prestige that he has gained and assures him the means of subsistence.

However, life in Granada is not easy. His friend and protector Don Iñigo López, now viceroy and governor of the kingdom of Granada, must control the situation in the conquered city, in the midst of people who are trying to defend their own traditional values; his friend Hernando de Talavera, named archbishop of Granada, tries everything to erase the Muslim traces and to create a Christian climate in the city, and thus demands the greatest dedication and the most exemplary conduct from the clergy. In fact, clergymen do not even enjoy complete safety, and must limit themselves to their religious functions. The Sovereigns, after their sumptuous triumphal entry into the city, retire to Santa Fe, which in reality is an entrenched camp, waiting to return to their own kingdoms until the most urgent problems are solved.

During those same days the long negotiations with Columbus are brought to an end, and on April 17, 1492 the *Capitulations of Santa Fe*, which constitute the first official act for the realization of the great voyage are signed. The last intensive stages — the absence of the Genoese from the Court, his personal and proclaimed decision to travel to France, his sudden unexpected recall, the quick conclusion of the agreements — have a singular analogy with the insistent letters that the Milanese humanist sends in those days to all those whom he considers his friends at Court in order that they manage to have him recalled; and in fact they have the same motivations: returning to their inherited states after the victory. Isabella and Ferdinand would have been entirely absorbed in the complex problems of their respective kingdoms entrusted for four years to their regents, and in all the problems they had promised to solve at the end of the war (of concern to us here is the preparation of Columbus's voyage and the opening of the school of *Bellas Artes* for the Court's noblemen) would maybe have had soon a new and indefinite delay.

The Sovereigns move in fact to Castile and then Aragon and Catalonia; Columbus journeys to Palos, where the ships must be equipped; Peter Martyr leaves the cathedral, where though by the Queen's request he has been named canon, he reached the wandering court and begins his activity.

The first official Spanish documents that concern him are dated precisely 1492:

1) Isabella's letter to the archbishop of Granada for the nomination of the Milanese orator *Pedro Martyl*, to canon of the cathedral on March 25, 1492;

2) the nomination to *contino* at the Spanish court (designating the position of one «attached permanently to the court without specification of a particular charge;

3) the «pay roll» of the stipends of the court of Castile in which also the name of Peter Martyr appears.

We must make clear that the earliest documents of the cathedral of Granada go back only to the year 1508, and, therefore, we do not have the official act of his being appointed to canon. On the other hand, the title of "Professor of Liberal Arts for the Nobles of the Court" first appears in the credentials given in 1501 to Peter Martyr for his mission to the sultan of Egypt: the beginning of his activity undoubtedly did coincide with his return to Court.

As is well known, there was not an official capital of the kingdom of Castile until the time of Philip II, and the Monarchs reside from time to time in different centers of the country, places where the problems are more urgent and where the courts convene, formed by nobles, clergy and citizen councils representing the people.

Thus, in addition to the difficulties of having his teaching accepted by the children of the nobility who, even though young, already have the prestige of the title and some of them that of warrior, Peter Martyr also has to worry about finding a dignified seat for his "school" in each locality, a seat for all the dignitaries of the Court that must be assigned by royal functionaries not always very well-disposed toward this foreigner who has become a first rank personality.

The beginning of his activity is very difficult, because of the lack of interest and discipline in his young students who, after the trying war years, seek rest and diversions, certainly not the severe and methodic study of Latin. Once again, Queen Isabella, with her feminine intuition, understands the distress of the humanist and finds the most appropriate solution: she orders her grandchildren to attend Peter Martyr's classes every day, and so the young noblemen feel obliged to follow her example. The climate changes completely and the first positive fruits are reaped.

It is not clear for how long he carried out his task. The title always appears in official documents, but we think that it became an excuse for retaining the stipend since he then undertook in succession new engagements more directly related to the political administration of power and closely connected with the royal household which required a great amount of time and discretion.

From 1492 to his death, except for brief periods during the absence of the Sovereigns or for diplomatic missions assigned to him away from the court, he lives almost always at the Court, and he becomes the interpreter of its political thought, trustee of the secret concerns of the royal family, historian of the great events of those years, occasionally a noted figure or the central figure in clamorous episodes.

To outline Peter Martyr's life means to recall the history of Spain from 1492 to 1526: more often he is an *èminence grise*, apparently reserved and irritable, who leads, however, a life full of meetings solicited by him because he needs to know everything, in particular what is happening in Italy and in the New World being directly involved in what happens in Spain. We can limit ourselves to recalling a few of the more significant career moments that are important events exemplifying the role he played as spectator, interpreter, and protagonist.

The year 1493 is a key moment: the humanist is in Barcelona at the Court when the news arrives of the return of Columbus, welcomed with every honor by the Catholic Monarchs. He is present at the feverish activity surrounding the departure of the second expedition of 17 ships loaded with soldiers and workers, plants and animals to be taken to the New Lands. His humanistic spirit and curiosity reach the peak of enthusiasm and after talking with the protagonists of the great adventure he writes about it to far away friends, tackling before anyone else the scientific issues raised by the discovery.

The attitude about the novel discovery and its implications vary. Already with the second expedition, Queen Isabella is concerned primarily with sending clergymen who can promote the conversion of new peoples to Christianity; Ferdinand worries instead about having the Church recognize the rights of Castile to the New Lands against every Portuguese claim, and he orders Columbus to take possession of as many lands as possible. The Genoese wants to reaffirm the rights he has acquired and demonstrate the validity of his own theories. A crowd of ambitious, avid people comes forward, eager to participate in the expedition in the hope of easily obtaining wealth and honors. Peter Martyr aims especially at forging a proper perspective for the new reality of the discovery and the related acculturation process: he gathers all the information available on the nature of places and people; through his letters, he poses scientific, political, and religious problems to himself and his friends (Ascanio Sforza, Pomponius Letus, Alonso Carrillo, Diego de Sousa, Bernardino Carvajal), and he keeps Tendilla and Talavera up to date on events, recalling also the role they played in the preparation of such an undertaking.

But he is not a withdrawn scholar seeking refuge in his culture, or the bookish treasures of past and present. He is a man who appreciates life, who suffers for the tragedies and losses of others, who gets angry about injustices and deceits and, in particular, about the blood that is being shed in the wars of Europe, the violence carried out in the New World, the unworthy actions of those who should be the highest representatives of morality and justice.

By consulting the letters and glancing at the documents, one can discover in him a temporary crisis in the years 1495 and 1496.

The letter of June 11, 1495 to Bernardino Carvajal is very bitter, with severe judgements about the pontiff's role and that of the Roman Curia, concerning what is happening in Spain; it even reveals doubts about the choice of Francisco Jiménez de Cisneros as the Queen's confessor.

We find also evidence of an attempted return to Milan in a letter by the Milanese ambassador Sfondrato to Ludovico il Moro which contains a proposal to nominate Peter Martyr ambassador of the Duke of Milan to the Catholic Sovereigns for a given period, so that he may then return to his homeland with great prestige. We do not doubt that the letter might have been solicited by the interested party in a moment of depression when all his ideals seem to collapse; the church appears more and more dominated by intrigues and greed; even the loyalty of the Spanish Sovereigns is failing (many captains sent to the New World are in actual violation of the *Capitulaciones*, an offense to the Genoese); Ferdinand weaves his plots, deceiving even his close relatives, and a man ignorant of political affairs is appointed to an extremely delicate post. It is likely that the humanist told the Queen of his desire to return to Milan, justifying it with the need to lend support to his family: one could account in this manner for Isabella's letter to Ludovico il Moro, previously mentioned (see p. 373), in which she recommends the relatives of Peter Martyr, particularly Giorgio d'Anghiera, his brother.

Highs and lows follow one another. Peter Martyr is told to ready himself to serve as an extraordinary ambassador to the King of Hungary: it is a cause of great joy, even though he knows the troublesomeness of a trip and the difficulty of the assignment; the chance of again seeing his homeland, relatives and friends is more important to him. However, the mission is cancelled, since it is considered totally unnecessary, given the attitude of the Magyar king, who has gained the pontiff's approval.

Our writer continues to be interested in everything pertaining to the discoveries and shares Isabella's keen and painful sense of distress whose triumphs as Queen have their counterbalance in her misfortunes as mother.

In 1501, a mission of great importance is entrusted to Peter Martyr. The fall of Granada and the policies of forced conversions or of expelling from the peninsula the non-converted provoke a profound reaction in the Islamic world. Christian monasteries in the Holy Land are damaged, pilgrims are persecuted, and the sultan of Egypt threatens major retaliations, including war, if the persecution of his co-religionists does not end.

The Catholic Sovereigns must avert this threat and look for an agreement, but it is not easy to find the right person among the high

Spanish nobility to deal with the Moslems, since all are directly involved in the war with Granada and in royal politics. The assignment is given to Peter Martyr of Anghiera, who is sent in his capacity as "Professor of Liberal Arts to the Nobles of the Court." For obvious reasons, his positions as chaplain of the Queen and canon of the cathedral of Granada are not mentioned. He goes as a man of culture, representing the human values that must be at the basis of all coexistence among men and states; his duty is to clarify that there are no Islamic persecutions in Spain and, therefore, that there should not be persecution of Christians in the Islamic lands.

Peter Martyr leaves, but the beginnings are not too auspicious: the regions he crosses are scourged by plague and therefore the ambassador and his retinue are not welcomed in the cities; often they find neither lodging nor food; some get sick. Finally, he arrives in Venice, where he will embark on ships of the Republic and head for Egypt. He had also received secret instructions from the Sovereigns to convince the Venetian government not to side with the French, but he arrives at the moment in which one doge is dead and the new one is not yet elected, and consequently his audience in the Senate is reduced to only a courtesy visit and his expression of gratitude for the support given him on his trip.

The convoy has gone ahead and he catches up in Pola, but the sea conditions are prohibitive; he takes advantage of this circumstance to visit the nearby Roman ruins. He finally leaves, but finds himself in the midst of storms and great danger of sinking. He arrives in Alessandria and, while waiting for the pass to proceed for Cairo, he visits the city and its surroundings. He then obtains permission to go to court, but he runs the risk of being robbed and lynched by a furious crowd. These are certainly not the best psychological conditions for someone who has to carry out difficult negotiations. However, the Islamic ruler accepts the report on the correct behavior of the catholic Sovereigns, accepts the request to have damaged buildings rebuilt and protect pilgrims, and dismisses the ambassador, loading him down with gifts for himself and his monarchs.

Peter Martyr returns to Venice, where this time he is welcomed by the new doge, but he realizes that the Republic of Venice is by now siding with the enemy camp and urges his Sovereigns to nominate a permanent ambassador to the Venetian Republic, advising that the person be a man of great experience and great culture (a possible reference to himself?).

He goes through Milan and stops for eleven days in his native Arona, days that remind him of his childhood and renew his ties with relatives and friends enjoying the marvelous views of Lake Maggiore. He also makes a substantial donation of sacred and profane items to the main parish church of the city, in solemn form, with a certificate drawn up by notaries in the presence of the Borromeos as witnesses. The church, however, is in a state of ruin, and, from that moment and for many years, he will insist on being nominated abbot so that he can restore it with the prebends owed to him.

But events are pressing: to return to Spain Peter Martyr must cross an Italy and France that are now at war with his Sovereigns. The French would be very happy to lay their hands on him, especially since they know he is loaded with precious gifts; so he turns for protection to the Borromeos, and especially to his relative, Giangiacomo Trivulzio, grand marshal of France, who finally accompanies him to a meeting with the powerful chancellor of Amboise, who, after a lively political-diplomatic discussion, all in Latin, secures for him a safe pass signed by the King, which places him in safety. He returns to Spain where he is welcomed with the greatest honors. Of this mission he will write his precious report, entitled *Legatio Babylonica.*

After his return from Egypt, even though we find in the records his nominations to Professor of Liberal Arts (December 15, 1502) and to prior of the cathedral of Granada (November 25, 1503), one can say that Peter Martyr, at least until 1508, is totally preoccupied with the tragic events of the royal family. Isabella declines rapidly, consumed by her sickness and even more by her sufferings, especially for the death of Prince John, the male heir, and more for the unstable psychological state of Juana, now become heir, madly in love with her husband Philip of Hapsburg nicknamed "Handsome." In 1504 the Queen dies and her faithful chaplain (there is a document of nomination dated May 8, 1501) escorts the remains to Granada, where she had arranged to be buried. It is a painful trip for one who owes so much to this Sovereign and has been so close to her.

A conflict explodes between King Ferdinand, who has proclaimed himself regent, and Philip, who claims the power which legitimately belongs to Juana, considered by both of them to be incapable of exercising it. The Castilian nobility believes that the right moment has arrived to recover their own autonomy from the king of Aragon, and they play on the ambitions of the young prince consort, who is accustomed to a very different dynastic tradition and unfamiliar with Iberian traditions and the relationships between the Crown and the citizens. The aged sovereign neither wants to give up the regency or tolerate being deprived of the lands of the kingdom of Castile and of the new wealthy regions of the New

World. Philip claims his own rights and is afraid the recent marriage of his father-in-law with Germana, sister of the king of France, might put in danger the rights of succession to the throne of his son, the infante Charles.

Spanish national unity, de facto achieved by the marriage of Isabella and Ferdinand, threatens to break up. The positions seem irreconcilable, and Peter Martyr, adviser to King Ferdinand and chaplain of Queen Juana, Philip's bride, continues to offer to both parties suggestions and advice. He is worried above all about the future of Spain, his country of adoption, and he also assumes, upon Ferdinand's request, an official mission of mediator. He is tied to the Aragonese king by gratitude, even if he has received greater benefits and honors from Isabella and has no affection for the French lady who has taken her place and is so different. Maybe he prefers young Philip who shows him affection and esteem and whom, in his heart, he recognizes to be more in the right, even if his humanistic formation will force him to think that young people should always show respect for their elders.

The mission is unsuccessful and in the end it will be Ferdinand who gives up. Peter Martyr will try to console the defeated with a little Latin poem, *Janus*, exalting his great glories and celebrating the achieved peace.

Ferdinand, who has conquered the kingdom of Naples, wants to go there and begs Peter Martyr to stay close to his daughter Juana, who is always afraid she will be locked up by her husband in some remote castle. The humanist, at that moment, is thinking once more about returning to Italy, but does not feel like turning down the assignment. He has known the unfortunate girl since she was a young child and feels great sorrow for her, although compelled and subject to her eccentricities.

Ferdinand leaves and while stopped at Portofino because of bad weather, the news of the death of Philip reaches him. "He felt not a little sorry or seemed sorry for his son-in-law, his daughter's husband; nonetheless he pursued the journey he had started..." Peter Martyr relates with these words to his friends Tendilla and Talavera how the father-in-law reacted to the news of the son-in-law's death.

Actually, Juana, legitimate queen of Castile, at the death of her husband seems to lose what was left of her equilibrium. She contemplates her husband's cadaver, has it embalmed and, already unstable, sets out on the tragic voyage through the regions of the peninsula with the coffin of her husband that she will allow no other woman to see. She has the procession stop far from every inhabited area. Once in a while she insists that they open the casket to verify her husband is still in it. Peter Martyr is one of the three prelates charged with escorting and keeping vigil on the corpse, and perhaps of the three he is the most capable of staying close to the mad queen. He tries to discuss with her problems of state, and she listens to him; she even seems to possess a moderate ability to make decisions, but then when documents are prepared, she refuses to sign, declaring that she wants to wait for her father's return.

The lack of effective power creates everywhere disorder and economic crisis; the always latent contrasts between the nobility and commoners surface again, with local administrators acting arbitrarily. Forced to put up with Juana's moods, Peter Martyr many times urges Ferdinand's return and he also writes him a rather critically harsh letter. Maybe he has gone too far: there is a moment of coldness between the Sovereign and his adviser, to whom everyone turns to find the solution to their problems, beginning with the clergy of Granada who, because of the death of Archbishop Talavera, consider him their highest authority. But the state is in crisis, money is lacking for the army, and the royal treasurers would like to get hold of the Church's funds.

The document of renunciation by Peter Martyr to a prebendary (*ración* or *nación*) in the Canaries is dated December 12, 1508. The document is not very clear, but it makes one think there might have been an attempt to remove the Milanese from the court by sending him to the Canaries. At the same time there are letters of his seeking to obtain the nomination to abbot of San Graziano of Arona, addressed to Trivulzio and also to the cardinal of Amboise. In these letters no mention is made of dissension with the King, but it is not hard to sense that he lacks that peace of mind which can allow him to frequent the Court. In addition, he confesses that he is not very accurate in his information because many letters that arrive at the Court are kept secret from him.

The years pass. The King is more and more isolated, less and less tolerated by the proud Castilian nobility and, little by little, there is a reconciliation with his foreign adviser, who writes that Ferdinand would like to have him constantly at his side and force him to endure an uncomfortable, nomadic life.

His uncontrollable passion for Queen Germana, so much younger than he, and his unrestrained passion for hunting accelerate the King's end. Peter Martyr notices that the King of Spain and the King of France are rather similar in forgetting that they are now rather old and behaving comically, like young people full of strength.

When Ferdinand dies, the humanist writes a positive review of him. In general, he tries to defend him from ongoing accusations of avarice, but he cannot help mentioning his ingratitude toward the Great Captain and the betrayal of his cousin, the King of Naples. He accompanies the casket to Granada where the King will be buried next to Isabella in the royal chapel still under construction, and turns all of his hopes toward young Charles who, in 1515, declares himself of age and claims power.

The internal political situation is more complex than ever because the new king is not only the legitimate heir of his grandfather King of Aragon, Valencia, Catalonia, etc., but the presumed heir to his mother Juana of Castile, who was also Queen of León, Asturias, Granada and of the lands of the New World, still official possessions with full royal rights; and, finally, Charles is the presumed heir as well of Maximilian of Hapsburg who holds the title of Holy Roman Emperor, a title to which the grandson could aspire.

In order to prepare his arrival, Charles sends ahead his Flemish advisers, who are preceded by their fame as rapacious vultures and make one think about the dark prediction that Spain will be devoured by the long-legged crane (Flemish courtiers wear long hose and short pants). The facts confirm these fears. Spain is, for Charles's emissaries, a land of conquest, and they worry not so much about the royal authority as about accumulating riches, granting adequate compensation to the nobles, even to the French, traditionally enemies of Spain. The discontent grows, and in Castile, once more, the specter of Juana, the mad queen, is evoked. The only remedy would be the coming of the King.

Finally, Charles arrives and the situation seems to improve a little, especially for the Kingdom of Aragon, even if in order to gain the favor of the people the new sovereign makes donations which exceed the royalties that he has to collect, so that he becomes poorer and poorer and, as Peter Martyr says, the Kingdom of Castile once again will pay for everyone. Among the men of court that arrive with Charles there is Adrian of Utrecht, bishop of Tortosa, who has to resort to Peter Martyr's Latin in order to learn Spanish and with whom he shall forge a great friendship. Two Lombards are also present: Luigi Marliani, doctor to the King and counselor, a relative of the humanist, and Mercurino Arborio da Gattinara, vice-chancellor and perhaps also a relative of the King. For Peter Martyr who had always been close to the Catholic Sovereigns, except for the duration of the war of Granada, while almost isolated from the other courtiers, and whose relations with Isabella and Ferdinand were almost always kept on the level of personal trust, with the new King and his court one can notice a considerable change of status: he will always remain at the side of the King when the latter is in Spain and when the King is away, the Italian will remain a trusted advisor to the king's ministers who manage the power in his absence. Charles, who has a vivid intelligence and, little by little, is converted to the love for culture, although still too dependent upon his Flemish and German advisers, sees in this humanist the person who had been close to his grandparents Isabella and Ferdinand, the one who was able to extend to his unfortunate mother the love and attention which even she occasionally realized.

The presence of Marliani and Gattinara had undoubtedly its weight, but we must admit also a deep affection and a great personal trust on the part of the King, who renews all his appointments and adds more.

Meanwhile, the death of Maximilian of Hapsburg raises the problem of the nomination of Charles as emperor. Both he and his advisers are deeply involved in serving the investiture.

But the King must obtain the official investiture of the Kingdoms of Spain before returning to Germany. Time presses. If the Courts of Catalonia recognize him as King, the Courts of the kingdom of Valencia, according to their statutes, demand that he appear in person to be proclaimed King. The zeal of Governor Cabanillas is of no account. The King first convenes the courts, then postpones the celebration, trying to obtain support; finally he sends Peter Martyr on a special mission, fully counting on his ability. The Italian accepts unwillingly because he does not consider the claim of the King to be legitimate and believes the King himself should be the first one to respect the statutes.

Charles leaves and his Flemish emissaries, in agreement with many nobles, resume their vexations. Besides, they have the full support of chancellor Chévres, who holds the power in his hands while the King and his advisers are busy gaining support for the election among the Great Electors.

Peter Martyr, who failed in his mission and who from Valencia must reach Valladolid, has the opportunity to notice the great commotion which is spreading in the councils. Charles I, needing soldiers in the battle against the French, has allowed the formation of a citizen army. The populace is armed and becomes less and less resigned to endure the oppression of foreigners and nobles. Alarmed, he writes to Marliani and Mercurino da Gattinara, and since not much weight is given to his information, he even goes so far as to accuse the two friends and relatives of complicity with the "goat," as he calls the chancellor. This time Mercurino replies, and rudely: "do not put your nose into other people's affairs and mind your own business." Probably the friend is afraid that the criticisms of the humanist might reach Chévres' ears who then might take revenge, as he had done before with others; but Peter Martyr will not let his lips be silenced, and thus replies that even if he has received much from Spain, he is ready to leave everything and go away, but he cannot remain quiet at any cost if things are not going well: he is a member of the royal council and cannot fail in his duty.

Chévres dies and Mercurino becomes the new great chancellor. The relations between the two Lombards are again characterized by the former friendship and trust. But what the humanist had anticipated comes true. The revolt of the *comuneros* explodes and Castile is put to fire and sword: the members of the royal government in Valladolid find themselves in the middle of the conflict between the nobles, who want to put down the populace once and for all, and the commoners, who feel stronger and believe they have the support of the Crown since they are claiming their own rights. Once again the legitimacy of the power of Charles is invoked since his mother, Juana — although mad — is still alive.

Peter Martyr is a member of the royal Council and, therefore, is in trouble like the others. He has friends among the heads of the city forces and among the nobles, and tries to calm down both. To the former he points out that if their reasons are valid, the way in which they are trying to uphold them is very wrong. He reminds the nobles that their demands go against an established tradition. By doing so, he makes himself unpopular with both factions and he runs the risk of getting killed. But, in the moments of greater danger, in spite of the fact that he is along in years and his health is poor, he finds again his old energy. He keeps in contact with both factions, trying to reach a compromise or a truce; he proposes that the apostolic legate Vinicio Albergati serve as a mediator and when Albergati, after having consented, out of fear backs down, Peter Martyr falsifies a document of proxy and obtains a meeting between the two parties. He still is not capable of bringing the conflict to a conclusion, but continues to inform Mercurino da Gattinara and Marliani of the situation and of its developments, insisting that they convince the King to return to Spain as soon as possible.

Having been elected emperor, Charles returns. Meanwhile the popular forces, ill-prepared militarily and politically, with leaders too presumptuous and often not united, right away suffer several defeats. The nobles, on the other hand, fear the reaction of the Sovereign king and emperor. The fire is going out. The *consejos* are satisfied because the Sovereign has accepted their requests, which, however, will remain a dead letter almost in their entirety. Similarly, many privileges of the nobles will decline during the authoritarian rule of the young Austrian sovereign.

Charles I of Spain and V of the Empire, does not forget Peter Martyr, who was so much involved with great personal risk and cunny ability in that difficult situation. Already in 1520 he nominated him "royal chronicler" (the positions of chaplain of the queen and Professor of Liberal Arts had been confirmed from the start); then he names him member of the Supreme Council of the Indies. Finally, accepting one of the Italian's specific requests, he names him abbot of Jamaica. Peter Martyr requested the nomination in recognition of his interest, but he declared that the income owed to him must be spent for the reconstruction of the church there destroyed by fire, so the Sovereign shows his affection by ordering that the royal treasury match his contribution so that the work might be realized.

The ailments of age force Peter Martyr to be carried on a stretcher when he has to move to follow the Court, but he does not give up his charges, as it is documented by the inspection certificate of May 5, 1526, the order issued in Seville for the inspection by the *Casa de Contratación*, overseer of the economic management of the lands of the New World.

But by now we are at the sunset.

In September of that year, Peter Martyr is with the Court in Granada, the city of his youth, where Isabella and Ferdinand, his friends Tendilla and Talavera, and many companions of wartime are buried. The landscape reminds him vaguely of the area of Verbano where he was born: he feels that his days are numbered.

On September 23, he draws up his will: he has always written in Latin, but he dictates this document in Spanish because, if he dies in Spain, he wants everyone to be able to understand it. It is a serene and detailed text in which he reaffirms his faith, recognizes that he has received benefits, arranges that his body be buried in the cathedral of Granada, of which he is still a prior, leaving bequests to the chapter to pray for the salvation of his soul, and mentioning all those who have helped him and his relatives with small donations.

Privileged, among all, is his niece Laura, posthumous daughter of his brother Giovanni Battista, to whom he leaves the greater part of his money, provided that she gets married, lives in Arona and reclaims the lands and the houses of the family so that the memory of the D'Anghieras shall remain alive.

He dies in Granada on October 30 or 31, 1526. The clergy of the cathedral, as Predaza witnesses, have this memorial stone put on his grave: "To the narrator of the events of our age and of the New World until now unknown, Peter Martyr Milanese, Roman senator, who left his country and fought in the war of Granada, then when the city was conquered was first canon and then prior of this church, the dean and the clergy erected this grave for a very dear colleague in the year 1526."

Another circumstance associates Peter Martyr to Christopher Columbus, the person of whom he was friend and first historian: nothing is certain about the actual location of their mortal remains.

Peter Martyr had quoted in his will a codicil for his burial in a specific place in the cathedral chapter but it seems that in 1526 the great cathedral had not yet been finished and the nearby church of Saint Francis served as cathedral. This church was later given to the order, which built a large convent around it. With the secularization of church properties in the eighteenth century, the complex was turned over to the military administration and at present it is the seat of the regional military headquarters.

It seems that in 1929, during some repair work, the remains of thirty buried bodies were found in a room that had been walled up, and among them must have been those of Peter Martyr and Hernando del Pulgar.

Research conducted in the archives of the cathedral has uncovered the authorization by Charles V to give burial in it to Hernando del Pulgar for having participated in the conquest of the city, but nothing related to Peter Martyr of Anghiera has been found, even though he had been prior and had left to the cathedral many bequests. Only his three stoles, made of precious fabrics that the sultan of Egypt had given him, are preserved, in the Treasury Room.

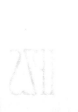

II. – OUTLINE OF PETER MARTYR'S THOUGHT.

The interest in the wealth of information contained in his *Decades* for the extraordinary events of the period and especially for the realities emerging from a New World has caused scholars to neglect the remarkable personality of Peter Martyr. Occasionally introduced as a historian or, sometimes, as a chronicler of the discoveries and conquests, and even recognized almost as the "first journalist of modern age," he has always generically been classified both a "humanist" — because he wrote everything in Latin — and a "courtier," as he lived at the court of the Catholic Sovereigns and Charles V. Almost no one has emphasized the originality of his thought and the novelty of his stance on various aspects of life and culture, when, indeed, he is one of the first and most authoritative representatives of a "new humanism," in tune with the new course of history, opened up by Christopher Columbus's enterprise.

He appears imbued with the spirit of the traditional humanism, that of his early years in Rome and with Pomponius Letus's circle: his first production, almost as a literary exercise, is in verse of good linguistic and metric construction, of a certain vivacity and some felicitous landscape depictions. More valuable are the compositions of the Spanish period, almost all done between 1487 and 1506, in particular some short poems.

The *Inachus*, composed in honor of the count of Tendilla, marks the transition from poems occasioned by circumstances, at times vivaciously satiric, to themes of greater demand which would reach epic dimensions.

The *Pluto furens* is of particular interest: the devil, angry because the Catholic Sovereigns continue to obtain triumphs for the Christian faith, urges the infernal forces against them. Hence the various attempts on their lives (instigated by the devils), among which particularly dangerous was that of October 1492 against King Ferdinand. But Christ and the Virgin are watching over him and the forces of evil are defeated.

In *Ianus* the poet celebrates the reconciliation between Ferdinand and his son-in-law, Philip of Hapsburg, for the rule of the Kingdom of Castile, after dramatic confrontation: in reality, the father-in-law had to give in to Juana's husband and the humanist tries to console the defeated king by recalling his past victories.

In *Victoria* are extolled, often with epic tones the deeds of the beloved pupil Pedro Fajardo during the revolt of Alpujarras.

We still have, among the short narrative poems, *Equestria*, in praise of the Venetian ambassador Pasqualigo, and *Convivium regum*, which recalls the sumptuous festivities in honor of the Queen of Naples, King Ferdinand's sister.

The learned traditional tone leaves perhaps very little room to the imagination: the moments of greatest tension occur when the poet relives in the "feats" of his "heroes" his own experiences as a soldier in the Granada war. All the poems, published illegally in 1511 in Seville by Lucio Marineo Siculo, were published again with the consent of the author in Valencia in 1520.

Much superior, though, is Peter Martyr's talent as a prose writer. The *Legatio Babylonica* is an ample report, divided into three books, on his mission as extraordinary ambassador to the sultan of Egypt, and he comes across to us as an acute observer of people and landscapes, capable of capturing the reality of little-known lands affected by prejudice. As a humanist, he also researches any evidence of the past wherever he goes, among the Roman ruins at Pola as well as among the Egyptian pyramids and in Alexandria, (which lost the old splendor), never hiding his admiration for Venice. Such work, whose first draft was contained in the letters sent during the trip to Ferdinand and Isabela and to friends, passed rather unnoticed, perhaps because everyone was now more interested in the news that was coming from the New World.

Among classical authors, his preference is clearly for historians like Livy, moralists like Seneca, and naturalists like Pliny. From the vague hints found in his epistolary and from references in the *Decades* is evident a certain dislike for erudition for its own sake, pure or empty form, and of language rigidity.

But it is above all with the extraordinary event i.e revelation of a "New World" (he — before anyone else — so labels the lands discovered by Columbus) that Peter Martyr develops his less traditionalist thought, moving toward a "new humanism" that rises with him and which will mature very slowly in the following centuries. If "man" was the exclusive focus of Humanism and Renaissance, Peter Martyr realizes that the new realities should call for reconsideration of the canons of human values as traditionally understood.

His concrete experiences during the war of Granada drive him away from the intransigent intolerance and near hatred for the enemies of the Christian faith, the Muslims: he sees in the soldiers of the half moon, who fight with great heroism, the defenders of their own families, lands, and traditions. He too is a brave soldier — he went to fight by his own choice — he faces the pain and risks connected with such a decision and bows with emotion to the defeated enemy, taking pity on the suffering population. And even earlier, although he came to Spain with the aristocratic pride of a man of letters so superior to the "ignorant population that does not count at all," he has discovered the genuine values of people that participate in the Spanish councils and take direct responsibility for the life of the nation while personally contributing to the armed struggle.

For the people in the New World he has no reservation: regardless of the fact their customs are so different from those of the Europeans, he actually, on occasions, exalts and defends them. In his reports of the very first news received from Columbus and his companions, Peter Martyr depicts a plain, good-natured population unaware of property, avarice, or corruption, although affected by real power struggles among their leaders. It would almost seem that he wants to make a precise distinction: men as individuals are good by nature; the state, as a political entity, always generates discord and wars, conquered and conquerors. So, typically, there is the recollection of the classic celebration of a tranquil private life contrasted with the anxieties of public life, and the vague nostalgia for the golden age, common to many humanists; but, atypically, there is also a taut condemnation of the "newcomers" who arrive and upset a world of contentment.

We can single out immediately two meaningful attitudes which show us a very "modern" outlook in Peter Martyr. First of all, we see that he does not pass any negative judgment on the "nudity" of the natives, since to him it does not imply per se an immoral condition: nudity is a custom, dictated by climate and simplicity of life, so it is a nudity without malice, without sin. The other perspective worthy of note concerns religion. Peter Martyr never charges the American Indians with being "infidels." Indeed, he tries to find out what religious beliefs they have; he says that they could easily be converted and for their customs could become good Christians, but their not being Christians is not for him a discriminating element between "good" and "bad."

If sometimes he uses the term "barbarians" he uses it in the sense of the Greek expression which meant "those who do not speak our language," he does not attribute to such a term a negative connotation. A clear confirmation is the fact that in the appendix of *Vocabula Barbara* which concluded the *Decades* we find as well Italian and Spanish words, proper names of cities and places, besides American Indian words, that is, "barbarian" in the sense of not belonging to the lexicon of classical Latin.

When Peter Martyr writes about American Indians' traditions and myths, he underlines their unaffected simplicity and sometimes their poetic qualities while recalling that the myths of classical peoples were as simple. It is evident that in religious matters, values different from those of one's own faith cannot be tolerated, but there is never any a priori condemnation of the people because of their nature as "infidels," that is, non-Christians.

Peter Martyr will continue in his pages to exalt the positive values of new peoples, and will offer information that is more realistic and less mythical, and certainly not distorted: his attention to every aspect of life, and especially to the expressions of cultural life, reinforces his original premise to recognize equal dignity for all men.

The "discovery" had probably caused a crisis regarding the achievements of many centuries of intellectual work, undermining the classical and Christian culture which Humanism was trying further to develop. But the very existence of new lands, of diverse peoples, of a vegetative and animal world which did not have equivalents in the regions until then known forced Peter Martyr to an "acknowledgement awareness," certainly not easy. The reticence to admit that the new lands did not belong to Asia had, perhaps, also a religious motivation: the continents were three, three the human races, as there were three persons in one God, and it was dangerous not to accept tradition. Let us remember that Leonardo da Vinci declared himself a "man without letters" and that he studied "in the great book of nature," avoiding any doctrinal framing of his own experiences, but having to hold this stance cost him dearly. The "new" aspects of the natural and human world had considerable implications that had to be incorporated somehow in political, economic and social structures, even on the juridical and doctrinal levels.

In Peter Martyr, the desire to be scrupulous in the search for truth was always present, but it was not easy for him to accept what seems to come out of the natural order: he called the discovered lands "New World," but "New" is for him "previously unknown," not "completely alien to the known world." We can say then that he reports news of strange things which are related to him "by duty of chronicle," but he always stresses that the responsibility for certain prodigious novelties (and these very often are echoes of medieval pseudoscience or fictions derived from the books of chivalry) should not be attributed to him. He is especially doubtful when the "new things" are associated or confused with extreme ease with reality or European cultural tradition: he doubts the existence of women warriors on the island of *Madanino* who live like the ancient Amazons, and of Sirens (which are the manatees); and if he recalls the Lestrigoni he does so in order that it may not surprise us that cannibals exist in the New World since they were also acknowledged in the classical tradition.

When the topic becomes more scientific, his language also becomes more precise: the huge quantity of fresh water in the mouth of the Marañón brings him to the conclusion that a river of such flow can only originate from a continental mass of enormous size with an adequate hydric basin.

His attention is never partial; it covers all the aspects of the natural and human world. So when the canoe of a wealthy merchant transporting goods of every kind is discussed, Peter Martyr observes that this fact implies the existence of a very organized and articulate society with an established practice of holding fairs to exchange products and transport them from the areas of production to those of sale.

The ever vaster expanses of land opened up by the conquests and the tumultuous developments that were associated with it, the simultaneous course of great events in Europe, (of which Spain is almost always the protagonist), and his obligations at the Court, perhaps prevented Peter Martyr from dedicating more time to the probing of scientific problems and the knowledge which enriched the cultural patrimony of his time; yet, we have much convincing evidence of his ability for research. He solves a problem which had excited with passion and troubled protagonists and scholars alike: upon the return of the flagship *Victoria*, having completed its three-year circumnavigation of the globe and the only ship that came back from Magellan's expedition, its crew noticed that their calculations were one day off; they thought they had arrived home on a Thursday, but they found out they had arrived on a Wednesday. The fact that going from East to West we gain time and going from West to East we lose time is obvious today, for it is a common experience of those who travel long distances by plane; but then it had not been experienced and it was not easily understandable, especially because of the apparent East-West course of the sun. Peter Martyr cannot accept the simple fact of the loss of a day without looking for a valid reason. He discusses it with others and then is able to give his explanation, which is a scientific one. His early doubt about the Asiatic nature of the islands discovered by Columbus and now his doubting the gain of one day circumnavigating the earth from East to West should be sufficient proof for us of the true dimension of Peter Martyr's scientific attitude.

A detailed examination of his contribution to the development of scholarly knowledge still remains to be made, but perhaps even more urgent is a re-assessment of him as a political figure. He is a «courtier» in the etymological sense of the word, from the time he joins the court of the Catholic Sovereigns as a *contino*, but nothing is less true of him than that he was a docile servant of his lords. We notice, in fact, that he always signs himself *Petrus Martyr Angleriae Mediolanensis* to emphasize that he is not a Spanish subject upon whom duties of obedience fall. He offers his arm in the fight for the defense of faith, he gives his services in the field of culture, he offers his advice and acts for the needs of the Crown, repaying the trust placed in him, but he wants to preserve his thinking autonomy and his freedom of choice.

The lucidity that Peter Martyr expects in science, and in the defense of equal dignity among all men constitute not only theoretical premises about which he writes willingly, they are also a way of life; he wants to apply to daily practice those moral teachings that he has emphasized in his lessons to the Spanish nobles. It is very important, in order to better understand Peter Martyr's psychology, to examine his relationships with the family of the Catholic Sovereigns.

Much has been written, even recently, on a special relationship of Columbus with Queen Isabella, mostly by twisting reality in favor of baseless deductions. The facts reveal only the constant and strong protection and liking of the great Queen toward the Genoese. Similarly Peter Martyr's epistolary could be distorted to imply a special relationship between Peter Martyr and Queen Isabella.

To the Lombard humanist the Queen personifies the highest feminine ideal, both as queen and a mother, endowed with intelligence, energy, goodness, tenderness and piety; when he speaks of her, one can sense his admiration and affection, which surpass by far the devotion of a man of court.

Isabella sees in Peter Martyr a figure of great culture and profound sensitivity, who shares her high ideals and who always knows how to find the most appropriate words to solve a thorny problem or to soothe a pain. The Queen, endowed with good cultural preparation, is most susceptible to the voices of ancient wisdom and of Christian authors both of which the humanist knows when to recall and in a manner that provides the best comfort.

There are some pages in his letters that document the torments of the Queen, such as when she refuses to intervene with her son John, who, moved by excessive passion for his bride Marguerita, consumes his already weak strength accelerating the end of his days. We are shown a pious Queen caught between her bashful modesty or concern about the health of her heir, and respect for the young man's feelings.

400

We also see, again through the writing of Peter Martyr Isabella's concerns for Juana, who must travel to meet her husband in Flanders: the already difficult undertaking of crossing the English Channel is made more arduous by an inclement season and the hostility of the French. The Queen turns to her Admiral of the Ocean Sea, begging him to point out the less dangerous route, information which Columbus offers immediately. The text of the Genoese has not survived, but we have the moving letter of thanks from the Queen for his extremely useful advice. We would almost like to say that the eager love of Isabella for her children is transmitted also to Peter Martyr, perhaps because he does not have a detached appointment with duties and restrictions but, rather, a closer familiarity with the Sovereigns and their family. Devotion and affection, therefore, characterize Peter Martyr's role, and this can be well explained knowing his personality; sometimes, though, the friendly attitude of the members of the royal family toward him is not as easily matched by other court officials.

Quite distinct is Peter Martyr's behavior toward young King Charles, who, in his view, is the true heir of the greatness of his ancestors, the Catholic Sovereigns, and especially Isabella. When the prince proclaims himself of age and claims the sovereign power, he is little older than a boy. Educated in Flanders and surrounded by advisors who pretend to guide him in their own way, he comes to Spain and discovers a different ambience; he is accompanied by two Italians related to Peter Martyr, Marliani and Gattinara, and finds again Peter Martyr, whom he had met when he was a young child and for whom he too feels instinctive trust being also aware of how close the humanist was to his grand parents and parents and thus values his unselfish loyalty.

At the court of Charles, king of Spain and emperor of the Holy Roman Empire, Peter Martyr acquires a more official role and a greater influence, given his strong friendship with the two Italian advisors of the Sovereign, but perhaps also because the King, on account of the great difference in their age, has toward him a more open trust, an almost filial respect, to which corresponds on the part of Peter Martyr a devotion which encompasses concern and affection.

Did Peter Martyr carry out concrete political roles while working and living in close, continuous contact with the Sovereigns?

Because he was very attached to his land of origin, Milan, and to Italy, which he considers his motherland (in the sense of literary tradition from Virgil to Petrarch), while in Spain he foresees the misfortunes that are about to fall on the peninsula and, particularly between 1493 and 1495, writing to Giovanni Borromeo and Ascanio Sforza, he urges them to implore Ludovico il Moro not to induce foreign interventions. The Italian events and the violence perpetrated by armies against the innocent populations always find a painful echo in his letters, but he is aware of not being able to intervene; even if in his heart he has reservations, moral ones especially, he cannot interfere with King Ferdinand's Italian politics.

He successfully performs his mission as extraordinary ambassador to the Sultan of Egypt, he writes the official correspondence as "Latin Secretary," he keeps in touch with the ambassadors from various countries who live at the Court, but he never adopts a "personal" position regarding foreign politics. So not even in this sense can one speak of him as a "courtier," because he never acted surreptitiously against anyone. Instead, one must have the greatest respect for his involvement in the internal affairs of Spain. We must also say that Peter Martyr is perhaps the first one to fully realize the birth of a nation with the marriage of Isabella and Ferdinand and always does his utmost to preserve this unity: in his habit of using at all times the term *hispani* he almost seems to want to deny every difference between Aragonese and Castilians.

We mentioned his attempt to reconcile father-in-law and son-in-law, and his trying time at the side of mad Juana, yet his role and intervention had determining weight and influenced the revolt of the *comuneros*. It is probably in this role that Peter Martyr most forcefully shows a definite political choice, for a stand that would like to be sincerely balanced between the opposite sides. He is a member of the Royal Council, does not belong to either the traditional nobility or the *Comunidades*; he feels that he represents the interests of the Crown, which for him coincide with those of the nation. As he already taught King Charles, at the basis of collective life he thinks there should be respect for the laws and customs consecrated by time, even when they have not been codified in written texts.

Without a doubt, present in him is the judicial Roman tradition, the concept of the state as a supreme organism in which everyone has a well-defined place, precise duties and inalienable rights. Justice, whose administration belongs to the State, must be always validated by the proper respect that those in a position of power must have for it. It is in this sense that one observes a difference of political views between Peter Martyr and his great friend Mercurino Arborio da Gattinara, advisor and then Chancellor of Charles V, the main inspiration for the Caesar style attitude of the young Hapsburg king. They both had a solid humanistic formation, a more strictly literary one in the case of Peter Martyr, more juridical in the case of Gattinara; for this reason one can perhaps justify a more ethical approach in Peter Martyr and a more practical approach (in other words, politically more realistic) in Mercurino da Gattinara.

As for most humanists, for Peter Martyr the ideal Rome was Republican Rome; for the Chancellor, however, the ideal was the restoration of the Roman Empire in a context that would include the whole world. But Mercurino needs to know better the Spanish environment in order to be able to perform well his duties as Chancellor, and Peter Martyr is certainly the most qualified person to help him. Foreign, Italian like him, honest, not tied to any faction, faithful to the Crown, for many years at the Court, expert in doctrine and of great experience, esteemed also by King Charles—Peter Martyr, by now older, feels flattered, certain that he can properly conclude his service to the monarchy at the side of the young grandson of his Sovereigns. The difference in political attitude between Peter Martyr's respect for the rights of the different social classes, consecrated in his view by tradition and Mercurino's belief in the absolute pre-eminence of the sovereign's will and of the interests of the Crown, from which to derive every political act, is hardly compatible, but it does not separate the two Italians, does not prevent their collaboration, which in effect will help Charles to overcome the opposition encountered in Spain because of his all too German formation.

Less documented, but certainly no less important, is his role in "Indian affairs," for which, from the beginning, the Catholic Sovereigns surely sought his collaboration. After the directives of the earlier phase, which were inspired in part by general principles set forth by Isabella but for the most part never enacted, there is a period of contingent and contradictory dispositions which deal especially with the relations between the conquerors and the economic interests of the Crown, since King Ferdinand had hardly paid attention to the high court functionaries, among them Peter Martyr, to whom Indian affairs were entrusted. The situation of the natives was becoming more and more tragic and the protests of religious authorities and the requests for legislative intervention which reached the Court, grew more and more numerous.

We remember, among all the others, the protestations of Bartholomew de Las Casas, but we must also say that neither is he the only one to feel the necessity to defend the American Indians nor are strong opponents of this position lacking: the latters had the advantage being supported by the conquistadors and the *encomenderos*, who do not want any restraints on their conduct and who want to reward adequately whoever supports them.

Only in 1523 is the *Consejo Supremo de Indias* formally established, as an autonomous agency composed in great part of prelates and jurists, of which Peter Martyr is also a member. References to the meetings of this Supreme Council are present in his writings, but the details about what is discussed are missing; however, we can suppose that he always sided with the defenders of the Indians, a stance taken by him from the beginning, even though that position was always that of the minority.

Peter Martyr speaks to us about it in his letter of February 20, 1525 addressed to the archbishop of Cosenza, in terms even too concise, that may make us think of his bitterness for a lost battle and his disapproval of the decisions adopted by the *Consejo*. The difference, on the one hand, between natural and ecclesiastical law, which state the principle that all men are equally free, and, on the other hand, the "imperial" law (that is, in this specific case, the law of the Spanish state of the time) which recognizes a "state" of freedom different for the various categories of men (citizens, foreigners, individuals belonging to distinct social classes or to different categories, etc.) is well stressed, and in Martyr's letter it is recognized that the right of the State prevails over the others, at least in practice, and consequently a different "freedom" for every group of people can be achieved within the State.

We mentioned that the jurists and theologians had declared to Queen Isabella that the people of the new lands could not be placed in a servile condition, but the need of a considerable work force for the Spanish settlements in the new lands and the institution of the encomienda had reduced the Amerindians, who were exploited beyond every limit of tolerance, to a practical state of slavery. The defense of the Indians had come especially from the "religious" sent to evangelize the new peoples, that is, Franciscans and Dominicans, who are summoned by the *Consejo* to give their opinion on the problem of the freedom of the Indians, but their intervention does not lead to improvement of the conditions of the Indians.

It was impossible to support the introduction of slavery as a general principle (but already a partial acceptance of it was inherent in the principle of "just war"), and therefore it became the "duty" of the Spaniards, in conformity with the papal bulls, to be concerned with the spiritual salvation of the natives. Only by subjecting the Amerindians to the tutelage of the "Christians" was it possible to avoid their return to vices and errors they previously lived with. It is evident that this was a religious justification of convenience that, at least to a certain extent, silenced the protests of the clerics and minimized the impact of the opinion of the jurists, since full freedom was denied in the name of the spiritual interest of the natives themselves. What Peter Martyr declares about the conclusion of the debate leaves no doubts about his negative judgement.

Some attempt to approach Charles V on behalf of the Amerindian was again made by the humanist in 1526, in Granada itself, the city which preserved the remains of the great Isabella. Not even one month after her death, the King was issuing a series of decrees to settle the relations between the natives and the Spaniards, decrees which unfortunately, as the following *leyes nuevas* showed, in great part were not enforced or were misrepresented.

While courteous and accessible, Peter Martyr had perhaps a character endowed with a coherence of its own and incapable of acquiescing to the will of the stronger. Sometimes, in fact, it seems that he went well beyond the limits allowed by the times in his conduct and judgements about the "grandees" with whom he came into contact, both on the political and the moral level: the "State" for which he was longing perhaps could not be realized, a state in which the classes might be active and in peace, in which honesty and justice might find support in the certainty of law guaranteed by the royal power.

An individual had to be good, understanding, not greedy, not ambitious, not meddling, able to hold fast to his opinions and faithful to the teachings of religion and morality. Still Peter Martyr was not a persistent critic of everything and everyone, nor did he like to insist on speaking about the triumph of evil. He very often acknowledged the conflict between loudly proclaimed principles and the reality of practical action, but he realized that unfortunately it is not possible to change the nature of things. Therefore, he preferred to remain silent: in his silence, as we have said, there is the bitter awareness of a just man who feels powerless.

III. – PETER MARTYR AND CHRISTOPHER COLUMBUS.

In the studies on Christopher Columbus, his milieu and undertaking, Peter Martyr d'Anghiera is frequently remembered, or, more precisely, the parts of his works which deal with the Genoese are remembered. Yet, research focused on illustrating the actual relation between these two, who lived in the same environment, albeit with different roles, at the court of the Catholic Sovereigns, and enjoyed the protection of Queen Isabella of Castile, is not really abundant.

Some scholars have pointed out that perhaps the Lombard humanist spoke little of Columbus, that he did not defend him in his writing from the lies of adversaries and from the unjust treatment received by the Spanish Crown, and that he did not mention his death because he did not understand the greatness of the Discoverer. Yet, theirs is a close relationship, marked by great friendship, born in the years just preceding the departure for the great voyage, as Peter Martyr states several times.

It has been observed that, although the humanist would continually send letters to his Italian friends telling all that was happening in Spain, he spoke for the first time of Columbus only in the letter of May 14, 1493 to Giovanni Borromeo, in other words, only after Columbus's return from the discovery crossing, and even on that occasion he omitted to report the particular circumstances in which the mission was carried out.

It is right to believe that Peter Martyr might have had good reasons to keep quiet until May 1493 about Columbus the man and his enterprise. First of all, there were the conflicts with the Portuguese, who claimed for themselves the exclusive right on the Atlantic navigations: the treaty of Alcobaza of 1480, between Portugal and Castile, ratified by the pontiff, limited the activity of the Castilians to navigations on the parallel of the Canaries, which were under their rule. The Portuguese, who had not supported Columbus's project and had almost surely tried to carry it out on their own, were decisively opposed to every Spanish initiative of this kind. Besides, we know that when Columbus finally left on his voyage, three Portuguese ships were crossing the waters of the Canaries in an attempt to stop him.

Even though the Genoese had lived in Spain for seven years, the *Junta*, convened by the Sovereigns to examine the project, had pronounced a negative decision: only the Queen, and not officially, had continued to support Columbus. When the war of Granada finally ended, the long negotiations concluded and the expedition left. Yet the outcome was uncertain, and therefore it was better to await its conclusion. Only after the victorious return could one talk about it, only when the Catholic Sovereigns had obtained the legitimation of the undertaking and of their right to Atlantic navigations from Pope Alexander VI.

Peter Martyr, living at the Court of Spain, could not betray that discretion and that reserve which protected the interests of his Sovereigns: for these reasons, one understands his silence on Columbus until that moment.

The letter of September 5, 1493 from Peter Martyr to Tendilla and Talavera is important evidence for the prior contacts between the two Italians. In it the humanist, announcing Columbus's successful return, reminds the two friends of the long discussions about the planned voyage they had held, when the Genoese insisted on obtaining the necessary means for the undertaking, and the crucial support given by them, as royal advisors. The letter seems to recall particularly the last period of the negotiations, toward the end of 1491, when, once the surrender of the city of Granada had been agreed upon by the king, the Sovereigns decided to support the voyage. It must be made clear that the negotiations ended at the camp below Granada, but the signature of the *Capitulaciones*, after the details were agreed on, took place in Santa Fe on April 17, 1492, when Tendilla, Talavera and Peter Martyr were in Granada.

The official discussions of Talavera and Tendilla in the Council of the Crown and their support to Columbus had certainly had their premise in previous thorough discussions, of a scientific nature, involving Columbus and Peter Martyr. Hernando de Talavera in the *Junta* he chaired had been the most determined to turn down the proposal, for doctrinal reasons, and finally changed his mind because of some newly submitted evidence which made him modify his previous convictions.

Columbus had gone to Spain with strong views derived from his experiences and his intuitions as a navigator, but he had clashed with the scholastic tradition of the scholars, experts in classical texts; after their negative assessment, he had to commit himself to searching works of cosmography, geography, philosophy, and natural sciences for those passages that could support his thesis. As Paolo Emilio Taviani maintains, the scholarly documentation for the project was missing before Columbus came to Spain, and in our opinion it was researched by him with more diligence only after the negative response of the Council.

But to whom could the navigator turn? Peter Martyr seemed to be the right person. He was very knowledgeable about ancient texts, he represented that Italian humanism that was more open to the issues of the present and to the critical interpretation of the past than to pure philological research, and he was always eager to learn new things. Peter Martyr could not help being fascinated by the Columbian project, which most opposed because of prejudice and deep-rooted fears. Moreover, he had friends at Court and contact with the Sovereigns, and he could exercise a positive influence. Perhaps less important for the beginning of their friendship was the common Italian origin: Genoese and Milanese belonged at that time to two different "nations," often hostile to each other, even if in Peter Martyr there was a certain sense of the "common country" clearly envisioned by literary tradition.

Without a doubt, of greater importance was the favorable attitude of the Queen, a keen admirer of Italian culture and who shared his faith and ideals. The Queen would help Columbus, when possible, with subsidies and would ask him to be patient; Peter Martyr probably helped him on a doctrinal level to prepare himself for a new examination of his project (the decision of the *Junta*, however, was not final being merely a consulting body).

The doctrinal problem of major importance was the relative distance between the extremes of Spain to the West and the extremes of Asia to the East, separated by the "Ocean" (only the Atlantic had this name): quotations from Aristotle, Seneca, Strabo, Pliny and others were being examined, quotations that seemed to confirm this thesis, and certainly Peter Martyr's judgement in those discussions had to carry remarkable weight.

For the period of preparation of the first trip, the relation Columbus-Peter Martyr-Talavera is especially well documented, leaving aside don Iñigo López de Mendoza, count of Tendilla, the other correspondent to whom the letter of September 5, 1493 is addressed. Don Iñigo, besides being a brave soldier, is also a man of great humanistic doctrine: he is the one who convinced Peter Martyr to go to Spain and introduced him as a great man of letters; therefore, in this matter he can only be on the side of his friend and protegee. He is also the commander of the Castilian forces on the Granada front. The continuous postponement of a definite answer to Columbus is tied to the proclamation of the ongoing war and to the danger of Portuguese intervention: when the result of the war can already be anticipated, from October 1491 on, the Count of Tendilla, who will remain in Granada as viceroy and governor with considerable military forces, is in a position to assure the Sovereigns that by now any Portuguese attack could easily be driven back.

This is another element in the Council of the Crown that favors the Genoese. We continue to use the term Genoese for Columbus, and with just reason. Indeed it is Peter Martyr who first confirms the Genoese origin of Columbus. It also seems strange to us that this particular testimony of the humanist may be forgotten or remembered only in passing, whereas it deserves particular emphasis.

In the first letter on the discovery, addressed to Giovanni Borromeo on May 1493, Peter Martyr writes *Cristophorus quidam Colonus, vir Ligur*, "a certain Christopher Columbus, man of Liguria"; in the letter to Tendilla and Talavera of September 5, 1493, he says, *meministis Colonum ligurem* "you remember the Ligurian Columbus"; in the letter to Ascanio Sforza, of the same date, he repeats "*Cristophorus Colonus, vir Ligur.*" The fact that Peter Martyr uses "man of Liguria" instead of "Genoese" can have a double explanation. First of all, the term "*Ligur*" is associated with the Vergilian "*ligurem adsuetum malo*" "I prefer an experienced Ligurian" and, therefore, can emphasize the tradition of industrious and strong people to whom Columbus belongs; or it could refer to the historical moment—the Genoese people were siding with the French against Ferdinand of Aragon, and it was not opportune to underline that the author of such a great enterprise was not only a foreigner but also a Genoese. The Lombard humanist certainly shared Columbus's secrets and, capable as he was to register the reactions of the human soul, quickly realized that the condition of foreigner would have represented a serious problem for his friend; for these reasons he also used the form "Colonus," Latinizing the Spanish "Colón" of the official documents.

Peter Martyr does not fail to emphasize, in the first book of the first *Decade*, a significant detail of the first voyage: in addition to the fears of the crew about the length of the trip, the lack of suitable winds on the route of return, and the calmness of the sea, there was, perhaps more predominant, their slight trust in the leader of the expedition, a foreigner whom no one knew: "they would say that the Ligurian had dragged them into a precipice from where they would never be able to come back." We can point out that Columbus in the letter to Sánchez does not speak of the hostility of the crew (in the log book, in the versions left to us by Bartholomew de Las Casas and Ferdinand Columbus, they are vaguely mentioned), but especially he does not mention any resentment toward him as a foreigner, since this would have certainly hurt him. We remember that the title of "Admiral of the Ocean Sea" and the appointments as viceroy and governor of the new lands had not been conferred on Columbus at the moment of departure. They would be awarded to him only after the discovery and, therefore, revealing the opposition of the Spaniards to being commanded by a foreigner could have brought into question the clauses of the *Capitulaciones.*

One can deduce that something of the kind might have been heard by the Court between the first and second voyage from the fact that the Sovereigns, in granting to Columbus the seventeen ships requested, arranged that men who enjoyed their full confidence be part of the mission, with important duties, in spite of the agreements that reserved for the Admiral the choice of his collaborators.

The most valid confirmation of Columbus's non-Spanish nationality is given by Peter Martyr when he speaks of the events of the second and third voyages, and in particular of the accusations that were put forward to the Court about the behavior of the Admiral and his brother Bartholomew, who, according to the charges, were using violence against the loyal subjects of the King because these "very proud enemies of the Spanish blood" were protecting the natives, barbarians and infidels, leaving their crimes unpunished, but not tolerating any little error of the Spanish soldiers. It is a clear denunciation of the resentment of the Spaniards against the two foreigners. It was not only the ascent of a man of exceptional merit to high honors that stirred up envy and hostility, because that still remained in the tradition itself of nobility; it was that Columbus was alien to that tradition, because he was not a Spaniard.

We do not doubt that the campaign mounted against Columbus was conducted with the agreement of his adversaries at Court. Father Boyl and Margarit, both Catalonian and, therefore, subjects of Ferdinand and not of Isabella, departed from the New Lands almost immediately to deliver in Spain the first attacks against the Navigator, while he, according to orders received, was exploring other islands. As the complaints and the lies against the Admiral increased, Roldán rose against him and found many followers. Peter Martyr tries in vain to defend Columbus in the letter of August 11, 1495, to Carvajal, insisting, naturally, on the greatness of the discovery, almost as an indirect censure of the attitude of the Crown which authorizes new expeditions without the knowledge of the Admiral. Probably Peter Martyr does not entirely share the ideas of the Genoese on the nature of the discovered lands, but for unresolved doctrinal reasons. The fact that those lands belonged to Asia or another continent takes nothing from the greatness of his friend whom he is the first to describe as *Colonus ille, novi orbis, repertor.*

Peter Martyr speaks frequently of the letters he receives from the Admiral: it is significant what can be learned from the letter of August 8, 1495, in which Columbus promises to meet with Peter Martyr and his friends to discuss extensively the "Continental" nature of the discovered lands. The meeting takes place, as the humanist says, but the participants do not reach an understanding and it seems that each one holds to his own position.

The whole question of "recognition of the continent" is at times confusing. Columbus maintains that it is Asia, Peter Martyr says, instead, that it is an *orbis novus*. We need to remember that earlier Columbus insisted that Cuba was a continent even if, as Taviani maintains, he knew it was a lie. Columbus made the crew swear, in front of a notary public, that the land was a continent, threatening serious consequences to those who denied it. Peter Martyr does not mention this in 1500, when he writes books three through nine of the first *Decade*, because the insular nature of Cuba could not be argued any more, and there were already enough accusations against the Genoese without adding to his charges scientific error and abuse of authority.

In the 1495 meeting did they want to take up this point? We don't know who the friends were that were supposed to participate in the discussion, but surely they included scholars, experts in cosmography and the natural sciences, since it is evident that the problem was considered relevant and they would have to compare the nature of the places, people, animals, and plants against the well-known nature of Europe and the rather uncertain data they had of a more distant Asia.

The explicit statement that a new continent was discovered is attributed to Columbus by Peter Martyr after the third voyage, even if for the Genoese it is no longer the Asia of the Ganges but one of its appendices, so to speak. In order not to risk the accusation of heresy, Columbus resorts to the hypothesis that that land was the Earthly Paradise, but refuses to pursue it so as not to give up his fundamental objective: to find the way to reach Asia, in particular, India. Only after his arrest in Santo Domingo, having lost all the privileges granted to him and, therefore, no longer responsible for the task of finding Asia, does the Navigator want at least to be credited with the glory of being, as Peter Martyr had said from the beginning, the "Discoverer of a New World." This is the time when the Genoese, after so much suffering, claims for himself the providential mission of the conversion of new people to the Christian faith by preparing the *Libro de las Profecias*.

What certainly binds these two characters together is Peter's admiration for a man of action and Christopher's for a man he views as a repository of high doctrine, and the mere differences of opinion cannot invalidate their relationship: the greatness of Humanism and of Italian Renaissance and their decisive role in the history of culture lies precisely with their eclecticism.

When harsher years come, and letters of accusations against Columbus reach the Court with greater insistence, Peter Martyr lacks the evidence to be able to refute them; noticing with bitterness that the Crown has changed its attitude, he, in his own interest, stops writing about the New World. The return of the Admiral, stripped of all power, bitterly concludes the seventh book of the first *Decade*, written in 1500, and for fifteen years, there is no more mention of Columbus in the writings of the humanist. In the fourth book of the third *Decade*, Peter Martyr relates the events of the fourth voyage with all the tragic ups and downs and the humiliations that the Discoverer had to endure, and summarily states he does not know how it all ended. It is too evident that this statement is not untrue: even if the events referred to occurred many years before, the humanist could not ignore the return of the Genoese to Spain, his last vain struggle for the vindication of his rights, or his death.

Perhaps Peter Martyr, as some say, did not attach much importance to Columbus? Or, as others say, did he behave like a courtier who does not know how to think except with his lord's head and does not side with Columbus because he would be going against the Crown? In our opinion, another reason is rather evident: a deep bitterness, combined with the knowledge of being unable to defend Columbus, now that all the "interests" have blended against him. And, besides, the rough and stubborn personality of Columbus, even if he was so great, prevented him from arriving at a compromise between the rights, that had been granted to him, when the success of the enterprise was still doubtful, and the new reality that demanded the exercise of sovereign power over infinite spaces and immense riches be returned to the Crown.

We can hypothesize that Peter Martyr, friend of Columbus but also a confidant of the Catholic Sovereigns, might have tried to convince the Genoese to give up his intransigent claim for the full respect of the clauses of the capitulations, and perhaps he might also have illustrated to him the dangers of exercising political, administrative, and judiciary power in areas so distant and over men so unruly and proud. Such an attempt, if it ever took place, more than a personal initiative, must have been a specific suggestion of the Sovereigns. Given the particular esteem and affection of Isabella of Castile for both of them, the trust of the Queen in Peter Martyr, and her difficulties in speaking with Columbus after all the public accusations made against him, one could also think, however,

413

27

that, the personality of the Genoese, — had such an attempt ever been carried out — might have produced the opposite effect and perhaps would have led to the estrangement between the two Italians.

In Peter Martyr there is not an open and uncompromising defense of Columbus, but only praise for the greatness of his enterprise. Nor is there in him any particular accusation. He merely reports the charges against the Admiral as advanced by his adversaries, whom he had characterized earlier as undisciplined, not too fond of work, violent, and greedy. Martyr, at most, charges Columbus for errors — error and not fault — that are of damage to him as when we are reminded that the Genoese did not stop to pick up pearls being too worried about returning quickly to the island of Hispaniola, thus allowing his merited claim of the discovery of those riches to go to somebody else, or again when it is implied that the Admiral placed too much trust in people ready to betray him.

It may seem strange that Peter Martyr never touches upon the capitulations of Santa Fe, the final moment of the long and tiring negotiations between Columbus and the Crown, to which perhaps he too had contributed, the point of departure for the realization of the grand voyage, the successful beginning for the Genoese and, in the end, of his ruin (which, really, has been much exaggerated, to the point of creating the legend of a Columbus dying as a destitute).

It is known that Columbus had asked for many privileges that greatly surpassed those enjoyed by the *Almirante de Castilla* for all the activities associated with naval affairs. He also claimed the hereditariness of the title, appointments and benefits. The Crown had accepted his requests, albeit with some reservation: first of all, title and appointments would be granted only after the "discovery of the islands and mainland" and therefore only in case of success; in addition, an apparently obvious but substantial specification was made: "all the islands and lands that will be discovered and conquered through you and by you" and not all "the lands that will be discovered and conquered." The conflict between Columbus and the Crown, in a nutshell, arises exactly over this point. When, beginning in 1495, "different sea captains are sent in different parts of the new hemisphere," Columbus protests, claiming his full jurisdiction over the entire *Orbis Novus*, as Peter Martyr calls it, but the Crown maintains the right to organize its own expeditions.

The accusations, unfounded or purposely exaggerated, and the unquestionable mistakes made by the Genoese in his government of the new lands provided an excellent excuse and the only option for resolving the conflict: the renunciation of power over the new lands by Columbus in exchange for a proposed Marquisate in Spain. This option turned out to be an unsuccessful attempt to remove Columbus's banners from the ships' masts and from the turrets built in the new domains and relocate them on the towers of a castle within Spain.

In our opinion, Peter Martyr had too much experience to side with abstract principles against the reality of politics. That is why, in speaking of the American Indians, he declares them happy because they live without laws and judges. When it became clear that Columbus would have surpassed the Sovereigns themselves in the extent of lands, and incalculable riches, on which he would have held rights, he himself should have agreed on a limitation of his own prerogatives. His reluctance to give up definitely put him on the losers' side and no one could support him any longer.

Once again everything proceeds *extra lege* more than *contra legem*: there was no trial for Columbus on the basis of the accusations brought against him, as would have been legally valid; dismissed from power, put in chains, and then quickly freed with many apologies, he was not, however, reinstated to office. They allowed him to lead a new expedition (the fourth voyage) but now—on a par with other navigators, indeed, with a more limited number of men and means. Peter Martyr finds himself powerless to attempt a defense of Columbus. That great man, who knew how to overcome waves and winds, the terrors of the unknown, and the limits of scientific knowledge, does not comprehend his isolation and that he cannot eliminate the wickedness, violence, or greed of those who are by his side.

One could observe, judging by today's mentality and writing with the conviction that justice must prevail even over power (a belief that in very few parts of the world, even in our days, is really supported in actuality), that Peter Martyr, after 1500, does not waste a word in defense of Columbus and nearly forgets him. But this silence can also be interpreted in the sense that Peter Martyr did not care to diminish the stature of the great navigator, who must survive in history for his extraordinary enterprise, notwithstanding a denunciation of his inability to accept the said reality that right itself is not legally binding when matched against preeminent interests of those to whom it is entrusted.

IV. – THE *OPUS EPISTOLARUM* AND THE NEW WORLD.

Peter Martyr's Epistolary or collection of letters covers events from 1488 to 1525; the author did not personally witness all of them, but he knew about all of them and informed his friends, obtaining news and sifting through it in an attempt to provide complete information for historical as well as geographical and scientific purpose.

The epistolary style was certainly congenial to him: it allowed him to keep contacts with friends, to roam freely over all topics, to express judgments with greater freedom in a language with which he was familiar and which, if at times seemingly lacking the *labor limae*, even in its expressive immediacy, it nevertheless signals his erudition and knowledge of the classics.

The collection of letters is a cross-section of history, not only European history, which narrates events in their essential historical specificity as interpreted by a man of culture, great curiosity, interest for every aspect of life, and remarkable spiritual fervor. Facts are the predominant element of his letters, but when he writes less hastily, one appreciates occasionally landscapes, historical references, descriptions of cities, monuments, and extraordinary natural phenomena.

But the greatest focus is always on man, as an individual or a group of individuals who find themselves in the same psychological situation when confronting an event, often reacting more by instinct than thought ful judgment. In his pages there is a constant reminder of the human suffering caused by wars sought by the ambition of the powerful, a sincere sympathy for the pain of others, and a sense of rebellion when the individual is forced to yield to the needs of society.

The *Opus* was printed for the first time in Alcalá de Henares in 1530 and then later in 1670 in Amsterdam; in this second edition some errors are corrected in the numerical progression, along with some typographical misprints present in the first edition. In spite of the numerous searches carried out in public as well as in private archives of the families of the recipients, no original letter has ever appeared: the only one found is in Italian, addressed to Gilberto Borromeo, and it is not part of the Epistolary.

A 1657 manuscript copy, preserved in the Vatican Library is, actually, a transcription of the 1530 edition and since it does not seem convincing that in Rome a text of the *Opus Epistolarum* would be missing, it leads us to believe that the Holy Office, on the occasion of the proceedings of the canonization of Cardinal Francisco Jiménez de Cisneros, about whom Peter Martyr speaks, wanted to verify whether the 1530 edition did match the text prepared for printing.

The letters distributed in thirty-eight books are divided in the index into two groups, *epistulae historiales* and *epistulae morales*, whereas in the volume they are sequenced in chronological order.

The *epistulae historiales* are letters commenting events or deeds of people who played important roles in the life of the time, not only historically but also on the moral level because a wicked behavior of high representatives of society may bear negatively on mankind.

The harshest censures are directed to the clergy: there is no justification for Alexander VI—for his simony in achieving the pontifical throne, and his bestowing the title of cardinal on his son Cesare and others in exchange for political support. The faults of political leaders are not downplayed: he is particularly grieved by the errors of Ascanio Sforza, the deceits of Ferdinand the Catholic against his grandson the King of Naples, the unjustified ingratitude toward Gonzalo Fernández de Aguilar de Córdoba, the Great Captain, conqueror of Naples, and severe is his criticism of chancellor Guillaume de Croy, harsh his reproach of Marliani and Gattinara, seemingly charged with conniving.

In the *epistulae morales*, events provide an opportunity for moral reflections, usually aimed at comforting a friend in a painful moment or showing the necessity of keeping in mind human values and doctrinal teachings. They recall Seneca's epistles: there is always an ethical formulation which derives from the classical world and agrees with Christian morality. Through them appears Peter Martyr's great desire to help those who suffer and need help or forgiveness; indeed, at times he intercedes for those who erred out of human weakness and deserve clemency—he never condemns too harshly.

On the one hand critics underline the exceptional importance of the letters as rich historical news sources, while on the other hand they convey reservations about the authenticity of the text, which appears imprecise and corrupt. The different positions can be summarized in the following manner:

1) many letters have undergone revisions, restorations, and additions by the author, who wanted to turn the collection into a work of

history; consequently, inaccuracies in the chronological succession — such as the anticipation of a later event — of events can be explained;

2) the letters are authentic, and for this reason any error, or inconsistency concerning their dating, as well as textual interpolations should be attributed to the editor, who did not carefully edit the printing.

The hypothesis of a subsequent intervention by the author on the Epistolary is not very credible because it is filled with letters and news involving important figures which would have been more prudent to eliminate. The possibility cannot be excluded, however, that Peter Martyr might have thought of collecting his letters. The first letter, of January 1, 1488 to Cardinal Ascanio Sforza, seems in fact drawn up at a much later time than the date registered on it: the author, mentioning the reasons for leaving his homeland, refers to events that will take place in the following years, with a foresight that leaves us perplexed. Therefore, this letter would have been added later. Yet, we do not believe that he carried out a plan of revision and integration of the texts, because usually he writes his letters in a hurry, when he has interesting news to communicate, knowing as well that a mail carrier is about to depart. When there is not a courier ready and the letter remains in his hands, he often added more news causing inconsistencies between the letter dating and the chronology of the events just described.

He complains often of the difficulty of being timely, of having remained for a long time without a courier to whom to entrust the letters, of being forced to send news perhaps already known and therefore not important anymore. Probably if Peter Martyr had reviewed his collection of letters, we might not find in them certain evident chronological errors, certain anticipations which appear prophetic and, above all, letters of greeting or of communication without documentary value. We can presume that he might have planned on reorganizing the letters, but that he did not have a chance to because of his advanced age and poor health, as well as because of his work at Court and the drafting of the *Decades* (V-VIII), written from 1521 to 1524. In fact, not only the presence of letters sent to the same addressee, especially in the last books, often without title, bearing progressive numbering, but also the presence of letters sent by other correspondents to Peter Martyr and of documents recorded in the body of the letters sometimes not marked by numbering—all of this makes one think that the author might have tried to arrange the letters, beginning with the last years, eliminating messages of little importance and inserting instead texts not written by him which would contribute to emphasize his role at the court. Especially the letters of the first years did generate the most objections when his position, even with the protection of Queen Isabella, was undefined.

Perhaps at the beginning Peter Martyr employed young clerics, recruited to help him, and he rewarded and fostered their career at Court or in the Church. Later he was able to count on the help of more experienced scribes often paid directly by him: from 1520 the humanist had the title of "royal chronicler" with a stipend of 80,000 *maravedís*, which allowed him to maintain in his service a staff that would provide him with information.

Consequently this also affects the degree of textual reliability of his letters that appears to be one of the distinctive characteristics of the author, namely, his being scrupulously truthful. Often when the information is not the fruit of his direct experience, he indicates with precision the person from whom he has received it or occasionally admits he is unable to verify contrasting versions of news reported to him. Given the vastness of his interests, in his letters one can find fairly abundant references about what is happening in Europe and in the New World. The inaccuracy of certain dates which some scholars attribute to Peter Martyr should probably be blamed on the editor who had the manuscripts arranged only approximately by year and by addressee, who dated undated letters and incorporated more than one letter in the same text, perhaps on account of mixed up sheets of papers. Notwithstanding the blemish of inaccuracies, in most cases due to a careless printer, the historical truth of the letters is not invalidated.

If the letters were grouped by historical themes, we would have a series of documents of exceptional interest, in that in them we can find richly detailed and colorful episodes that presuppose first-hand knowledge. A first group might be constituted from letters written to his Italian friends from the war zone of Granada (1488-1491); another could include the correspondence from 1502 to 1508 about the painful events of the family of the Catholic Sovereigns, when Peter Martyr first lived next to Isabella as her chaplain and then next to Juana, her daughter. Peter Martyr's pages, on account of his pechant for details, have shed new light on Juana, harassed since her childhood by parents who denied her any autonomy, and considered incapacitated by her father and her husband Philip so that they might strip her of any power.

The letters of the first years of the reign of Charles, son of Juana and Philip of Hapsburg, give us a precise and dramatic picture of the conditions in Spain; the revolt of the *comuneros* finds in Peter Martyr a precious witness. The wars of Italy and the continuous changes in

Italian politics are reported by him with a precision no less reliable than that with which he describes the Navarre and Rossiglione wars which he witnessed at the side of the King.

It might seem surprising that Peter Martyr, in spite of the fact that from 1487 to 1536 did not leave Spain, except for his mission to Egypt, was so well informed about events in Italy, yet it should be kept in mind that the court of Spain was perhaps the most dynamic center of European politics in those years and that Peter Martyr, given his position, was well informed about everything. "Latin Secretary" to the Sovereigns and enjoying very good relations with ambassadors at the Court, he could access most information of interest to him. For example, he had direct contact with the Borromeos in Milan, with his brother Giovanni Battista, who served Venice, with Ascanio Sforza, Alonso Carrillo, Diego de Sousa, Pomponius Letus, Bernardino de Carvajal, Giovanni Ruffo in Rome, Luigi Marliani and Mercurino Arborio da Gattinara at the Imperial Court, and with Gian Giacomo Trivulzio and Teodoro of Pavia at the French court; he was friendly with navigators and conquerors, especially with Columbus, and also officially in charge of reporting to the Sovereigns about the New World.

On the validity of the historical, political and moral assessments of men and events made by the author, it seems, on the contrary, that critics have often been hasty and never attempted to identify his philosophy, presenting him rather as a courtier incapable of ideas and values of his own, concerned only about pleasing his master in order to receive favors and prebends. His strength as a humanist, his vast experience of men and political problems, his constant thinking about his faraway homeland afflicted by wars, his attachment to Spain, his country of adoption, seen by him — likely from its inception — as a united country, his loyalty to his friends—all this has not been placed in the right light. In reality he shows himself to be a man of his time, an expression of the "New" humanistic concern that went beyond the study of the past, to look at a present full of ferments and events, lived day by day since man is the *faber fortunae suae*. Unlike Machiavelli and Guicciardini, theorists and historians of politics of the first part of the sixteenth century, Peter Martyr is but a diligent and accurate chronicler: historical and political facts are to him caused only by human competence or ineptitude. He limits himself to reporting the facts and the political programs of the powerful, without forcing them to fit some political or historical theory. More of a chronicler than a historian, Peter Martyr is at times considered, not incorrectly, the first journalist since to the stringent account of events he addresses their resonance among men. In his pages live on with the reputed protagonists, all those affected by the events, especially the populations that end up enduring violence without any fault of their own or any chance to defend themselves. Living at the Court of Spain he succeeds in fore-seeing political upheavals: he would like to be able to avoid them for the common good, but he knows that ambitious men thirsty for power do not listen to the advice of wisdom.

Our main interest is here especially for the letters from 1495 to 1525, that deal closely with the news about the New World, in particular the first years in which is relayed news of the discovery and of the implications the new geographical reality poses. They represent more than rich information, they also help to document the psychological impact such "unveiling" had on Europe, which was experiencing a time period full of tension and problems. And among the selected letters presented in this book, some in particular deserve to be highlighted.

The letter to Giovanni Borromeo of May 14, 1493 speaks for the first time of Columbus' enterprise: only a few lines are dedicated to the discovery, but all-encompassing as they span from the drama of seven long years of waiting, to the actual triumph. The Navigator is cited as *vir ligur* and not *Genuensis* probably because Genoa was, at that time, on the French side and the author prefers not, even indirectly, to speak of it so as not to touch upon a subject unpleasant to the Court. Great relevance, perhaps insufficiently stressed by scholars, should receive the letter addressed to the Count of Tendilla and to the archbishop of Granada dated September 13, 1493 as it contains very precise accounts of the preparation of the first voyage, and mentions directly two people who played a relevant role in such a circumstance: Iñigo López de Mendoza, Count of Tendilla, at the moment viceroy and governor of the Kingdom of Granada, and Hernando de Talavera, archbishop of the conquered city, two witnesses and supporters of Columbus's requests. It should be noted that while in the letter to Giovanni Borromeo Peter Martyr had written *Christophorus quidam Colonus, vir Ligur*, in the letter to Tendilla and Talavera he speaks of Columbus as a person they are well acquainted with, someone they could not have forgotten even if met during the harsh days of the war in Granada; in fact, at the camp below Granada, Tendilla was head of the Castilian forces, commander of the royal guard in which Peter Martyr served and royal advisor, and Hernando de Talavera, confessor of the Queen. Columbus used to go often to the camp below Granada in the hope of obtaining what he had been seeking for years.

Their contribution in siding with the Navigator must have been crucial: expressions like *actum est*, and *consilio*, seem to imply evidence not of informal suggestions but of a formulation for a deliberation to be adopted by an official body. Peter Martyr states that without the support of these two illustrious members Columbus would have not been able to make his voyage, mentioning this deliberation made by the Royal Council, i.e. a collegial provision of which Isabella was the most convinced supporter with most other members, including the recipients of this letter, as shown by the capitulations of Santa Fe and other documents drawn up by the Crown to organize the expedition. This means that the decision on Columbus's enterprise was decided two years earlier at the camp in Granada: while the war against the Islamic Kingdom was moving toward its close, albeit among unforeseen events and dangers (the fire at the camp being one of the most clamorous episodes), Isabella continued to support Columbus more or less openly and, amid the clanging of arms, the project of the voyage had been re-evaluated.

It must be remembered that Hernando de Talavera had been the President of the Council of Salamanca and the most decisive adversary of Columbus's project; but, according to the evidence of this letter he had totally modified his stand on account of doctrinal reasons dictated by a cultural tradition which had its cradle in Spain, right in Salamanca, as well as perhaps because of political reasons. At the camp below Granada, in a totally different atmosphere, the change of Talavera's stand toward Columbus was probably determined by his friendship with Peter Martyr, who represented, at that time in the Court, the expression of Italian humanism in its most dynamic aspect, i.e. the interest for scientific issues; in his writings, in fact, one can see not only a mastery of the great classical naturalists (Pliny, Strabo, Ptolemy, etc.) but find evidence of knowledge of cosmographic and astronomical theories. If Peter Martyr by *actum est* implies, as in all likelyhood he does, a reference to meetings of an official character, one can also imagine that they were preceded by discussions by few intimate people under the tent. In the letter a triumphal tone is evident: the enterprise has succeeded, the *vir Ligur* has won, but with him also prevailed all those who believed in him and allowed him to go through with the enterprise. Historical evidence supports this interpretation: the capitulations were signed in Santa Fe on April 17, 1491, when Talavera, Tendilla and Peter Martyr were in Granada, engaged in establishing a new order in the subdued city, and the Sovereigns were preparing to return to their ancestral kingdoms. Tired of waiting, Columbus left, proclaiming that he would go to France, but was called back to conclude the negotiations: obviously the signing of the capitulations is only a formal act which completes detailed negotiations concluded long before, but whose drafting by a notary had been postponed for convenience or circumstances. The letter, therefore, clarifies some essential facts:

1) Peter Martyr's presence at the camp, at the moment when Columbus's project was being re-evaluated, must be considered very important to the achievement of a positive solution. His prestige as a man of doctrine and his knowledge of cosmography probably helped present the voyage in a more favorable light and obtain the full support of Talavera and of Cardinal Pedro Gonzáles de Mendoza, who was also an admirer and friend of the Lombard humanist;

2) Peter Martyr had already met Christopher Columbus at camp in Granada and had become his friend and supporter;

3) From this psychological state and his humanistic restlessness, is born in him the obligation to communicate to the world of culture all news concerning the new horizons revealed to man's intellect.

The letter to Ascanio Sforza of September 13, 1493 relates some particulars of the trip, among others a reference to the sighting of the New Land which provoked several discussions about a possible embezzlement on Columbus's part of the reward established by the Queen for the first person to sight land. In fact, for this a life annuity of 100,000 *maravedís* had been assigned to Columbus; in any case, presumably, although the Admiral was on board he was not on the crow's nest scrutinizing the ocean. It is the apex of the crossing, with the detail of the crow's nest, even if it refers to a real event, is perhaps still poetic fiction, because after Columbus saw a light in the night (and to be sure he had called Pedro Gutiérrez), land was actually sighted first by Rodrigo de Triana, who was traveling on the Pinta, that was sailing ahead of the Santa María. In addition, Peter Martyr gives information on the political "structure" of the new people while emphasizing with regret that even among those people the drive for power leads to internal wars and the submission of the conquered to the victors.

The letter to the archbishop of Braga, Diego de Sousa, of October 1, 1493, has a scientific theme, as shown by the author's digression on the location of the discovered islands. Yet, it must be pointed out that these observations also have a political implication, since Peter Martyr concludes his argument by saying that, what really matters is that the still uncharted half of the earth be discovered and maintains that this will take place also thanks to the activity of the Portuguese and the competition between the two countries. Moreover, one can observe that the author seems to want to stress his personal conviction, namely, that the discovered lands are not Asia, in order to remove any reason for conflict with the Portuguese, who were involved in the attempt to reach Asia by circumnavigating Africa. The Catholic Sovereigns in 1493 had prevailed upon Pope Alexander VI to draw the *raya* line to separate the areas of influence between the Spaniards and the Portuguese in order to avoid a conflict. The *raya*, however, was almost a mockery to the Portuguese, so a new demarcation had to be established much farther to the West, with the treaty of Tordesillas of 1494, agreed upon by the two powers.

The letter to Ascanio Sforza at the beginning of November 1493 announces that Columbus has departed on a second expedition. The fact that Peter Martyr, writing to Ascanio Sforza, also mentions Diego de Sousa, archbishop of Braga, without writing directly to him, makes one suspect that the author might have wanted De Sousa to know, even if indirectly, this news, which perhaps would not have pleased him too much.

In fact, the Portuguese, who had had a monopoly on the Atlantic navigation, certainly could not accept being surpassed by a foreigner, who, according to them, had snatched away from them the secret of navigating the "Dark Sea." It is a historical fact that Columbus made his first proposals to the Portuguese king, and that he had been turned down. After the already mentioned letter of October 1, 1493, there is an interval of more than a year in the correspondence with Diego de Sousa; the letter of October 31, 1494 is simultaneously directed to the archbishops of Braga and Pamplona. In it the news of the New World is meager and, according to the author, no longer interesting because the news is "old."

In the letter to Giovanni Borromeo of October 20, 1494, the news of the New World is attributed to Columbus, who states that from the island of Hispaniola he has traveled through so many land toward the West that he has almost touched the Golden Chersonese, the last boundary of the eastern part of the known world, and that he stopped two hours short of the full solar cycle. Peter Martyr reports, having begun to write books about those discoveries, that will leave out nothing worthy of memory, so as to offer a wealth of material to historians. This is the first announcement of the composition of the *Decades*, and it is not without significance that he gives the first news of his intention to his friend and protector, the one who first led him to humanistic studies, quite modestly saying that he wanted to gather all the news so that it might be used by scholars.

In the already mentioned letter of October 31, 1494, to the archbishops of Braga and Pamplona, Diego de Sousa and Alonso Carrillo, Peter Martyr reports concerning the New World only the news of the departure of a fleet of eighteen ships to Hispaniola (from other sources it appears that there were seventeen) and of the return of most of them, sent back to Spain by Columbus, who remained in the new lands to conduct other explorations. One notices a certain embarrassment on the part of Peter Martyr in providing these lean details to the Portuguese Diego de Sousa: even if the Portuguese had by now accepted the conditions of the Treaty of Tordesillas, the humanist, perhaps understanding the state of mind of his friend, avoids insisting on this topic.

With the letter of December 5, 1494, Peter Martyr begins the correspondence concerning the New World with his humanist friend Pomponius Letus and he contrasts the anguish of Italy overcome by domestic feuds and foreign invaders, with the greatness of Spain, which extends as far as the Antipodes. Referring to what he has already written to the archbishops of Braga and Pamplona about the New World, he adds some clarifications learned from those who came back with twelve of the eighteen ships sent on the second voyage. He ends the letter referring one more time to the archbishop of Braga, whom he mentions when he speaks of the death of John, King of Portugal, and of his successor. Probably here there is an attempt to resume contacts with his Portuguese friend, contacts perhaps somewhat damaged by the Columbian events, as the fact that we possess only two letters to Diego de Sousa before this one seems to show, unless we hypothesize that there might have been other pieces of correspondence that have not come down to us.

The second letter to Pomponius Letus about the New World, dated December 29, 1494, expresses the joy of the humanist in learning for the sake of learning. We learn from Peter Martyr that Pomponius had rejoiced and nearly cried when he found out, from his friend's letters, the news of the discoveries: it is the very attitude of a man of great learning. The author confesses to feeling the same way when he speaks with those who come from the new lands, called upon not only because of the friendship that he had been able to establish with some of them (among them, Columbus, already his friend from times preceding the discovery), but also because of his position. In fact, he had to deal with those who were leaving and coming back; he read their reports and shared them with the Sovereigns, who, even though they had not given him a formal appointment, did avail themselves of him because of a great esteem for his culture. In this letter are narrated the events of the second voyage up to the return of the first twelve ships. We must emphasize his references to an idyllic vision of the new people, which gave rise to the literary theme of the "good savage."

Peter Martyr also cites a letter written to him by Columbus in which the Navigator tells him he has begun to raise animals in those lands and sow plants from Europe. There remains no trace of this letter and others about which specific references are found in the epistolary but, no doubt, the humanist used them in drafting his letters and in editing the already begun *Decades*.

Finally, the geographical latitude and longitude data relative to Hispaniola are reported, provided to the author by experts in surveying. Peter Martyr then reports the episode of the slaughtered Spaniards who had been left on the island of Hispaniola entrusted to the protection of cacique Guacanagarí, who declares that they had been killed by a king of the interior, Caonabó. Columbus, even though tries to obtain precise evidence, is not able to find out the truth and, despite the contrary opinion of his people, he does not believe that he should punish Guacanagarí (whose claim that he had been wounded in the leg while fighting to save the Spanish turned out to be clearly false). Simone Dal Verde says that he found out from Alfonso Torres and two other participants in the second voyage that the Spaniards, each of whom had taken four wives, had fought among themselves and had one another massacred. Alfonso Torres, Michele da Cuneo, Bartholomew de las Casas, and Ferdinand Columbus speak of the slaughter of the thirty-eight Spaniards without giving explanations of the fact, but all emphasize that Columbus did not want to punish the Indian king because he did not want to alienate the people.

In the letter of June 11, 1495 to Bernardino de Carvajal, one notices a reference to the ambiguous conduct of the Crown and especially of King Ferdinand (even if the full jurisdiction of the new lands belonged to Isabella), who avoids compliance with the terms of the capitulations signed by Columbus and authorizes expeditions of new and sometimes inexperienced navigators, who search for wealth and glory and promise to send the Sovereign a great quantity of that gold which he needs to support with arms his policy against the French. The attack on Christopher Columbus and his brother Bartholomew, named *Adelantado*, begins; it will reach its peak with the return to Spain of the two Genoese in chains, stripped of all responsibilities.

The letter of August 9, 1495 sent to Bernardino de Carvajal is full of enthusiasm. The details about the discovered lands are numerous and precise: it describes the exploration by Columbus of a new land called Cuba, the discovery of fresh and salt water, and speaks of shells with pearls and of turtles with large carapaces. Peter Martyr recalls the doctrine of the ancients on their knowledge of Asiatic lands; since he is not convinced, he only gives brief mention that the new lands belong to Asia, and thus aligns himself with the official version.

On October 5, 1496, Peter Martyr informs Carvajal of the report that Columbus, back in Spain, delivered on the lands and things found and on the discussion that the news of the Navigator stirred among friends of the humanist. He does not mention them by name, but one can assume that they were the humanist Antonio de Nebrija, Alessandro Geraldini, perhaps Lucio Marineo Siculo and others, scholarly people who were at the Court and who had a fair knowledge of classic cosmography to which they wanted to relate the new experiences from overseas.

It is significant that there is not a hint of the slanderous charges against Columbus which were persistently reaching the court and of which probably the Queen had disposed. We know that she had called upon her Admiral for information on the dangers of navigation in the North Sea and in the English Channel, asking him to indicate the best route, since she was worried about the trip that her daughter, Juana, was going to take to reach her spouse, Philip of Hapsburg. In fact, Peter Martyr writes about the marriage and the trip, in the second part of the letter. Columbus's letter to the Queen has not been found, but the letter of thanks for the information given exists.

The date of this letter has raised several problems on which it is necessary to dwell. The text presents clear references to a voyage to the land of *Paria*, to the encounter with more developed peoples, and to the finding of a great quantity of pearls. From all the other sources, however, it seems that Columbus reached the coast of *Paria* and found the pearls during his third voyage, not during the second as should be inferred from the date of the letter; it is an obvious case of wrong dating. The problem in this case is complicated by the fact that the entire second part of the letter contains specific references to events of 1496; indeed, the departure of young Juana to meet her spouse in Flanders is also specified. The passage has aroused a heated debate between two great scholars of Columbus, Taviani on one hand, and Manzano Manzano on the other, since the latter, accepting the date without reservation, relies on the letter to confirm that Columbus reached the continent during the second voyage, while Taviani maintains that the date of the event must be changed to at least 1498, that is, after the return from the third voyage.

In support of Manzano's thesis there is only one testimony, not very trustworthy, of a sailor from the expeditions, an eighty-year-old man about whom Bartholomew of las Casas says that he usually made up things and falsified news; in favor of Taviani's thesis there are all the other texts concerning the two voyages. The great majority of European Columbian scholars, (including the Spanish), South Americans, North Americans, and Japanese have not accepted the Manzano thesis, who, on the other hand, remains always authoritative for his work on the seven or eight decisive years of Columbus's life in Spain.

Reservations have been expressed about the accuracy of some dates in the Epistolary, as has been said; but while errors in dating usually are contained within a margin of a few weeks, here it would be an error of at least two years, which is more incomprehensible if one considers that in the second part of the letter the related events agree with the date placed at the end of the message. Besides, it must be noted that Peter Martyr for this matter refers to the *Decades of the New World* which he is writing on the discoveries and that the reference to the land of *Paria* is found in the sixth book of the first *Decade*, which deals with the third and not the second voyage of Columbus. In the *Decades*, therefore, he agrees with all the other sources.

So it is very probable that a transposition of sheets might have occurred in the manuscript delivered for printing, and that the first part of the letter originally preceded the second; or perhaps one could suggest that the printer might have purposely displaced the pages. In fact, one must not forget that in the campaign of false charges against Columbus, the following were recurrent: accusations of having hidden the truth many times, of wanting to keep for himself wealth as well as power, of imposing on everyone his own view purposely adulterated. Keeping silent about the discovery of pearls was for his slanderers a proof of his lack of loyalty to the Sovereigns, a good reason to deprive him of power. It was a clear strategy that served to justify, at least in appearance, the unfair treatment inflicted on the Admiral and to justify the decision of the Crown not to award him rights and privileges initially granted him.

Moreover, it is known that Columbus himself, when he discovered the "pearls"-country, instructed the natives to gather a great quantity of them for his return and he left without harvesting any, unintentionally leaving himself open to accusations of not having acted in the interests of the Crown. Already, however, the news of the existence of pearls in those areas as well as of gold-bearing lands had reached Spain, even before the discoverers had arrived in person.

In the letter to Pomponius Letus of November 7, 1497, special emphasis is placed on the direction taken by the politics of exploration of the Portuguese and Castilians. In fact, the former had always tried to maintain the maximum secrecy, especially about their routes, and they had limited themselves in the long and tiring circumnavigation of Africa to secure areas of support for their ships. Once they reached the spice markets, the reasons for secrecy were no longer valid because the spices were exported by them to European markets and also because word about their ruthless repressions in Calicut had spread.

The Spaniards, instead, had made their undertaking public from the first moment, eager to have their rights immediately recognized by the papal bull. Aside from Isabella's religious purposes, a desire to expand the political domain is clear: new cities are founded and the work of the native people is exploited to the maximum in order to obtain as much wealth as possible.

In the letter to Pomponius Letus of December 18, 1497 (1597 is clearly a typographical misprint) there is an ambiguous expression, *quae de homine garriant, ne feceris participem*. Even if it is probable that it might refer to the beliefs of the natives regarding the creation of man, Peter Martyr could have alluded to the accusations against Columbus or he could have played on the ambiguity of these words. These rumors had also reached Rome from Spain and the writer considered them so unjust that he despised even talking about them. However, he did not ignore that there was a vast maneuver in Court against the Navigator, but had not opportunity to present the truth and did not want to antagonize everyone.

In the letter to Luis Hurtado de Mendoza of July 23, 1514, Peter Martyr relates the extraordinary initiative of Vasco Núñez de Balboa, who, having usurped power in Darién, throwing out Diego de Nicuesa and Martín Fernández de Encis, crosses the mountains and reaches the Pacific Ocean. It is evident that the writer refused to express a moral judgment or, better still, in what he writes he wants to emphasize that traditional values are not respected anymore and that the Crown is ready to adapt itself to these circumstances and even to reward those who offended the Crown when it might gain from such situations.

However, that the undertaking might have aroused enthusiasm in the Spaniards is shown in the pages of the third *Decade*, in which this venture is narrated in detail and sometimes with epic tones, since it noted the extraordinary discovery that between the lands until now known and the most remote part of Asia there is a Pacific Ocean. This discovery was made possible by the heroic effort and untold sacrifices of those who followed the rebel Balboa.

In the letter of December 13, 1514, to the same addressee or the preceding one, there is a rather explicit reference to the lack of initiative on the part of the colonists who have settled in a native village after throwing out the leader. Moreover, while in the above-mentioned letter of July 3, 1514, the impartial and extremely strong personality of Vasco Núñez de Balboa stood out; trampling on royal dispositions, he had been able to find the Pacific Ocean in his extraordinary feat, with a handful of men on whom he had imposed enormous sacrifices; in this letter the inhabitants of Darién show that they are not even able to provide for their own health by moving away from an unpleasant and unhealthy residence.

In the letter of July 21, 1518 to Marquises Luis Hurtado de Mendoza and Pietro Fajardo, Peter Martyr severely castigates in detail the greed of the people who rotate around the Court. In fact, he reports about the great quantity of pearls that arrives from the new lands and that immediately becomes prey of the Flemish and the French, who take advantage of the King's indulgence. He reports that the wife of the chancellor Guillaume de Croy, called Chévres, was able to secure for herself 160 pounds of pearls, leaving not even one for the King's sister who had just married. On this occasion, Peter Martyr assumes the attitude of the majority of the Spaniards, decidedly hostile toward the Flemish, but he seems to defend King Charles, because he considers him unprotected from the usurers who surround him.

With the letter of December 1, 1519, to the Marquises, appears for the first time in the collection of letters the name of Hernán Cortés, who, deserting Diego Velásquez, the governor of Cuba who had sent him to explore new lands rich in gold and jewels, settles there and organizes the territory, assuming full power.

In the last part of the letter dated March 6, 1521, to the Great Chancellor Mercurino Arborio da Gattinara, Peter Martyr reveals that in the New World there have been found fortified cities, large houses and temples, people well-dressed and adorned, and he promises to speak about this at length at another time. The location of these cities is, however, inaccurately given since it would seem that they are located in the southern part of Cuba, while in reality they are west of the island, indeed, in Mexico.

In the letter of March 7, 1521 to the Marquises, he corrects the inaccuracy of the preceding letter to the Great Chancellor. He speaks of a big lake of salty water several miles from the sea, of a city that rises in that lagoon, Tenustítan (Mexico City), and of the extraordinary greatness and wealth of King Montezuma. If in the previous letter the news is reported briefly, because the Chancellor must concern himself with facing the revolt of the *comuneros*, here with his two favorite pupils he can speak more elaborately of the great discoveries and also of the important cultural implications they raise. In fact, the New World is inhabited also by people who possess a great civilization.

In the letter of August 30, 1522 to Giovanni Ruffo, archbishop of Cosenza, Peter Martyr reports that the ship *Victoria*, the only one of the five entrusted to Magellan, who was killed by the natives, has finally returned after having gone around the world.

From a reference to the *Consejo Supremo de Indias* it can be inferred that this body did not have a stable seat, but would follow the movements of the Crown. On the other hand, the *Casa de Contratación de Indias* had a stable seat in Seville capable of managing all economic problems, even if, given the more intense development of the movement of ships to and from the New World, the peninsular port of arrival and departure became in practice Cádiz with Seville keeping the title of metropolitan seat of the Admiral of the Ocean Sea.

In the letter of November 4, 1522 to the Marquises, after having spoken of the controversy between Spain and the King of Portugal about the islands of the spices that the latter considers to belong to him because they are near the Moluccas, Peter Martyr gives an interesting explanation about the loss of one sun-day experienced by the crew that went around the world in three years. This confirms the unusual preparation of the writer, who for this reason had been appointed by the Sovereigns to follow the events of the explorations.

In the letter of November 19, 1522 to the archbishop of Cosenza, Peter Martyr speaks of the arrival at the Azores of three ships sent by Cortés, loaded with great wealth, artistic objects, clothes and decorations; he talks particularly of three "tigers" transported on the ships, one of which broke the cage and hurled itself against the men, wounding some, and, when struck, was thrown in the ocean; the second one was killed as a precaution, and only the third one arrived in Spain. It must be noted that Peter Martyr uses the term tiger to indicate the American jaguar. In fact there are no tigers in America, but even today in Latin America the jaguar is called "tiger." The animal was considered a divinity or a personification of the divinity in all of Mesoamerica. The Mayas used to say that men of the second age had been transformed into jaguars by the gods; this tradition is in part still alive among the farmers of Mayan origin in Guatemala and Honduras.

The author further reports on the treasures sent by Cortés in the letter of June 11, 1523 to the archbishop of Cosenza, but adds that little of it arrives in Spain due to the attacks of the French pirate Florin. It should be pointed out that privateering was in a certain way complementary to warfare between armies and rival fleets and, in addition, privateering was the most practiced at sea and it always had the open or secret support of the Sovereign. At the beginning it was only the French, in European waters, who plundered the Spanish ships arriving with the riches of the New World; later it would be mainly the English and the Dutch, who would operate on islands and coasts, especially those of the Caribbean Sea.

The motive for the conflict between the Spaniards and Portuguese over the respective areas of influence resurfaces in the letter of June 20, 1524, in which Peter Martyr deals with the expedition that the Spaniards plan to make along the route of Magellan to the land of spices. Following the protests of the Portuguese, the mixed commission meets at Badajoz to reach a decision on the question, but it dissolves without concluding anything.

With the treaty of Tordesillas, the *raya* mapped out by Alexander VI had been moved 270 miles to the West, and as a consequence the Portuguese obtained Brazil (not limiting themselves only to the coastal area, but penetrating much in the interior). In theory, since they had crossed the Pacific, the line agreed upon at Tordesillas should have also been valid for the corresponding meridian and, in other words, left to the Portuguese what was placed East of the line, namely, the spice islands. One more time, however, right was overpowered by force: the Portuguese certainly could not think of opposing Charles V with arms, even if for the moment he was engaged on many fronts. Besides, the Portuguese expansion had begun as a search for bases of support of trade and, therefore, they had no desire for territorial conquests, while the Spanish expansion had aimed from the beginning at taking possession of new lands.

The central part of the letter dated August 3, 1524, to the archbishop of Cosenza, refers to the nomination of the writer to be abbot of San Jacopo of Jamaica. Appointment to ecclesiastical offices in the New World was controlled by the Spanish Crown, but it then required the approval of the pontiff; thus, Peter Martyr writes to his friend so that he might speed up the matter. At the time of Leo X, Martyr was forced to keep one of his men at the Holy See to look after his interests, but now that does not seem necessary anymore if he turns directly to the archbishop, Giovanni Ruffo. He probably hopes that what he writes is reported to the pontiff and he, therefore, confirms that he has never been eager for honors and wealth. However, he gives three motivations for his request to the Emperor about the above-mentioned nomination, among them the pledge to spend the revenues from the appointment to build in stone the wooden church which burned. This intention is expressed as well in the letter of June 13, 1525, addressed again to Giovanni Ruffo, but here we learn that the Sovereign, to show his affection for the writer, has arranged that the royal treasury intervene to match and cover the necessary expenses.

In the letter of November 18, 1524 to the archbishop of Cosenza, Peter Martyr gives news of the conflicts between Cristóbal de Olid, an agent of Cortés, Gil Gonzales, representative of the King, and Pedro Arias for power in Cuba, of Garay, governor of Jamaica, who had fallen into the hands of Cortés and then died. The fighting among the conquistadors is mentioned without much comment. However, it is evident that the *Consejo Supremo de Indias*, of which Peter Martyr is part, does not have the power really to impose the royal rule in those far away lands.

In the letter of February 22, 1525 to the archbishop of Cosenza, the writer reports, among other things, the discussions held in the *Congreso Supremo de Indias* about the freedom of the natives. For this purpose it is necessary to emphasize that when in the collection of letters Peter Martyr has resumed talking about the events of the New World, after the silence of the years 1499-1513, even though he dwells upon the greatness of the Aztec empire, he reports especially on the fighting among the Spaniards and gives few details on the warfare between Cortés and Montezuma.

The conquistadors seem to be fighting among themselves out of lust for power and wealth in a conquered land whose inhabitants do not even seem to exist. But the problem exists and it is very serious: on the one hand, there is the evangelizing mission, entrusted by the pontiff to Spain, or better still to its Sovereigns; on the other hand, there is the desire to take possession of enormous wealth which must go to the leaders of the expeditions, their men and to the Crown, which recognizes the power, often usurped by the conquistadors, only if it receives great treasures.

So the natives become souls to be conquered, but especially laborers to be exploited: the situation becomes so serious that those who evangelize are forced to intervene, at least as far as possible, to save the survivors. The intervention of the Sovereign and of the body that represents him, that is, the *Consejo Supremo de Indias*, is requested. The natives are assigned to conquistadors turned colonists with the institution of the encomienda, but the *encomenderos* do not tolerate the interference of members of the religious orders who protest against the inhumane treatments (Bartholomew of las Casas, who had begun his activity in the new lands as *encomendero*, will arrive as bishop of Chiapas to threaten with excommunication those who do not give up the encomiendas and do not return the natives to freedom).

Reading the Epistolary one discovers a progressive distancing of the author from the subject, a transition from the account of the particulars of the discoveries to a description of the peoples, their customs, their beliefs, sometimes a certain irritation, a lack of interest, as if the New World by this time had lost its fascination. The great undertaking accomplished by Columbus with the support of the Catholic Sovereigns had raised many hopes, but it had also created envy, fear, greed, contrasts more or less evident, as the deterioration of the relations between Columbus and the Sovereigns also showed. The greatness of the empire had given Columbus such power that it would not have been possible to restrain him, but the Genoese Navigator had a strong and stubborn character, which did not want to accept compromises, and perhaps he was too proud of his victory. From this arise the false accusations, the exaggeration of his mistakes, the coalition of all interests against him. Peter Martyr cannot intervene in his favor, however. As he has demonstrated in his activity at the Court, he has a clear vision of politics and of human nature, of the limits beyond which no one is allowed to go; he does not believe the false charges, but still he cannot force Columbus to change an attitude which makes him more and more unpopular.

Therefore, the humanist avoids the issue as much as possible, because he would have to report the wrongs of both parties and choose the side on which to stand, but without any justifiable proofs. He knows the conflict between Columbus and the royal power, and he knows that not even Isabella, as Queen, could have agreed to relinquish the royal privileges or her own freedom of action in choosing men or to neglect the great wealth about which people fantasized.

V. – *DECADES DE ORBE NOVO.*

The war in Granada prompted Peter Martyr to think of moving from the fragmentary information of his Epistolary i.e. topically diverse news in the form of letters, temporally constrained to the moment of their drafting, to editing an ample historical work on the subject, which he had thought of titling *Diaria Castrensia*. The dramatic fall of the last Islamic kingdom in Spain, which ended a war that had lasted eight centuries, as well as the magnificence of the scenery, the spiritual tension, the heroisms and sufferings to which he had been a direct witness were deemed by the writer a topic worthy of history.

However, in 1493 a new, immense horizon suddenly opens: Christopher Columbus returns from the western antipodes. The news appears almost in a flash; then the scopes of the enterprise are specified, with few particulars of a voyage begun in the face of the incredulity of many; Peter Martyr in his letters already spoke of a certain Columbus as discoverer of a New World.

Having provided some details to his correspondents, he is constantly urged by them to give new information. In communicating to his friends news about the new lands he shows he realizes that the subject is so broad and of such importance as to merit a specific treatment, not only desultory references, and he says so openly in the letter of October 20, 1494 to Borromeo. Therefore, he sets about the drafting of the first book of the first Decade, dedicated to Ascanio Sforza, concerning the first voyage of Columbus and his departure on the second voyage. In reality this book is dated November 13, 1493, while the second, also dedicated to Ascanio Sforza, which relates the first part of the second voyage up to the return to Spain of the first twelve ships, has the date of April 29, 1494. Although the idea for the work had been conceived very early, the drafting was slow and it was carried out very fittingly over time.

Books I 3-9 are dedicated to Cardinal Ludovico d'Aragona and deal with the second and third voyages of Columbus and with the events taking place in the New Lands from 1494 to 1498, namely, the undertakings of Bartholomew, brother of Columbus, the rebellion of Roldán Jiménez, and the return of the Admiral and his brother to Spain, devoid of their commission and in chains. In I 8-9 the events of the voyage of Alonso Niño and of Vincenzo Yáñez Pinzón are narrated and others until 1500. The tenth book, which closes the first Decade, is dedicated to the Count of Tendilla; in actuality it is a new draft of a shorter text offered by Peter Martyr to Ludovico d'Aragona, who wanted to take the writings to Rome in 1500, but which was later expanded to include news up to 1510.

The first Decade is important because it embraces the first years of the discovery and three voyages by Columbus; it was published in Spain, at Seville, in 1511, without the consent of the author by initiative of Lucio Marineo Siculo, who had taken it from his friend, although partially reduced and altered texts of it were already circulating. Angelo Trevisan, secretary to Pisani, ambassador to Spain, had made a summary of it in 1501 and had mailed it to the reporter Domenico Malipiero. It appeared in Venice in 1504 with the title *Libretto de tutta la navigazion de re de Spagna de le isole e terreni novamente trovati*. The text appears later, in 1507, in Chapter IV of the book *Paesi novamenti retrovati et Novo Mondo di Alberico Vesputio, fiorentino*, by Fracanzio da Montalboddo, and in 1508 a Latin translation was published.

It is not clear how Trevisan might have come into possession of Peter Martyr's work: we could assume a theft of manuscripts or an illegal copying ordered by him, who frequented the writer's home as secretary of the Venetian ambassador to Spain; perhaps Peter Martyr, who was leaving then for Venice, from where he was going to embark on his mission to Egypt, had requested the ambassador to secure for him an audience with the doge. The writer, when informed of that arbitrarily printed edition, complained about it, but, as he writes at the end of the tenth book to the count of Tendilla, he did not have the courage to revise the work. It is probable that Lucio Marineo Siculo, having published Peter Martyr's *Carmina*, the *Legatio Babylonica* and the *Decas Prima*, published on his own initiative, might have wanted to urge his friend to resume the interrupted work. The years 1500 to 1510 had been full of obligations and worries for Peter Martyr, but certainly even in that period he continued to gather information about the New World, both from the protagonists that he was able to approach, and from the reports arriving at Court.

In 1514 he edited the second Decade, and in 1516 the third one, both dedicated to Pope Leo X; so that the work might be properly published, he turned for its printing to his friend Antonio de Nebrija, the humanist philologist, who in 1516 published the three Decades and the *Legatio Babylonica*.

438

The fourth Decade, also dedicated to Leo X, was written in 1519 and published separately in Basel in 1521, with the title *De insulis nuper inventis liber*; the fifth, begun in 1529, dedicated to Pope Adrian VI, except for books 7-10 which were dedicated to Clement VII, was finished in 1522; while the sixth, sent to Cardinal Giovanni Ruffo that he might present it to the pontiff, was written in 1522. The seventh, dedicated to Francesco Maria Sforza, duke of Milan, and the eighth dedicated to Clement VII, were written in 1525.

The eight *Decades de Orbe Novo* were then printed in one volume in Alcalá de Henares in 1530 by M. de Eguía, who also supervised the printing of the *Opus epistolarum*.

The thirteen years interval between the drafting of the first and second *Decades* finds an explanation in that lack of enthusiasm for writing about which he himself hints to the count of Tendilla; morever, the disgust that he feels for what is happening in the New Lands and in Spain, in that Court which he had exalted as a seat of virtue and justice, very probably constitutes a further reason for restraint by the writer.

The 1495 letter to Carvajal is the first testimony to a certain uneasiness: the news that Columbus has returned to Spain in chains and devoid of all power bothers him. The grand, extraordinary discovery that had stirred excitement in the most noble hearts, was transforming those lands in which the men used to live contented in a natural state, into a horrible environment.

Peter Martyr realized that he was in a particularly delicate situation: he did not forget (and certainly others would not let him) that he was a foreigner, even if he was favored by the Queen. He was in a situation very similar to that in which Columbus found himself: able to speak openly in his defense, but without an official political office that would give weight to his judgement; little appreciated at Court for his dislike of Queen Germana de Foix, wife of King Ferdinand after the death of Isabella; involved in not-so-easy relations with Cardinal Cisnéros; and, as a clergyman, obliged to watch out for the Inquisition.

But the fundamental reason Peter Martyr interrupts his writing of the *Decades* very probably is an inner rebellion against the illegality which prevails in all the complex world of discovery and conquest, where everything is from the beginning *extra lege*, sometimes even *contra legem*. We could offer the hypothesis that in the period from 1501 to 1513 Peter Martyr might have been prohibited from writing about the New World, because there are no references to it in his Epistolary, but perhaps this never happened. Involved with the mission to Egypt and troubled by the painful problems of the royal family, perhaps he willingly abstained from writing. In particular, his urging in every way the nomination to abbot of Saint Graziano of Arona makes us think that he might have wanted to have an excuse to get away for a certain period and to return to his country, with some proof of the prestige he had obtained.

We cannot think that the solicitations of the Italian ambassadors and of Leo X were sufficient to make him resume the interrupted work. Once the historical situation changed, he was hoping that young Charles, aware of the tasks that were his as sovereign, would have brought back to the New Lands the authority of law and justice.

The problem of the validity of the *Decades of the New World* as a source for the history of the discoveries and the conquest was discussed extensively from the very first publication of the work, in that it was often adduced as evidence in disputes between the heirs of the discoverers or of the conquerors. Some have advanced reservations on the basis of the not always objective judgements of the first reporters of America, near contemporaries of the writer, for whom Peter Martyr, not knowing the New World, could not offer an accurate picture of the events. According to this view we should reject a good part of the historical writing of the 1500s and accept as valid only the reports of the protagonists; many of them edited their writings, even falsifying or concealing facts in order to evidence their worth and denounce the deceits and misdeeds of their adversaries.

Even if in the writings of Peter Martyr there are faulty details that arise from a certain taste for the marvelous, one can also see evidence of a searching soul, a critical capacity, a deep knowledge of men and things. Sometimes he seems to indulge in astrological interpretations of natural phenomena, but he always doubts fantasies, claiming that he deals with news received from others and reporting it as such.

He is most attentive to the phases of the developing geographical knowledge about the New Lands, the stages of the conquest, the unhappy condition of previously free people forced into slavery. More as chronicler than as historian, he gathers witnesses of distant events from sources not always written, impartial and documented, trying to capture the dynamics of events from comparison between written and oral accounts. Decades II-VII in particular are rich in precise details, since from 1513 the writer again held an important assignment in the Royal Council.

As much as he wants to be objective, he sometimes lets himself be swayed by affection and admiration for the characters who respond to his humanistic ideals, like Columbus or Hernán Cortés, whom he admires for his geniality and great courage as well as his political ability.

He understands the importance of Columbus's discovery, and realizes that a new continent was forcefully changing the opinion that people had about the shape of the Earth. The term *orbis novus* that he had introduced in 1493 puts him, at least on a theoretical level, in opposition to the Discoverer, but he never enters into controversy with him; rather, he tries to justify his thesis with the support of scholarship, always mentioning his reservations. Many times his contacts with Columbus are mentioned. At least until Columbus's departure for the third voyage, Martyr never criticizes the skill of the navigator, even if at times he does not accept his geographic, astronomical and cosmographical considerations.

It is interesting to note that for *Decade* I 1, Peter Martyr profited especially from what he had directly learned from the Navigator and from his companions' description of the adventure, since the Admiral's journal was a text that had to remain secret, especially because it contained precise nautical references. Also for *Decade* I 2, he certainly made use of letters addressed directly to him personally by Columbus and of the report of Antonio Torres and his companions.

However, the references to geographical positions in the ocean reveal themselves to be completely useless, not because the author is imprecise but because political considerations require him to keep information vague, even if news of the discovery is divulged for reasons of prestige. In the background of the undertaking which, in any case would become well known among mariners, there was a high ideal (which should have been welcomed by all of Europe and which, so to speak, minimized the motive of competition with the Portuguese for the spice trade), that is, the diffusion of the Christian faith among new people, following the conquest of Granada.

There is no doubt that from the beginning Spaniards realized the exceptional importance of the discovery and the necessity to affirm the preeminence of Spain over other powers.

It seems useful, therefore, in this study which prefaces texts and translations of parts of the Decades (I 1-7; III 4) concerning the discovery and voyages of Columbus, to better emphasize those passages that offer, beyond more or less exact data, the possibility of singling out the most significant episodes, the profiles of the protagonists, the importance of certain events, and finally the effects of the information he gathered on him as a humanist, a politician, a clergyman, a person of great learning, but, as also in the case of his contemporaries, a heir of classical and medieval knowledge.

In *Decade* I, responding to the wish of his friend Ascanio Sforza, he sends news about the discoveries and their participants, giving information in a meager and imprecise manner about the preliminaries of the undertaking (information perhaps dimmed by the greatness of the event itself). Instead he elaborates on the description of the Canaries, which he considered to be still a little unknown, and especially on the events of the voyage, providing news not documented by other texts. He does not fail to underline the resentment of the sailors toward a foreign captain, but also their subsequent awareness that Columbus is the only one in a position to bring them back; even those who have no more faith in the success of the expedition realize that the only possibility of salvation consists in trusting Columbus's ability.

Particularly interesting is Peter Martyr's information about the cannibals and about the food of the natives, especially corn. The statement that this grain was abundant in Lombardy and in the fields of Granada cannot be accepted. Thorough studies have revealed that the plant originated in Central America. For that reason we believe that Peter Martyr in all probability confused corn with the *coix lacrima jobi*, that has black kernels, brought to Europe by the Turks, and used for rosary beads and, during periods of famine, for making bread, when wheat was lacking. (Corn instead has white, red, orange, blue, gray, or black kernels). The description of parrots found in those islands offers an opportunity to discuss whether the discovered islands belonged to India, because of characteristics similar to those of the Indian soil. Although the ancients acknowledged the proximity of Spain to India Peter Martyr seems to realize that they are New Lands.

Reporting then on the return of Columbus to Spain and on the honors bestowed upon him, he also alludes to the nomination as *Adelantado* of Columbus's brother Bartholomew a man who revealed himself to have great military and political ability but whose nomination was one of the causes of the resentment the Spaniards had toward the Navigator.

In *Decade* 12, on the basis of the report by Torres and of the information obtained from other crew members, he reports particulars about the cannibals' huts, the human remains found in them, the women of the island of *Madanino* who have customs similar to those of the Amazons, the encounter between the Spaniards and the canoe of the queen of the cannibals who was captured and sent to Spain where the writer confirms to have seen her in Medina. He narrates with many particulars the episode regarding the slaughter of the thirty-eight men (or thirty-nine, according to other sources) left by Columbus on the island of Hispaniola. Peter Martyr points out the approach of the Admiral, who, in order not to provoke the natives with an immediate punishment of the responsible Guacanagarí, instead accuses another cacique, Caonabó, and represses his personal resentment and does not allow himself to get involved through the impulsiveness of his comrades.

These two books of the first *Decade* are full of the spirit of adventure and of the discovery of an unexpected reality: not everything is always positive, but the negative facts seem more the consequence of fear of the unknown (the murmurs and the threats of the crew against Columbus in the first voyage, the emotional reaction of the first encounter between the native populations and the Spaniards). Although the books are full of details, they reflect just the same the spirit of the letters written during the years 1493-1494, the spirit of the humanist moved by the emotions of Columbus, who sees his plans realized.

In the subsequent books one notices a more detached tone suited to a work of history, with a clear separation between the account of the facts and the description of natural elements, customs, and beliefs of a new people, without an attempt to provide, as he does in the letters, the correct location of the New Lands.

From the preface to *Decade* I, dedicated to Cardinal Ludovico di Aragona, in which Peter Martyr remembers having suspended the drafting of the work after the misfortunes of Ascanio Sforza and having resumed it upon the exhortation of the King of Naples, Federico, one can deduce that Columbus kept track of what was happening in the New World, and that the writer might have had free access to that information. In this book the island of Hispaniola is described and geographically located; the writer pauses with pleasure to describe the fertility of the land and the abundance of gold found in the sand of the rivers which is only appreciated by the natives if it is artistically worked. There is also a brief mention of the conflict with the Portuguese, of Alexander VI's papal bull, and of the treaty of Tordesillas in 1494 concerning the division of the ocean. Once again arises the problem of identifying the New Lands with those that were thought by scholars to be East of the Ganges in India. On this point Peter Martyr continues to have some reservations, but again avoids controversy with Columbus; in the later books he will report that once the Admiral found the new continent he thought that it was not the true India "of the Ganges," but a new land, almost an appendix of it, and that on the fourth voyage he would try to find a passage to Asia.

The hospitality of the natives toward the Spaniards is then an object of attention: they cheerfully accept that their roasted fish be eaten but the snakes (or better, the iguanas erroneously believed to be serpents) ignored, although their exquisiteness will be appreciated later. Then, fishing in deadwater is described, and the episode of the archer who met with men dressed in white, and the tale of the very old man who addresses Columbus with a very impressive speech on the necessity of acting well to assure oneself a happy fate after death. This encounter closes the book with a mythical vision of the golden age.

The topics of *Decade* 14 are mostly the maneuvers against the two Columbus brothers. Pedro Margarit and Father Boyl return to Spain with the intention of stirring up serious accusations against them. Bartlomew Columbus had tried to maintain discipline among the men who, instead of devoting themselves to work, were giving themselves to abusing their power over the native population, provoking reaction and revenge from them. As Peter Martyr specifies, the men who left with the second expedition were, for the most part, adventurers, desirous of becoming wealthy without work; their behavior pushed the natives to rebel and to try to drive them away, for they resorted to burning their lands, a practice which backfired with considerable damage for them. According to Peter Martyr, the unsown fields, destroyed harvest, and shortage of food caused more than fifty thousand deaths. After losing a battle to the Europeans, Caonabó and his subjects were forced to come to terms, or, in other words, to make tribute in gold, provisions, spices and other products, depending on the resources and provided that Admiral's men not wander in their lands without authorization. Peter Martyr describes the natives as lovers of their freedom; he dresses in grandeur, so to speak, the strongest opponent to the Spaniards, Caonabó, but he also shows the natives to be aware of the impossibility of sending the foreigners away and ready to give tributes in order to guarantee their lives and dignity. These pages implicitly defend the behavior of Columbus and his brother against insubordinate and savage men, and they exalted the person of Alonso de Hojeda, a bold, knowledgeable companion during the second voyage, a person always faithful to the Admiral.

Decade 15 constitutes an extensive report on the activity of Bartholomew Columbus in Hispaniola. It is also rich in details that seem to have been obtained from a particular text, perhaps from the memoirs of the *Adelantado* himself about the customs and the food of the natives and about the painful events that followed the departure of the Admiral.

The natives appear to be struck by the superiority of the Spaniards and they wish to make friends with this advanced people, favoring a peaceful assimilation. They suppress the attempts at rebellion provoked by the violence of Roldán, in whose presence Bartholomew, having pledged to maintain an attitude worthy of restraint suited to his position, finds himself almost a prisoner waiting for the arrival of his brother. Peter Martyr lets us understand that it was not the discontent of the sailors, somewhat justifiable because of their fear of the unknown, which seems to prolong itself too much, but the revolt of violent men, far away from every control of the sovereign power, free from every bond of obedience, keen to upset and compromise a situation already difficult on its own.

In *Decade* I 6 the events of the third voyage of Columbus are narrated, from the departure from Spain to the arrival at the island of Hispaniola. The encounter with twenty-four young men of neat appearance and white complexion travelling in a canoe is described. Peter Martyr reports the particular that Columbus gives assurance that he never went off the parallel of Ethiopia and that, therefore, the physical difference from the Ethiopians must not be attributed to the climate, given the same latitude, but rather to the diverse nature of the soils.

A detail that reveals itself as important is the statement of Columbus who relates the fear he felt before arriving to the *Boca del Dragon* in front of a water spout: "from which point he began to navigate as a child; in no place had he been so afraid."

Here therefore, is a detail particularly revealing of the first years of the Discoverer. The son of Domenico, a miller, he did not always remain in his father's shop, but took advantage of all the opportunities that presented themselves, and he sailed several times. We can suppose that these first voyages "as a child" were probably made on small wooden vessels which engaged in trade between Genoa and Savona or pushed as far as the ports of Corsica and Sardinia (and let us not forget that one of the most difficult passages of navigation for sailboats in the Mediterranean is the Bocche di Bonifacio).

Naturally, of these navigations of the first years there has not remained any documentation since the young Christopher could have hardly been registered among the members of the crew. In the seventh chapter of the first volume of his *Christopher Columbus* Taviani recalls what was stated by Ferdinand Colombo (and which can be found repeated in the *Libro de las Profecías*) about the activity of his father when he was still very young, facts that are repeated and confirmed by Genoese historians.

In the passage mentioned here, though, there is something more: a recollection of all his own experiences of storms at sea, compared with the most recent one, and it is natural that those he faced in adolescence would occur to him because they were the first ones and, therefore, those which stay more engraved in his memory. Other items of interest are the opinions of Columbus on the duration of the day in those lands, and on the position of the polar star (a matter disputed by Peter Martyr who follows the opinions of the astronomers and does not want to discuss fantastic statements. The explanation that the discovered lands in this voyage are a continent and that they are not joined to Cuba, which was thought by many to be an island, deserves attention. There is the reference to the widespread desire to discredit Columbus, to discredit his views, but at the same time one notices in Peter Martyr the will to support his friend at least morally, if not on the scientific level, deferring to history every judgment on truth.

In the first part of *Decade* I 7, Peter Martyr reports to the Admiral and his brother on the serious situation created by the rebellion of Roldán and his men. Their accusations of violence, cruelty and disloyalty toward the Sovereigns were aimed at removing all authority and power from Columbus. Once more the policy of moderation shown toward the natives now exasperated by the oppression of Roldán, seems to bear fruit: the behavior of the two Columbus brothers, energetic but not ruthless, convinces the population to accept the new arrivals. With bitterness, then, Peter Martyr reports the capture of Columbus and his brother, who are stripped of their power and taken away in chains after the nomination of a new governor, Francisco de Bobadilla, who was sent by the Sovereigns to investigate the rebellion and to find out why such a scarce quantity of gold and local products were being brought back to Spain. The writer does not fail to point out the speed with which the decision of dismissal was carried out, a decision that could not have been an arbitrary initiative of the new governor; but being well acquainted with the context of the Court he knows that, in spite of the Sovereigns' ordering freedom for the two brothers, Columbus will not be reinstated in his privileged position. Peter Martyr is left with the consolation, typical of a man of learning, of hoping that history, at least on the moral level, will restore the truth.

In *Decade* III 4 Peter Martyr narrates the events of Columbus's fourth expedition. After sixteen years of silence, not even interrupted to give the important news of the death of the Discoverer (there is only one hint, in Decade II:... *Colono iam vita functo*), he feels the necessity to speak of it, even if it is in a harsh manner, which lets his disapproval be known for those who treated Columbus in a disrespectful manner. Described here are the departure from Spain and the encounter with a canoe of a rich merchant, loaded with various objects, but especially with cotton blankets woven in different colors, with a richness of particulars that emphasize the developed conditions of that people. During this voyage his brother Christopher is accompanied by Bartholomew the *Adelantado*, a title he had in the previous expeditions. One can suppose that even if the exercise of power had been taken away from him, the title would not have been revoked (indeed, the children of Columbus themselves continued in court as pages even when the opposition against the Admiral reached its pitch). The natives are not surprised at their arrival, and they introduce themselves as friends; but they are not ready to tolerate the Spaniards' staying in their territories, and they force them to abandon Hispaniola and to move to Jamaica.

In this island the already uncertain health of the Admiral grows worse, although thanks to the intervention of Diego Mendez he is able to return after ten months of privation to Hispaniola. Peter Martyr interrupts his account of the events concerning Columbus with this information, preferring even in the following years to ignore facts known from other sources, but he continues the narrative, describing the coast of the mainland explored by the Admiral during the fourth voyage and expounding on the geographical facts (longitude and latitude) of the region of Veragua.

We wonder in all this about Peter Martyr's silence concerning the events and the attitude of the Spaniards toward a man who had accomplished such a great undertaking, but we must consider that no one would have been interested in defending his position. Even if most of the privileges granted to him by the Capitulations of Santa Fe institutionally already belonged to the *Almirante de Castilla*, the immense size of the land and riches acquired by Spain had made the negotiated agreements unacceptable to the Crown.

Besides, because of their policy of respect for the native people and peaceful penetration, Christopher and Bartholomew had sometimes intervened against the Spaniards who had abused power and commited crimes in the New Lands, and, behaving in such a manner, foreigners that they were, they had offended Spanish pride. These considerations could not have been reported by Peter Martyr, and his not having done so certainly does not diminish the historical value of his work. Tied to the Court of Spain, he could not defame people who had become powerful, especially the Crown, which seemed to have betrayed and abandoned in misery that man who had been the progenitor of its power and the one he considered the greatest man of his time. His scruple and his accuracy in description, and his wealth of information seem to diminish somewhat just as he is narrating the activities involving Columbus, the real hero of those events, thus revealing, according to some, a respect for power and a preoccupation with his own interests. However, it is necessary to keep in mind the time in which he lived: the Inquisition went so far as to accuse a man of great learning and exemplary life like Hernando de Talavera, confessor of the Queen and archbishop of Granada of having little zeal in defending the values of faith, and it was at a time in which the Catholic Sovereigns and the very Christian King of France, Francis I, slaughtered people for their ambitions in Europe and in the New World, a time finally in which books were printed only with royal permission and numerous works about the New World remained in manuscript form for centuries because the authorities did not want them to be known.

APPENDICES

edited by

ELISA MAGIONCALDA and ROSANNA MAZZACANE

Note: The appendices concern annotations critical to the text, formulated with the following criteria: the numerical references refer to the page and line of the Latin text; the first reading is the one marked with the symbol of the initial or initials corresponding to the collected texts, followed by others; the abbreviations *corr., coni, om*, correspond to "correxi," "conieci," "omisit" and indicate emendation of the text. In particular, in Appendix II, before the square parenthesis, the reading accepted in the text is given, and, after the parenthesis, the equivalent from the Seville edition of 1511.

Collated Editions (identified by full title):

C = *Opus epistolarum* PETRI MARTYRIS ANGLERII Mediolanensis Protonotarii Apostolici atque a consiliis rerum Indicarum: nunc primum et natum et mediocri cura excusum quod quidem praeter stili venustatem nostrorum quoque temporum historiae loco esse poterit. Compluti Anno Domini .M.D.XXX. cum privilegio Caesareo. Colof.: Excusum est hoc volumen Epistolarum Petri Martyris Mediolanensis citra controversiam eruditissimi in celeberrima et in omni literarum genere maxime florenti. Academia Complutensi in aedibus Michaelis de Eguia anno a Christo nato M.D.XXX. (rist. an. Graz 1966 = *G*).

A = *Opus epistolarum* PETRI MARTYRIS ANGLERII Mediolanensis Protonotarii Apostolici, Prioris Archiepiscopatus Granatensis atque a Consiliis Rerum Indicarum Hispanicis, tanta cura excusum, ut praeter styli venustatem quoque fungi possit vice Luminis Historiae superiorum temporum. Cui accesserunt Epistolae Fer!dinandi de Pulgar. Editio postrema. Amstelodami, apud Danielem Elzevirium M.DC.XX.

H = PETRI MARTYRIS Angli Mediolanensis *Opera. Legatio Babylonica. Oceani Decas. Poemata. Epigrammata.* Cum privilegio. Impressum Hispali cum summa diligencia per Jacobum Corumberger Alemanum, anno millesimo quingentesimo XI, mense vero aprili, in folio.

C¹ = *De Orbe Novo Decades.* Cura et diligentia Antonii Nebrissensis fuerunt hae tres protonotari PETRI MARTYRIS decades impressae in contubernis Arnaldi Guillelmi in illustri oppido Carpetaneae provinciae, Compluto quod vulgariter dicitur Alca. Factum est nonis novembris, anno 1516, in folio.

C² = *De Orbe Novo* PETRI MARTYRIS ab Angleria Mediolanensis protonotarii Caesaris senatoris *Decades.* Cum privilegio imperiali. Compluti, apud MICHAELEM DE EGUÍA, anno .M.D.XXX., in folio (rist. an. Graz 1966 = *G*).

B = PETRI MARTYRIS ab Angleria Mediolanen. oratoris clarissimi, Fernandi et Helisabeth Hispaniarum quondam regum a consiliis, *de rebus Oceanicis* et *Orbe Novo Decades* tres: quinbus quicquid de inventis nuper terris traditum, novarum rerum cupidum lectorem retinere possit, copiose, fideliter, eruditeque dcetur. Eiusdem praeterea *Legationis Babylonicae* libri tres: ubi praeter oratorii muneris pulcherrimum exemplum, etiam quicquid in variarum gentium moribus et institutis insigniter praeclarum vidit, quaeque terra marique acciderunt, omnia lectu mire iucunda, genere dicendi politissimo traduntur, Basileae qpud Ioannem Bebelium. M.D.XXXIII.

P = *De Orbe Novo* PETRI MARTYRIS ANGLERII Mediolanensis, Protonotarii, et Caroli quinti senatoris *Decades* octo, diligenti temporum observatione, et utilissimis annotationibus illustratae, suoque nitori restitutae, labore et industria RICHARDI HAKLUYTI Oxoniensis Angli. Additus est in usum lectoris accuratus totius operis index, Parisiis, apud Guillelmum Auvray, via D. Ioannis Bellovacensis, sub insigni Bellerophontis coronati. M.D.LXXXVII. Cum privilegio Regis.

ms. = *ms. Barb. Lat.* 2117.

450

Appendix I: Critical Notes to the *Opus epistolarum*

ep. 131 C = 130 *A* = 129 *ms.* (pp. 34, 36)

4 exolveret *C ms.*: exsolveret *A*/5 Iudaeis *C A*: Iudeis *ms.*/7 religiosissimi *A*: religiossimi *C ms.*/9 extructum *C A*: estructum *ms.* /12 provinciam* *A*: provintiam *C ms.*/19 haec *A ms.*: hec *C*/fervent *C A*: ferbent *ms.*/22 Britanniae *A*: Britaniae *C ms.*/23 irruperunt *C A*: irrumperunt *ms.*/24 quaeritant *A ms.*: queritant *C*/genitrix *C ms.*: genetrix *A*/26 misera *C A*: missera *ms.*/27 praedam* *A ms.*: predam *C*/ilia in *C A*: illiam *ms.*/28 sustinete *CA*: substinete *ms.* infoelices* *C*: infelices *A ms.*/30 comitatum *C A*: commitatum *ms.*/31 caeteri* *A*: coeteri *C ms.*/32 arbitror *A*: arbitror *C ms.*/34 miserae *A*: misere *C ms.*/37 prospectus *A*: porspectus *C ms.*/38 Cleofae *A*: Cleofe *C ms.*

ep. 134 *C* = 133 *A* = 132 *ms.* (pp. 36, 38)

1 Attollite *A*: Atollite *C ms.*/4 hemispherio* *corr.*: hemisperio *C ms.*, hemisphaerio *A*/4 quia *C ms.*: qua *A*/6 rediit *C A*: reddit *ms.*/8 gossampium* *corr.*: gosampium *A*, gosamium *C ms.*/10 milia* *C ms.*: millia *A*/11 milia**C*: *A ms.*/19 ages *corr.*: agies *C A ms.*/20 caetera* *A*: coetera *C ms.*/21 immensos lacertos *C ms.*: immensas lacertas *A*/22 noxios *C ms.*: noxias *A*/23 aemulatur* *A*: emulator *C ms.*/26 coeli *C ms.*: caeli *A*/28 amisit *A ms.*: amissit *C*/31 provinciae* *A*: provintiae *C ms.*

ep. 135 *C* = 134 *A* = 133 *ms.* (pp. 38, 40)

4 quattuor* *corr.*: quatuor *C A ms.*/8 quae *A*: que *C ms.*/14 miliaria* *corr.*: miliana *C ms.*, milliaria *A*/milia* *C ms.*: millia *A*/15 coelo *C ms.*: caelo *A*/18 aequore *A*: equore *C ms.*/20 gossampium* *corr.*: gosampium *C A ms.*/21 cinnami* *corr.*: cinami *C ms.*, cinamoni *A*/24 tulit *A*: tullit *C ms.*/30 parere *C A*: parare *ms.*/33 caetera* *A*: coetera *C ms.*/permittent *C A*: permitent *ms.*/34 Carolum *corr.*: Karolum *C A ms.*/Perpiniano *A ms.*: Perpeniano *C*

ep. 136 *C* = 135 *A* = 134 *ms.* (pp. 40, 42)

3 littus* *C A*: litus *ms.*/5 extra oceanum *C*: extra occeanum *A*, ex occeanum *ms.*/Indie *A*: Indie *C*, indiem *ms.*/9 praedicant *A*: predicant *C ms.*/11 aequinoctiali* *A*: aequinocciali *C ms.*/12 littora* *C ms.*: litora *A*/13 aemulatione* *A*: emulatione *C ms.* 14 caetera* *corr.*:

coetera *C A ms.*/15 Carolus *A*: Karolus *C ms.*/16 misit *C A*: missit *ms.*/Perpinianum *C A*: Perpilianum *ms.*/20 Ambasia *C A*: Ambassia *ms.*/21 provinciam* *A*: provint[iam *C ms.*/24 Carolo *A*: Karolo *C ms.*/27 Caesar *C A*: Caessar *ms.*/caeteri* *A ms.*: coeteri *C*/29 obcaecatis* *A*: obcecatis *C ms.*/31 coepit *C ms.*: cepit *A*/casuras *C A*: cassuras *ms.*/33 quom *C ms.*: quum *A*/36 Kalendis *corr.*: Kalendas *C ms.*, Calendas *A*

ep. 139 *C* = 138 *A* = 137 *ms.* (pp. 44, 46)

1 Alfonsi Cagnas *C A*: *om. ms.*/3 chirographum* *A*: chyrographum *C ms.*/4 Teve Ardales *corr.*: Teverdale *C A ms.*/5 siti *corr.*: site *C*, sitae *A ms.*/6 praestimonialibus *C A*: praetimonialibus *ms.*/10 querellae *C ms.*: querelae *A*/12 vigesimum *A*: vigessimum *C ms.*/15 premebatur* *A*: praemebatur *C ms.*/18 supraemam *C ms.*: supremam *A*/22 caeteri* *A*: coeteri *C ms.*/23 sacculo *C A*: saculo *ms.*/25 dicit vulgus *C ms.*: vulgus dicit *A*/29 aequum* *A*: equum *C ms.*/viderint *ms.*: videritu *C*, videritis *A*/30 querella *C ms.*: querela *A*/precio* *A*: praecio *C ms.*/33 architalassus *C ms.*: archithalassus *A*/34 admiraldum *C A*: almiraldum *ms.*/37 generis *A*; ganeris *C ms.*/39 Kalendas *C ms.*: Calendas *A*

ep. 141 *C* = 140 *A* = 139 *ms.* (p. 46)

2 huiuscemodi *A*: huiusce *C ms.*/5 maris *C A*: mari *ms.*/7 supraemum *C ms.*: supremum *A*/7 benivolentiae *A ms.*: benivolentie *C*/11 referri *A ms.*: refferri *C*/13 propiores *A*: propriores *C ms.*/14 Valdoleto *corr.*: Valleoleti *C ms.*, Valleoleto *A*/Kalendas *C ms.*: Calendas *A*

ep. 143 *C* = 142 *A* = 141 *ms.* (pp. 48, 50)

1 nonagesimi *A*: nonnagessimi *C ms.*/quadringentesimo *A*: quadringentessimo *C ms.*/2 millesimum *A*: millessimum *C ms.*/benignissime *A*: benegnissime *C ms*/4 Rosilionis *C A*: Rossilionis *ms.*/9 quo *A*: qui *C ms.*/11 vigesimus *A*: vigesssimus *C ms.*/12 ad veteres *C A*: adverteres *ms.*/15 tunc *C A*: ut *ms.*/18 provinciam* *A*: provintiam *C ms.*/19 Alfonsus *C A*: Alphonsus *ms.*/23 impraesentiarum *A*: impresentiarum *C.*, impraessentiarum *ms.*/24 hymeneos *C ms.*: hymenaeos *A*/26 despondent *C A*: respondent *ms.*/30 superficie* *A*: superfitie *C ms.*/32 Chersonesum *C A*: Chersonessum *ms.*/33 quattuor* *C*: quatuor *A ms.*/37 perscribere *C A*: prescribere *ms.*/38 praetermittan *C A*: praetermitam *ms.*/40 aggredientibus *A*: agredientibus *C ms.*/41 Kalendas *C ms.*: Calendas *A*

ep. 145 *C* = 144 *A* = 143 *ms.* (pp. 50, 52)

7 antequam *C A*: anteque *ms.*/detractaverit *C ms.*: detrectaverit *A*/10 Gonsalo *A*: Goncalo *C ms.*/12 Emanuelem *C ms.*: Emmanuelem *A*/13 provinciam* *A*: provintiam *C ms.*/17 expectare *C ms.*: exspectare *A*/20 conclusum *C A*: conclussum *ms.*/22 dedentque *C ms.*: dentque *A*/23 ex *A*: et *C ms.*/quattuor* *C A*: quatuor *ms.*/24 hemispherii* *corr.*: hemisperii *C ms.*, hemisphaerii *A*/25 Praefectus *A ms.*: Prefectus *C*/28 caeteraque* *A*:

coeteraque *C ms.*/littora* *C ms.*: litora *A*/29 remisit *C A*: remissit *ms.*/31 Methymnae*
A: Methymne *C ms.*/33 perniciem *A*: pernitiem *C ms.*/36 Kalendas *C ms.*: Calendas *A*

ep. 147 *C* = 146 *A* = 145 *ms.* (pp. 52, 54, 56)

2 tanquam *C A*: nunquam *ms.*/4 rerum *C ms.*: veram *A*/6 dissidiis *A*: disidiis
C ms./7 perniciem *A*: pernitiem *C ms.*/8 hac *corr.*: ac *C A ms.*/9 tyrannus *A*: tiranus
C ms./11 dammas *corr.*: damas *C A ms.*/molossos *A ms.*: molosos *C*/13 maiorum ad
libertatem C: ad libertatem maiorum *A ms.*/15 caeci* *A*: ceci *C ms.*/18 prostrent *C ms.*:
prosternant *A*/20 Pampilonensi *C ms.*: Pamplonensi *A*/22 occidente *A ms.*: occidete
C/hemispherio* *corr.*: hemisperio *C ms.*, hemisphaerio *A*/28 tellurem *A*: tellurrem
C ms./29 silvas *C ms.*: sylvas *A*/gossampium* *corr.*: gosampium *C A ms.*/preciosa *C A*:
praeciosa *ms.*/30 caetera* *corr.*: coetera *C A ms.*/36 Poliphemos *C ms.*: Polyphemos
A/37 aristae *A*: ariste *C ms.*/40 ad meridiem *A*: ad me meridiem *C ms.*/41 Canibales
A: Caniballes *C ms.*/42 sunt *C A*: sun *ms.*/47 pinguioresque *A*: pingioresque *C ms.*/49
Canibales *A*: Caniballes *C ms.*/50 canibalium *A*: caniballium *C ms.*/51 sphericas *C ms.*:
sphaericas *A*/appensas *A ms.*: appenssas *C*/53 occisi *A*: occissi *C ms.*/aspersum *C ms.*:
adspersum *A*/54 psittacinis *A*: psitacinis *C ms.*/56 canibalicam *C ms.*: cannibalicam
A/comitatam *A*: commitatam *C ms.*/57 apprehenderunt* *A*: appraehenderunt *C ms.*/59
comedendas *A*: commendendas *C ms.*/63 commercio* *A*: comertio *C ms.*/66 Emanuelem
C ms.: Emmanuelem *A*/69 Portugaliae *A*: Portugalicae *C ms.*/72 Emanuel *C ms.*:
Emmanuel *A*/76 procellosas *C A*: procellossas *ms.*

ep. 153 *C* = 152 *A* = 151 *ms.* (pp. 58, 60)

2 literas *C A*: litteras *ms.*/3 Pomponi *C A*: Pomponii *ms.*/6 prestari *C ms.*: praestari
A/7 facio: *A* fatio *C ms.*/9 aliquos *A*: alliquos *C ms.*/provincia* *C A*: provintia *ms.*/18
praefectus *A*: prefectus *C ms.*/20 provincia* *corr.*: provinciam *C A ms.*/21 quom *C ms.*:
quum *A*/25 Caunaboam *corr.*: Cannaboam *C A ms.*/28 de *C A*: om. *ms.*/Caunaboa
corr.: Cannaboa *C A ms.*/30 satius *A*: santius *C ms.*/34 reperiendorum *corr.*: reperien-
darum *C A ms.*/operum *C ms.*: plurium *A*/36 referunt *C A*: referant *ms.*/37 sementes
C A: sementes et *ms.*/43 tubarum *A*: turbarum *C ms.*/44 tonitruis *C ms.*: tonitrua *A*/46
coelo *C ms.*: caelo *A*/50 castaneae *C A*: castanneae *ms.*/51 aemulatur* *A*: emulatur
C ms./arcticum *A*: articum *C ms.*/53 sphericae *C ms.*: sphaericae *A*/59 Kalendas *C ms.*:
Calend. *A*

ep. 157 *C* = 156 *A* = 155 *ms.* (pp. 62, 64)

1 capacioribus *A*: capatioribus *C ms.*/9 decimum nonum *C ms.*: decem et novem
A/15 stellae *C A*: stele *ms.*/polaris *A*: pollaris *C ms.*/17 preciosis *A*: praeciosis
C ms./19 tritico *C ms.*: triticeo *A*/26 ad iter illas *C ms.*: iter ad illas *A*/30 cucurbitae
A: cucurbite *C ms.*/31 trigesimum *C A*: trigessimum *ms.*/32 lactucae *A*: latuce
C ms./rafani *C ms.*: raphani *A*/caeteraque* *A*: coeteraque *C ms.*/34 saccarum* *A*:
sacarum *C ms.*/36 in *C A*: om. *ms.*/37 gossampinis* *corr.*: gosampinis *C A ms.*/38
sphericas* *C ms.*: sphaericas *A*/40 herbarum* *corr.*: haerbarum *C A ms.*/41 aemulentur*

corr.: emulentur *C ms.*, aemulenter *A*/43 gossampinis* *corr.*: gosampinis *C A ms.*/45 gossampio * *corr.*: gosampio *C A ms.*/tenacioribus *A*: tenatioribus *C ms.*/48 Ianuarii *corr.*: Ianuarius *C ms.*, Ianuarias *A*

ep. 159 *C* = 158 *A* = 157 *ms.* (pp. 64, 66)

5 aequo* *A*: equo *C ms.*/10 colebat *C A*: collebat *ms.*/11 ordo *A*: hordo C, horda *ms.*/12 viciam *A*: vitiam C, vitam *ms.*/13 expectas *C ms.*: expectes *A*/aequum* *A*: equum *C ms.*/14 Helisabetha *C A*: Helissabetha *ms.*/15 haerede *A*: herede *C ms.*/19 astringemur *C ms.*: adstringemur *A*/25 praetermitto *A*: praetermito *C ms.*/26 milia* *C A*: millia *ms.*/27 coenae* *C ms.*: caenae *A*/29 Kalendas *C ms.*: Calendas *A*/M.CCCC.XCV *A*: M.CCCC.XCVIII *C ms.*

ep. 161 *C* = 160 *A* = 159 *ms.* (pp. 66, 68)

2 visum *C A*: vissum *ms.*/3 scilicet *A*: silicet *C ms.*/6 gratulabimar *C A*: gratulamur *ms.*/eundem *A ms.*: eundem *C*/servaveris *C A*: serbaberis *ms.*/13 Laetum *A*: Letum *C ms.*/14 Pampilonensemque *C ms.*: Pampelonensemque *A*/22 caetera* *corr.*: coetera *C A ms.*/23 velim *C A*: vellim *ms.*/25 hemispherii* *corr.*: hemisphaerii *A*: hemisperii *C ms.*/28 caeteris* *A*: coeteris *C ms.*/30 mense *C A*: mensse *ms.*/31 Castella *A*: Castellam *C ms.*/32 Ximenez *C ms.*: Ximenes *A*/33 confessorem *C ms.*: vocat confessorem *A*/39 saevientis *A*: sevientis *C ms.*/47 provincia* *A*: provintia *C ms.*/48 Caesareaugusta *C ms.*: Caesar Augusta *A*

ep. 165 *C* = 164 *A* = 163 *ms.* (pp. 70, 72)

1 ad *A*: om. *C ms.*/2 Laetum *A*: Letum *C ms.*/Pampilonensem *C ms.*: Pompelonensem *A*/5 quae *A*: que *C ms.*/6 littora* *C ms.*: litora *A*/7 Ophiram *corr.*: Offiram *C A ms.*/8 provinciam* *A*: provintiam *C ms.*/10 milia* *C ms.*: millia *A*/passuum *A ms.*: passum *C*/11 incolae *A* ms: incole *C*/terrae *A ms.*: terre *C*/13 littora* *C ms.*: litora *A*/14 nuncios* *A*: nuntios *C ms.*/15 littora* *C ms.*: litora *A*/16 terrae *A*: terre *C ms.*/17 aequinoctio* *A*: equinoctio *C ms.*/laeva *A*: leva *C ms.*/narrabat *A*: narrat ab *C ms.*/18 magnae *A*: magne *C ms.*/19 plaeraque* *C ms.*: pleraque *A*/20 plaerisque* *C ms.*: plerisque *A*/21 ulla coni.: nulla *C ms.*, multa *A*/conchilia *C*: conchylia *A*, conchillia *ms.*/25 coenosaque *A*: cenosaque *C*, coenossa *ms.*/alia *C A*: alioque *ms.*/31 hemispherium* *corr.*: hemisperium *C ms.*, hemisphaerium *A*/34 Arisoteles *A*: Aristotiles *C ms.*/35 coelo *C ms.*: caelo *A*/36 littoribus* *C A*: lictoribus *ms.*/41 interpretes* *A*: interpraetes *C ms.*/49 Tortosiae *corr.*: Tortosie *C ms.*, Tertosiae *A*

ep. 169 *C* = 168 *A* = 167 *ms.* (pp. 72, 74, 76)

1 fasciculo *A*: facisculo *C ms.*/3 impraesentiarum *A*: in praesentiarum *C*, in praessentiarum *ms.*/6 plaeraque* *C ms.*: pleraque *A*/7 adhaerentes *A*: adherentes *C ms.*/Indiae *A*: Indie *C ms.*/8 continens *C A*: contines *ms.*/11 conchilium *C ms.*: conchylium *A*/12

454

plaerisque* *C ms.*: plerisque *A*/13 gossampinis* *corr.*: gosampinis *C A ms.*/15 caeterum* *A*: coeterum *C ms.*/21 tintinnabulis *A*: tintinabulis *C ms.*/24 si *C ms.*: si nostri *A*/33 comitia *A ms.*: commitia *C*/34 Matthaeo *A*: Mattheo *C ms.*/36 dissovunt *A*: disolvunt *C ms.*/39 reginae *A ms.*: regine *C*/45 oceanum *A*: occeanum *C ms.*/portuosum *C A*: portuossum *ms.*/missura *A*: misura *C ms.*/47 classis *C A*: clasis *ms.*/49 aliae *A*: alie *C ms.*/caveatae *A*: caveatae *C ms.*/50 milia* *C A* millia *ms.*/littora* *C ms.*: litora *A*/52 tandem *C A*: tamen *ms.*/54 collachrymata *A ms.*: collachrimata *C*/visuram *C A*: vissuram *ms.*

ep. 177 *C* = 177 *A* = 176 *ms.* (pp. 76, 78)

3 coelestium *C ms.*: caelestium *A*/6 coeli *C ms.*: caeli *A*/8 Ramonus *corr.*: Remonus *C A ms.*/13 precio* *corr.*: praecio *C ms.*, pretio *A*/19 auricalco *C ms.*: aurichalco *A*/21 formosa *C A*: formosia *ms.*/22 visam *A*: visani *C ms.*/24 praetermitto *A ms.*: pretermitto *C*/27 Methymnae* *corr.*: Methinnae *C A ms.*

ep. 180 *C* = 180 *A* = 179 *ms.* (pp. 78, 80)

2 assequutus* *corr.*: assecutus *C A ms.*/3 rithmos *C ms.*: rhythmos *A*/5 praegnantes *A*: pregnantes *C ms.*/6 suaemet *ms.*: suemet *C*, suimet *A*/frater *C A*: fratrer *ms.*/10 haec *A ms.*: hec *C*/14 inclusit *C A*: inclussit *ms.*/15 mirabolano *C ms.*: myrobalano *A*/16 affixam *C A*: afixam *ms.*/17 aperuisse *A*: apperuisse *C ms.*/18 aequorea *A*: equorea *C ms.*/19 balenarum *C ms.*: balaenarum *A*/20 semina *C A*: saemina *ms.*/23 deprompsisse *C A*: depronsisse *ms.*/aperirent *A*: apperirent *C ms.*/25 te *C ms.*: te fluctus *A*/obruant *A*: obrruant *C ms.*/29 ortum *A*: hortum *C ms.*/30 divisam *C ms*: divissam *ms.*/31 patriam *C A*: patria *ms.*/34 Methymnae* *A*: Methinnae *C ms.*/Kalendas *C ms.*: Calendas *A*

ep. 181 *C* = 181 *A* = 180 *ms.* (pp. 80, 82, 84)

1 aequa* *A*: equa *C ms.*/2 Carvaiali *corr.*: Carvaialli *C ms.*, Caravaialli *A*/forte *C A*: sorte *ms.*/7 caeterisque* *A*: coeterisque *C ms.*/9 scrutati *C A*: scruptati *ms.*/10 ultra *C A*: intra *ms.*/11 antarcticum *A*: antarticum *C ms.*/quam *C ms.*: quamque *A*/arctico *A*: artico *C ms.*15/superarunt *C A*: supperarunt *ms.*/16 littora* *C ms.*: litora *A*/19 peritissimis *C A*: peritissimum *ms.*/directi *C A*: directum *ms.*/20 sirtes *C ms.*: syrtes *A*/vadosas *A*: vadossas *C ms.*/21 laevam *A*: levam *C ms.*/23 Callecutum *corr.*: Callequutum *C A ms.*/25 Callecutus *corr.*: Callequutus *C A*, Callequtus *ms.*/lapideis *A*: lapideiis *C ms.*/26 grandius *C A*: gradius *ms.*/27 Egipto *C ms.*: Aegypto *A*/28 Siria *C ms.*: Syria *A*/30 laeti *A*: leti *C ms.*/tantae *A ms*: tante *C*/32 commercia* *A*: comertia *C ms.*/33 amicitiam *A*: amiciciam *C ms.*/35 commercio* *A*: commertio *C ms.*/36 Callecuteum *corr.*: Callequuteum *C A ms.*/37 exorto *C A*: exolto *ms.*/39 penitus *A*: poenitus *C ms.*/40 plaerasque* *C A*: plerasque *ms.*/42 caeteraque *A*: coeteraque *C ms.*/44 nolis *A*: nollis *C ms.*/45 prestare *C ms.*: praestare *A*/48 nos his *C A*: his nos *ms.*/50 atque *C A*: nanque *ms.*/51 antarcticos *C ms.*: antarticos *A*/52 sollicitudinibus *corr.*: solicitudinibus *C A ms.*/53 praebeamus *A ms.*: prebeamus *C*/54 Methymnae* *corr.*: Metinnae *C A ms.*/Kalendis *corr.*: Kalendas *C ms.*, Calendas *A*

ep. 185 *C* = 185 *A* = 184 *ms.* (pp. 84, 86)

2 immo *A*: ymmo *C ms.*/3 iudicio *A*: iuditio *C ms.*/10 Emanuel *C ms.*: Emmanuel *A*/Portugaliae *A ms.*: Portugalliae *C*/internicie *A*: internitie *C*, intericie *ms.*/12 ubi *corr.*: ubi ubi *C A ms.*/13 caravelas *C A*: caravellas *ms.*/15 ostia *A*: hostia *C ms.*/16 exuperant *C ms.*: exsuperant *A*/Callecutum *C ms.*: Calecutum *A*/17 Cochini *corr.*: Cocini *C A ms.*/littoribus* *C ms.*: litoribus *A*/21 Cochini *corr.*: Cocini *C A ms.*/plaerasque* *corr.*: plerasque *C A ms.*/23 apparant *C A*: apparat *ms.*/24 Portugallicam *corr.*: Portugalicam *C A ms.*/25 penitus *A*: poenitus *C ms.*/28 Callecutea *C ms.*: Calecutea *A*/29 Portugallicis *corr.*: Portugalicis *C A ms.*/30 Callecutei *C ms.*: Calecutei *A*/33 plaeraque* *C A*: pleraque *ms.*/36 indidere *C ms.*: edidere *A*/37 Callecuteae *corr.*: Callucuteae *C ms.*, Calecuteae *A*/38 combussisse *A*: combusisse *C ms.*/Callecuteorum *corr.*: Callucuteorum *C ms.*, Calecuteorum *A*/43 arctici *A*: artici *C ms.*/46 assequuntur* *A*: assecuntur *C ms.*/48 quando *C ms.*: quoniam *A*/49 quando *C ms.*: quoniam *A*/quando *C*: quoniam *A ms.*

ep. 189 *C* = 189 *A* = 187 *ms.* (pp. 88, 89)

2 conquereris *A*: conquaereris *C ms.*/8 velis *C A*: velles *ms.*/illa *C ms.*: illi *A*/mensura *C A*: messura *ms.*/13 insedisse *A*: insidisse *C ms.*/14 archano *C ms.*: arcano *A*/16 quaerendarum *A*: querendarum *C ms.*/18 mirabolanos *C ms.*: myrabolanos *A*/19 plaerasque* *C ms.*: plerasque *A*/22 verterentur *C ms.*: reverterentur *A*/26 mamma mamma *corr.*: mama mama *C A ms.*/27 haereditariam* *A ms.*: hereditariam *C*/28 commercio* *A*: comertio *C ms.*/29 mirabolanos *C ms.*: myrobalanos *A*/aemulantia* *A*: emulantia *C ms.*/30 plaeraque* *C*: pleraque *A ms.*/33 femora *C ms.*: foemora *A*/35 foeminas *C A*: foemineas *ms.*/nefarium* *A*: nepharium *C ms.*/38 tantae *A ms.*: tante *C*/40 Matutae *A*: Matute *C ms.*/41 archanis *C ms.*: arcanis *A*/42 rithmos *C ms.*: rhythmos *A*/44 Kalendas *C ms.*: Calendas *A*/MCCCCXCVII *A ms.*: MCCCCCXCVII *C*

ep. 190 *C* = 190 *A* = 188 *ms.* (pp. 90, 92)

1 infoelici* *C ms.*: infelici *A*/3 rettulit *corr.*: retulit *C A ms.*/4 detrectaturum *C A*: detractaturum *ms.*/12 autoritate *C A*: authoritate *ms.*/13 ignominiam *A*: ignomiam *C ms.*/15 summam *A ms.*: sumam *C*/19 egre *C ms.*: aegre *A*/22 quae *C A*: quem *ms.*/26 gossampio* *corr.*: gosampio *C A ms.*/gossamipoque* *corr.*: gosampioque *C A ms.*/27 simulacra *C ms.*: simulachra *A*/29 simulacra *C ms.*: simulachra *A*/34 foeminas *A ms.*: feminas *C*/37 velitis *A*: vellitis *C ms.*/40 Nonis *corr.*: Nonas *C A ms.*

ep. 201 *C* = 202 *A* = 199 *ms.* (pp. 92, 94)

2 milia* *C*: millia *A ms.*/4 opinio *C A*: oppinio *ms.*/7 scintillanti *A*: scinitilanti *C ms.*/12 plaerisque* *C ms.*: plerisque *A*/16 gossampina* *corr.*: gosampina *C A ms.*/19 commercia* *A*: comertia *C ms.*/23 Babilonico *C ms.*: Babylonico *A*/25 ostiis *A*: hostiis *C ms.*/27 protendere *C ms.*: portendere *A*/28 aemulatur* *A*: emulatur *C ms.*

ep. 205 *C* = 206 *A* = 206 *ms.* (pp. 96, 98)

4 futurae *A*: future *C ms.*/ascribebant* *C ms.*: adscribebant *A*/5 floccifacere *A*: flocifacere *C ms.*/7 oceaneis *corr.*: occeanis *C A ms.*/14 Egiptios *C*: Aegyptios A, Egyptios *ms.*/15 Saporem *corr.*: Saborem *C A ms.*, Savorem *ms.*/19 huiuscemodi *C A*: huiusmodi *ms.*/22 eget *C ms.*: aeger *A*/23 hymno *A*: himno *C ms.*/33 emito *C A*: emitto *ms.*/precio* *corr.*: prescio *C*, pretio A, praescio *ms.*/assequutus* *corr.*: assecutus *C A ms.*

ep. 247 *C* = 248 *A* = 245 *ms.* (pp, 98, 100, 102) (in *C* there is a typographical error in the progressive numeration: 266)

1 literas *C A*: litteras *ms.*/2 genealogice *A*: geneologice *C ms.*/5 epigrammate *A*: epigramate *C ms.*/7 Madriti *corr.*: Matriti *C A ms.*/caeterique* *A*: coeterique *C ms.*/12 semilachrymans *A ms.*: semilacrimans *C*/nonnulli *A ms.*: nonulli *C*/13 tamen *A ms.*: tame *C*/17 satiata* *A*: saciata *C ms.*/21 plaeraque* *A*: pleraque *C ms.*/27 Elveteiis *C ms.*: Helvetiis *A*/29 saepe *A ms.*: sepe *C*/30 commercio* *A*: commertio *C ms.*/Elvetiorum *C ms.*: Helvetiorum *A*/32 milium* *C ms.*: millium *A*/35 eas *C ms.*: eius *A*/36 provincia* *A*: provintia *C ms.*/40 deuncialium *corr.*: doncialium *C A*, doncalium *ms.*/49 vicina *A*: vicinia *C ms.*/50 dulcium *A*: dultium *C ms.*/51 nullibi *corr.*: nullubi *C A ms.*/57 lassitudo *A*: lasitudo *C ms.*/58 caetera* *A*: coetera *C ms.*/61 sint *C ms.*: sunt *A*/aequum* *A*: equum *C ms.*

ep. 529 *C* = 532 *A* = 503 *ms.* (pp. 102, 104)

5 Cauhietum *A*: Cauchietum *C ms.*/7 praeterea *C A*: praepterea *ms.*/littora* *ms.*: litora *C A*/12 miliarium* *corr.*: milliarium *C A ms.*/13 maris *A*: marii *C ms.*/14 oceanum *A*: occeanum *C ms.*/15 caravelis *corr.* caravellis *C A ms.*/17 amicitia* *A*: amicicia *C*, amicitiam *ms.*/26 plaeraeque* *C A*: plaereque *ms.*/27 Elisias *C ms.*: Elyisias *A*/28 harenosasque *C*: arenosasque A, arenossasque *ms.*/29 helluonum *corr.*: eluonum *C ms.*: heluonum *A*/35 beate *C ms.*: beatae *A*/39 Urabae *corr.*: Urabe *C A ms.*/43 littorum* *ms.*: litorum *C A ms.*/infoelici* *C ms.*: infelici *A*/44 commilitonum *A*: comilitonum *C ms.*/46 edemus *corr.*: aedemus *C A ms.*/49 Valdoleto *corr.*: Valledoleto *C A ms.*

ep. 537 *C* = 540 *A* = 510 *ms.* (pp. 104, 106, 108)

1 Nuñez *C ms.*: Nunnez *A*/2 designatis *A ms.*: dessignatis *C*/4 Anziso *C A*: Ancisso *ms.*/7 assequutus* *C*: assecutus *A ms.*/10 defensores *A ms.*: deffensores *C*/12 eas *C ms.*: eos *A*/14 milites *C A*: millites *ms.*/15 Nuʃez *C ms.*: Nunnez *A*/17 Kalendas *C ms.*: Calendas *A*/25 Pannonia *A*: Panonia *C ms.*/29 occasione *C A*: occassione *ms.*/33 milia* *corr.*: millia *C A ms.*/37 aggressi *A*: agressi *C ms.*/40 Valdoleto *corr.*: Valleoleto *C A ms.*/Kal. *C ms.*: Calendas *A*

ep. 542 *C* = 545 *A* = 515 *ms.* (pp. 108, 110)

3 nitentem *C A*: nitere *ms.*/4 Borystenem *A*: Boristhennem *C ms.*/9 immaturum *A*: in maturum *C ms.*/11 Iulianum fratrem *A ms.*: Iulianu fratre *C*/12 Sabaudiae *A*:

Sabaudie *C ms.*/17 circunsepti *A ms.*: circunpseti *C*/20 culmina *A ms.*: culmima *C*/21 ventis *A ms.*: vetis *C*/22 Elisiae *C ms.*: Elysiae *A*/23 oceanum *A*: occeanum *C ms.*/egestas *A*: aegestas *C ms.*/24 applicati *C A*: aplicati *ms.*/27 Elvetii *C ms.*: Helvetii *A*/30 immurmuratur *A*: immurmurantur *C ms.*/31 nihil *C A*: nil *ms.*/33 Methymnam* *corr.*: Mentinnam *C* A, Methimnam *ms.*/34 Valdoleto *corr.*: Valleoleto *C A ms.*/35 hydropisim *corr.* hidropesim *C*, hydropisin A, hidropessim *ms.*/37 Methymna* *corr.*: Metinna *C* A, Methinna *ms.*/Kal. *C ms.*: Calendas *A*

ep. 544 *C* = 547 *A* = 517 *ms.* (pp. 110, 112)

1 Ieronymorum *C*: Hieronymorum *ms.*: Jeronymorum *A*/2 Methymna* *corr.*: Methimna, *ms.*, Metinna *C A*/3 miliaria* *corr.*: milliaria *C A ms.*/7 silvas *C ms.*: sylvas *A*/11 aliquando *C ms.*: aliquandiu *A*/12 Placentiam *A ms.*: Placenciam *C*/13 exarcatus *C ms.*: exarchatus *A*/14 Elvetii *C ms.*: Helvetii *A*/18 stratagema* *A*: stratagemma *C ms.*/21 misit *C A*: missit *ms.*/literis *A*: literas *C ms.*/22 minime *A ms.*: mimine *C*/25 literas *C A*: litteras *ms.*/27 torum *corr.*: thorum *C A ms.*/28 coeant *C A*: queant *ms.*/queat *C A*: quaeat *ms.*/31 misisse *A*: mississe *C ms.*/32 littore* *corr.*: litore *C A ms.*/34 abundaret *C ms.*: abundare *A*/continentis *A*: continentes *C ms.*/40 silves- tribus *C ms.*: sylvestribus *A*

ep. 548 *C* = 551 *A* = 521 *ms.* (pp. 114, 116)

1 siderum* coor.: syderum *C A ms.*/2 Kalendas *C ms.*: Calendas *A*/5 literales *C A*: litterales *ms.*/mamillas *C ms.*: mammillas *A*/6 Orduñae *corr.*: Orduniae *C A ms.*/7 addiscenti *A*: adiscenti *C ms.*/11 licentiatus *A ms.*: licenciatus *C*/Agui£iga *C ms.*: Aguinniga *A*/15 licentiatum *A ms.*: licenciatum *C*/17 Elvetii *C ms.*: Helvetii *A*/20 milia* *corr.*: millia *C A ms.*/22 Elvetii *C ms.*: Helvetii *A*/26 calamitosi *C A*: calamitossi *ms.*/31 Elvetios *C ms.*: Helvetios *A*/35 Guelforum *A*: Gelforum *C ms.*/Gibellinorum *A*: Gebellinorum *C ms.*/38 Phoebeio *corr.*: phaebaeo *C*, phoebaeo A, phaebeo *ms.*/rabidum *A*: irabidum *C ms.*/41 Valdoleto *corr.*: Valledoleto *C A ms.*/47 Kalendas *C ms.*: Calendas *A*

ep. 557 *C* = 560 *A* = 530 *ms.* (pp. 116, 118)

1 Veh tibi veh *C ms.*: vae tibi vae *A*/3 appellatus *C A*: apellans *ms.*/10 Kalendas *C ms.*: Calendas *A*/12 visum *C A*: vissum *ms.*/14 ociosum *C A*: ocium *ms.*/16 licentiatus *A ms.*: licenciatus *C*/17 Aguiñiga *C ms.*: Aguinniga *A*/Orduñae *C ms.*: Ordunnae *A*/19 sorori *C A*: sororii *ms.*/20 plaerisque* *corr.*: plerisque *C A ms.*/24 appulso *corr.*: apulso *C ms.*, apulso *A*/26 Nunez *C m.*: Nunnez *A*/Gaspar *C ms.*: Gasper *A*/28 amicitiam *A ms.*: amiciciam *C*/30 silvestribus *C ms.*: sylvestribus *A*/32 tintinnabulis *A*: tintinabulis *C ms.*/38 Darienis *C A*: Dariennis *ms.*/39 effectum *C*: affectum *A ms.*

ep. 558 *C* = 561 *A* = 531 *ms.* (pp. 118, 120)

3 Plasentiam *C A*: Placentiam *ms.*/procelloso *C A*: procellosso *ms.*/4 Torillum *corr.*: Torrillum *C A ms.*/7 valitudinis *C ms.*: valetudinis *A*/8 secessit *A*: secesit *C ms.*/9

praetextu *corr.*: pretextu *C A ms.*/17 quindecenne *C ms.*: quindecenni *A*/sit *C A*: sic *ms.*/20 Caesarem *C A*: Caessarem *ms.*/21 milia* *corr.*: millia *C A ms.*/23 Caesareo *C A*: Caessareo *ms.*/24 Caesari *C A*: Caessari *ms.*/26 reppulit *corr.*: repulit *C A ms.*/Caesaris *C A*: Caessaris *ms.*/28 miserunt *C A*: misserunt *ms.*/29 Henricum *corr.*: Enrichum A, Enrrichum *C*, Enrricum *ms.*/29 stemmata* *A ms.*: stemata *C*/30 posteritas *A*: potesteritas *C ms.*/34 quattuor* *C ms.*: quatuor *A*/sagittarum *C A*: sagitarum *ms.*/38 Plasentiae *corr.*: Placentiae *C A ms.*

ep. 559 *C* = 562 *A* = 532 *ms.* (pp. 122, 124)

6 primiciae* *C ms.*: primitiae *A*/vicarium *A ms.*: viccarium *C*/7 deserebantur *C A*: deserabantur *ms.*/primiciae* *C ms.*: primitiae *A*/10 contra tuae sanctitatis *C A*: contra sanctitatis tuae *ms.*/12 plaerisque* *A ms.*: plerisque *C*/19 impressorum *A*: impraessorum *C ms.*/20 permisi *C A*: premissi *ms.*/25 autores *C*: auctores *A ms.*/26 Babilonica *C ms.*: Babylonica *A*/28 in religione nostra *C A*: in nostra religione *ms.*/29 beatitudo *C A*: valitudo *ms.*/30 stratus *C A*: stractus *ms.*/31 Catholici *A*: Catholicis *C ms.*/34 Guadalupe *ms.*: Guadaluppe *C A*/Kalendas *C ms.*: Calendas *A*

ep. 624 *C* = 623 *A* = 591 *ms.* (pp. 124, 126)

4 milia* *corr.*: millia *C A ms.*/precium* *corr.*: praecium *C ms.*, pretium *A*/5 Valdoletanum *corr.*: Valloletanum *C A ms.*/7 rettulit *corr.*: retulit *C A ms.*/Croi *C ms.*: Croy *A*/9 archanis *C ms.*: arcanis *A*/13 tractantur *A*: tractentur *C ms.*/15 chalcographos* *A*: calchographos *C ms.*/fabulosos *C A*: fabulossos *ms.*/18 Zemibus coor.: cemibus *C A ms.*/aemulantibus *A*: emulantibus *C ms.*/19 precio* *C ms.*: pretio *A*/21 remitto *C A*: remito *ms.*/22 neophitaeque *C ms.*: neophytaeque *A*/29 arpiarum *C ms.*: harpyarum *A*/30 quod *C ms.*: ut *A*/34 neophitas *C ms.*: neophytas *A*/39 Caesarea *C A*: Caessarea *ms.*/Kalendas *C ms.*: Calendas *A*

ep. 630 *C* = 629 *A* = 597 *ms.* (pp. 126, 128)

1 Selimsachus *A*: Selimpsachus *C ms.*/2 stratagemate* *C*: strategemate A, stratagemmate *ms.*/7 reddat *C A*: redat *ms.*/15 veneficia *C A*: beneffitia *ms.*/18 perniciem* *A*: pernitiem *C ms.*/19 typhonibus *A*: tiphonibus *C ms.*/21 conclusum *C A*: conclussum *ms.*/24 Callecuto *corr.*: Collocuto *C A ms.*/26 Chersonesum *A*: Chersonessum *C ms.*/septennio *A*: septenio *C ms.*/27 illis insulis *C A*: insulis illis *ms.*/28 quattuor* *C*: quatuor *A ms.*/milia *corr.*: millia *C A ms.*/31 effoeminantium *C A*: et se effoeminantium *ms.*/Magallanes *corr.*: Magalianes *C A ms.*/34 Gattinara *corr.*: Gatinera *C A ms.*/36 Caesare *C A*: Caessare *ms.*/38 Scyllam *A*: Sillam *C ms.*/Caribdim *C ms.*: Charybdim *A*/40 classis *C A*: clasis *ms.*/42 Caesarea *C A*: Caessarea *ms.*/Kalendas *C ms.*: Calendas/octobris *A*: om. *C ms.*

ep. 635 *C* = 634 *A* = 602 *ms.* (pp. 130, 132)

2 autoribus *C A*: auctoribus *ms.*/3 littoribus* *C ms.*: litoribus *A*/9 praedam* *A*: predam *C ms.*/12 rabiosum *C A*: rabiossum *ms.*/15 comitiis* *A*: comiciis *C ms.*/19

milia* *corr.*: millia *C A ms.*/25 Caesare *C A*: Cassare *ms.*/26 nobili *A ms.*: nobilli *C*/relatum *C A*: datum *ms.*/27 Casarem *C A*: Caessarem *ms.*/29 Ebuso *C A*: Ebusso *ms.*/30 iam *C A*: ad *ms.*/34 miserunt *C A*: misserunt *ms.*/lachrymis *C A*: lacrimis *ms.*/37 urbe *A*: urber *C*, uber *ms.*/Ilerda *corr.*: Illerda *C A ms.*/Kalendas *C ms.*: Calendas *A*

ep. 650 *C* = 649 *A* = 617 *ms.* (pp. 132, 314)

1 Thabarca *corr.*: Tabraca *C A ms.*/2 obsessis *C A*: obsesis *ms.*/praesidiis* *A*: presidiis *C ms.*/herbis *C A*: hervis *ms.*/7 anhelante *C A*: anelante *ms.*/9 summulam *corr.*: sumulam *C A ms.*/10 quo *C ms.*: qui *A*/11 leviter *C A*: laeviter *ms.*/aerumna *C A*: erumena *ms.*/12 quanta *C ms.*: quanto *A*/14 Iamaicae *A*: Ianiaicae *C ms.*/15 Cubae australis *C A*: australis Cubae *ms.*/16 Iamaicam *A*: Ianiaicam *C ms.*/26 dent coni.: dat *C A ms.*/30 Kalendas *C ms.*: Calendas *A*

ep. 650 bis *C* = 650 *A* = 618 *ms.* (p. 134)

2 Cozumellam *A*: Gozumellam *C ms.*/6 miserat *C A*: misserat *ms.*/7 diviserunt *C A*: divisserunt *ms.*/8 aptantes *A*: optantis *C ms.*/14 de *C A*: om. *ms.*/16 impraesentiarum *A*: in praesentiarum *C ms.*

ep. 715 *C* = 715 *A* = 683 *ms.* (pp. 136, 138)

2 literae *C A*: litterae *ms.*/chalcographorum* *A*: calcographorum *C ms.*/19 amygdalis *A*: amigdalis *C ms.*/20 e pansis ficubus coni.: epansis e ficubus *C ms.*, e pansis e ficubus *A*/24 precia* *C ms.*: pretia *A*/25 praetermisi *C A*: pratermissi *ms.*/26 concussura *C A*: concussuram *ms.*/28 caeci* *A*: coeci *C ms.*/30 clausula *C A*: clausa *ms.*/36 Indiis *C A*: Indis *ms.*/oceaneis *corr.*: oceanis *C A ms.*/39 ac ornatas *C A*: ac coronatas *ms.*/42 Valdoleto *corr.*: Valleoleto *C A ms.*

ep. 717 *C* = 717 *A* = 685 *ms.* (pp. 138, 140, 142)

11 aquaticis *C A*: aquatibus *ms.*/est in eius lacunae *C A*: in eius lacunae est *ms.*/15 millium* *corr.*: millium* *C A ms.*/23 ipsae *C A*: ipse *ms.*/in aqua *C A*: in qua *ms.*/24 milium *corr.*: millium *C A ms.*/29 circunseptas *C A*: circunpsetas *ms.*/pulchrae *A*: pulchre *C ms.*/31 milia* *corr.*: millia *C A ms.*/33 supellectilia *C ms.*: suppellectilia *A*/34 gossampio* *corr.*: gosampio *C A ms.*/38 gossampium *corr.*: gosampium *C A ms.*/41 amygdalae *A*: amigdale *C ms.*/45 atrocibus *C A*: attrocibus *ms.*/50 preciosiores* *A*: praeciosiores *C ms.*/52 nucleosa *C A*: nucleossa *ms.*/53 amygdala *A*: amigdala *C ms.*/54 tamen *C ms.*: tantum *A*/60 simulacra *corr.*: simulachra *C A ms.*/61 variis deorum statuis *C A*: statuis variis deorum *ms.*/immolant *A*: imolant *C ms.*/62 alii *C A*: allii *ms.*/69 Valdoleto *corr.*: Valleoleto *C A ms.*/millesimo quingentesimo vigesimo primo *C*: MDXXI *A*, millessimo quingentessimo vigessimo primo *ms.*

ep. 758 *C* = 755 *A* = 725 *ms.* (pp. 142, 144)

2 desiderat *C A* : dessiderat *ms.*/4 facinorosus *C A* : facinorossus *ms.*/deprehensos*
corr.: depraehensos *C A ms.*/7 impraesentiarum *A* : in praesentiarum *C*, in praessentiarum
ms./10 composito *C A* : compossito *ms.*/persuasit *C A* ms2.: om. ms1./11 exercitui *A* :
exercitu *C ms.*/14 opprobria *C A* : opprobia *ms.*/15 Caesarem *C A* : Caessarem *ms.*/17
Mendocium *C A* : Mendozium *ms.*/18 miliare *corr.*: milliare *C A ms.*/29 pressi *A* : praessi
C ms./31 saccareisque *C ms.*: sacchareisque *A*/32 littoribus *C ms.*: litoribus *A*/appropin-
quabat *C A* : apropinquabat *ms.*/pyrata *C ms.*: pirata *A*/35 Bobadillam *corr.*: Boadillam
C A ms./36 littora* *C ms.*: litora *A*/39 littoralibus *C*: litoralibus A, littoribus *ms.*/40
Britanni *A* : Britani *C ms.*/41 pariturum *A* : paritura *C ms.*/42 premebamus *C A* :
praemebamus *ms.*/prememur *C A* : praememur *ms.*/43 obiices *C A* : obices *ms.*/44 nobis
facultas est *A* : nobis est *C ms.*/impraesentiarum *A* : in praesentiarum *C*, in praessentiarum *ms.*/47 Valdoleto *corr.*: Valleoleto *C A ms.*

ep. 766 *C* = 763 *A* = 734 *ms.* (pp. 146, 148, 150)

1 Caesarem *C A* : Caessarem *ms.*/2 Britannia *A* : Britania *C ms.*/literis *C A* : litteris
ms./4 vadosus *C A* : vadossus *ms.*/ceperunt *A* : coeperunt *C ms.*/8 Alburquerchi *C A* :
Alburcherqui *ms.*/13-14 copias...tribus *C A* : copias ex ipso oppido fontis rabidae oppido
Germanorum circiter mille a praessidiis exierunt pedites. Ex ipso fontis rabiae oppido
Germanorum circiter mille a praesidiis exierunt pedites tribus *ms.*1, copias Germanorum
circiter mille a praessidiis exierunt pedites. Ex ipso fontis rabiae oppido Germanorum
circiter mille a praesidiis exierunt pedites tribus *ms.*2/14 praesidiis *C A* : praessidiis *ms.*/15
cannono *corr.*: canono *C A ms.*/20 ascenderunt *C ms.*: adscenderunt *A*/23 ceperunt *A* :
coeperunt *C ms.*/31 cannono *corr.*: canono *C A ms.*/32 simulacro* *corr.*: simulachro
C A ms./33 millies *C A* : milites *ms.*/37 raptata *C ms.*: rapta *A*/38 pyratis *C ms.*: piratis
A/39 milia* *corr.*: millia *C A ms.*/46 aemulatus* *A* : emulatus *C ms.*/48 Pyrenaeorum
A : Pyrenneorum *C ms.*/49 cepit *A* : coepit *C ms.*/52 subvexit *A* : subnexit *C ms.*/54
ascendere *C ms.*: adscendere *A*/64 Atlantis *A ms.*: Athlantis *C*/67 preciosa *C A* :
praeciosa *ms.*/Caesari *C* A.: Caessari *ms.*/71 et *C ms.*: ac *A*/Cortesius *C A* : Cortessius
ms./78 Caesaris *C A* : Caessaris *ms.*/79 visam *C A* : vissam *ms.*/80 praegnans *ms.*: pregnans
C A

ep. 770 *C* = 767 *A* = 738 *ms.* (pp. 150, 152)

1 Kalendarum *C ms.*: Calendarum *A*/4 fasciculo *C A* : faciculo *ms.*/Turcarum *A* :
Turcharum *C ms.*/5 Rhodon *A* : Rhodo *C ms.*/ad medullam *A* : ad me medullam
C ms./10 Dertosia *corr.*: Detursia *C A ms.*/Tarraconem *corr.*: Terraconem *C A ms.*/15
exerere *C ms.*: exserere *A*/19 deprehensi *A* : depraehensi *C ms.*/20 levitatis *C A* :
laevitatis *ms.*/21 Methymnae* *corr.*: Methinae *C A* : Methinnae *ms.*/25 Kalendis: Calendis *A ms.*/26 Caesar *C A* : Caessar *ms.*/32 Callecuteis *corr.*: Collocuteis *C A ms.*/33
aequatori *A* : equatori *C ms.*/34 Magallano *corr.*: Magagliano *C A ms.*/35 quattuorque*
corr.: quatuorque *C A ms.*/38 ac diffusam *C A* : ad diffusam *ms.*/41 Kalendas *C ms.*:
Calendas *A*

461

30

ep. 773 *C* = 770 *A* = 741 *ms.* (pp. 154, 156)

3 inclusus *C A*: inclussus *ms.*/cedit *C A*: caedit *ms.*/4 Turcarum *A*: Turcharum *C ms.*/6 Graeciae *A*: Greciae *C ms.*/14 sollicite *corr.*: solicite *C A ms.*/16 quae *C ms.*: qui *A*/18 caritate *C A*: charitate *ms.*/23 Chersonesum *A*: Chersonessum *C*, Cherssonessum *ms.*/26 Caesar *C A*: Caessar *ms.*/27 assignatos *C A*: asignatos *ms.*/Portugaliae *corr.*: Portugalliae *C A ms.*/34 gariophillis* *corr.*: gariophilis *C ms.*, garyophylis *A*/39 chalcographorum* *A*: calcographorum *C ms.*/41 Valdoleto *corr.*: Valleoleto *C A ms.*

ep. 774 *C* = 771 *A* = 742 *ms.* (pp. 156, 158, 160)

1 Kalendis *C A*: Calendis *ms.*/2 Caesar *C A*: Caessar *ms.*/7 casu *C A*: cassu *ms.*/8 laesae *C A*: lessae *ms.*/12 Garci *C A*: Garssi *ms.*/14 assequuti* *corr.*: assecuti *C A ms.*/15 doña *C ms.*: donna *A*/23 Caesar *C A*: Caessar *ms.*/Cabrensem *corr.*: Caprensem *C A ms.*/25 doñam *corr.*: donam *C ms.*, donnam *A*/26 Cabrerum *corr.*: Caprerum *C A ms.*/33 Caesarem *C A*: Caessarem *ms.*/36 nares *coni.*: aures *C A ms.*/Portugalensium *corr.*: Portugallensium *C A ms.*/37 Cortesio *C A*: Cortessio *ms.*/41 precio* *C A*: praecio *ms.*/43 duae *A*: duas *C ms.*/reliquae *A*: reliquas *C ms.*/pyratarum *C ms.*: piratarum *A*/49 Florinus *A*: Florenus *C ms.*/pyrata *C ms.*: pirata *A*/53 Cortesii *C A*: Cortessii *ms.*/55 munerum *A*: numerum *C ms.*/58 fortunam *A*: fortuna *C ms.*/62 oceano *C A*: occeano *ms.*/68 pyratarum *C ms.*: piratarum *A*/69 alia *C ms.*: illa *A*/71 oceanum *C A*: occeanum *ms.*/73 oceano *C A*: occeano *ms.*/74 Kalendas *C*: Calendas *A ms.*/Millesimo Quingentesimo Vigesimo *C A*: Millessimo Quingentessimo Vigessimo *ms.*

ep. 782 *C* = 779 *A* = 750 *ms.* (pp. 160, 162, 164)

1 Caesari *C A*: Caessari *ms.*/2 molestissimum *C A*: maelestissime *ms.*/10 coelorum *C ms.*: caelorum *A*/hae minae *C*: heminae *A ms.*/11 embrionem *C ms.*: embryonem *A*/pepererunt *C A*: pererunt *ms.*/12 mille militum *A*: mile militum *C ms.*/14 seditio *C A*: saeditio *ms.*/16 ausus *C A*: aussus *ms.*/Caesar *C A*: Caessar *ms.*/20 infoelix* *C ms.*: infelix *A*/21 quas *C ms.*: quos *A*/22 Cortesius *C A*: Cortesius *ms.*/23 pyratarum *C ms.*: piratarum *A*/Cassiteridibus* *corr.*: Casiteridibus *C A ms.*/25 caravelarum *corr.*: caravellarum *C A ms.*/tutelam *A*: tutellam *C*, tutela *ms.*/26 Ioannis *A ms.*: Ioanis *C*/27 praetoria *C A*: praeptoria *ms.*/preciosis* *A*: praeciosis *C ms.*/29 tigrium *C A*: trigrium *ms.*/30 precio* *corr.*: praecio *C ms.*, pretio *A*/31 Caesar *C A*: Caessar *ms.*/33 gazophylacio* *A*: gazophilatio *C ms.*/35 milium ducatorum *corr.*: millium ducatorum *C A*: ducatorum millium *ms.*/39 Caesari *C A*: Caessari *ms.*/44 politici *C A*: pollitici *ms.*/45 Henricus *corr.*: Enrricus *C A ms.*/46 requisitus *C A*: requissitus *ms.*/Caesare *C A*: Caessare *ms.*/49 nisi *C A*: nissi *ms.*/50 universum *C A*: unibersum *ms.*/51 Caribdi *C ms.*: Charybdi *A*/52 decidet *C ms.*: decidit *A*

ep. 786 *C* = 782 *A* = 753 *ms.* (pp. 164, 166)

1 Charites *C A*: charites *ms.*/2 archipresbyteratum *C*: archiepresbyteratum *A*, archpraebsyteratum *ms.*/5 Caesarem *C A*: Caessarem *ms.*/11 inclusos *C A*: inclussos

ms./12 Turdesillarum *C A*: Turdesssillarum *ms.*/arce *C A*: arcem *ms.*/13 catholica *A ms.*: chatholica *C ms.*/maiestatis *A ms.*: miestatis *C*/16 Caesareis *C A*: Caessareis *ms.*/20 Caesaris *C A*: Caessaris *ms.*/21 prosequar *C A*: prossequar *ms.*/tuae *C ms.*: suae *A*/22 oceanus *C A*: occeanus *ms.*/23 permittit *C A*: permitit *ms.*/sumam *C A*: summam *ms.*/28 Tenustitanam *C ms.*: Thenustitanam *A*/29 Caesari *C A*: Caessari *ms.*

ep. 791 *C* = 787 *A* = 758 *ms.* (pp. 166, 168, 170)

5 propiora *A*: propriora *C ms.*/10 Lipuscae *C A*: Lipuzcae *ms.*/11 plebeio *C A*: om. *ms.*/15 usa *C A*: ussa *ms.*/17 Caesare *C A*: Caessare *ms.*/18 praecedente *A*: praecedenti *C ms.*/22 casum *C A*: cassum *ms.*/26 impetenda *A*: impeteda *C ms.*/29 oppositas *C A*: oppossitas *ms.*/cathenas *C A*: catenas *ms.*/32 plaerisque* *corr.*: plerisque *C A ms.*/34 evasi *C A*: evassit *ms.*/littora* *C ms.*: litora *A*/37 resinae *C A*: ressinae *ms.*/stipandarum rimas *A*: stipendarum *C ms.*/41 causa *C A*: caussa *ms.*

ep. 801 *C* = 797 *A* = 760 bis *ms.* (pp. 170, 172, 174)

1 Panama *corr.*: Pannama *C A ms.*:/3 Egidius *C ms.*: Aegidus *A*/6 visa *C A*: vissa *ms.*/8 optare *A ms.*: optraem *C*/14 Caesare *C A*: Caessare *ms.*/16 Garaiana *C ms.*: Geraiana *A*/Cortesio *C A*: Cortessio *ms.*/Tenustitani *corr.*: Temistitani *C A ms.*/17 stratori *corr.*: strator *C A ms.*:/19 accessum *C A*: haeccessum *ms.*:/onustae *A*: onusta *C ms.*/23 perniciosum *C A*: perniciossum *ms.*/25 Caesar *C A*: Caessar *ms.*/26 differre *C A*: inferre *ms.*/28 Portugalensium *C A*: Portugallensium *ms.*/29 quattuor* *corr.*: quatuor *C A ms.*/30 syllogismatum *C ms.*: syllogismatum *A*/31 Caesare *C ms.*: Caessare *ms.*/33 Caesaream *C A*: Caessaream *ms.*/35 Portugalenses *C A*: Portugallenses *ms.*/40 Caesarem *C A*: Caessarem *ms.*/44 Caesaris *C A*: Caessaris *ms.*/46 vigesimi *C A*: vigessimi *ms.*/47 vadosus *C A*: vadossus *ms.*/54 ordeaceaque *C*: hordeaceaque *A*, ordaceaque *ms.*/55 plaeraeque* *A ms.*: pleraeque *C*/57 littora* *C ms.*: litora *A*/58 plaerasque* *A*: plerasque *C ms.*/59 littora* *C ms.*: litora *A*/61 Kalendas *C*: Calendas *A ms.*/Millesimo Quingentesimo Vigesimo *C*: MDXXIV *A*, millessimo quingentessimo vigessimo *ms.*

ep. 804 *C* = 800 *A* = 763 *ms.* (pp. 174, 176, 178, 180)

1 Caesarem *C A*: Caessarem *ms.*/2 misimus *C A*: missimus *ms.*/4 fretum *A*: fretrum *C ms.*/quaesiturus *C A*: quaessiturus *ms.*/8 intelligam *C A*: intelligant *ms.*/9 Portugalensium *corr.*: Portugallensium *C A ms.*/14 ministram *corr.*: minastram *C A ms.*/freilam *corr.*: freiram *C A ms.*/17 invasit *C A*: invassit *ms.*/18 cerebri *A*: cerebris *C ms.*/21 divino iudico *C ms.*: iudico divino *A*/23 Caesareo *C A*: Caessareo *ms.*/Rosilionem *C A*: Rossilionem *ms.*/26 ambitiosi *C A*: ambitiossi *ms.*/miserear *C A*: misserear *ms.*/28 illud *C A*: illum *ms.*/29 assequutus* *C A*: assecutus *ms.*/31 Caesarem *C A*: Caessarem *ms.*/32 verbis *A*: virtus *C ms.*/34 designatio *C A*: dessignatio *ms.*/35 Caesarea *C A*: Caessarea *ms.*/48 Caesari *ms.*/49 foelicissimae* *C ms.*: felicissimae *A*/50 foelicissimam* *C ms.*: felicissimam *A*/52 autumno *C A*: authumno *ms.*/aequinoctio *A*: equinoctio *C ms.*/53 literas *C A*: litteras *ms.*/54 Caesareas *C A*: Caessareas *ms.*/55 casu *C A*: cassu *ms.*/Caesarem *C A*: Caessarem *ms.*/56 repetii coni.: repetiit *C A ms.*/57 miscui *A*: miscue

C ms./60 Caesar *C A*: Caessar *ms.*/61 Subrisit *C A*: Subrisset *ms.*/63 incoeptum *C ms.*: inceptum *A*/65 ab *C A*: a *ms.*/66 quattuor* *corr.*: quatuor *C A ms.*/70 Caesare *C A*: Caessare *ms.*/73 Rosilionis *C A*: Rossilionis *ms.*/74 Caesar *C A*: Caessar *ms.*/79 Caesareo *C A*: Caessareo *ms.*/80 Portugaliae *C ms.*: Portugalliae *A*/81 pyrata *C ms.*: pirata *A*/83 milium* *corr.*: millium *C A ms.*/85 Caesaris *C A*: Caessaris *ms.*/88 Valdoleto *corr.*: Valeoleto *C A ms.*

ep. 806 *C* = 802 *A* = 765 *ms.* (pp. 180, 182, 184)

1 Catherinam *C ms.*: Catharinam *A*/Caesaris *C A*: Caessaris *ms.*/Portugaliam *corr.*: Portugalliam *C A ms.*/2 misimus *C A*: missimus *ms.*/4 Portugalensis *corr.*: Portugallenses *C A ms.*/5 properaverit *C A*: properavit *ms.*/7 quam *A*: quod *C ms.*/12 quattuor *corr.*: quatuor *C A ms.*/13 literas *C A*: litteras *ms.*/15 Cortesio *C A*: Cortessio *ms.*/17 Cortesio *C A*: Cortessio *ms.*/Christophorum *A ms.*: Christoforum *C*/18 Cortesio *C A*: Cortessio *ms.*/22 Ariam *A*: Ariem *C ms.*/28 infoelix* *C ms.*: infelix *A*/31 quattuor* *ms.*: quatuor *C A*/35 Cortesii *C A*: Cortessi *ms.*/41 Dominici *C*: Domini *A*, Dominicis *ms.*/50 foelicibus* *C ms.*: felicibus *A*/51 Caesar *C A*: Caessar *ms.*/55 abrasurum *C A*: abrassurum *ms.*/60 langorem* *C ms.*: languorem *A*/Caesar *C A*: Caessar *ms.*/62 Italae *C A*: Italiae *ms.*/Iacobus *A*: Iacobum *C ms.*/63 construxerat *C A*: construxerant *ms.*/64 pyratarum *C ms.*: piratarum *A*/66 milium* *corr.*: millium *C A ms.*/68 Oceanum *C A*: Occeanum *ms.*/71 uno *A*: una *C ms*/pyratarum *C ms.*: piratarum *A*/72 pyratae *C ms.*: piratae *A*/74 abduxerunt *C A*: eduxerunt *ms.*/78 Kalendas *C*, Calendas *A ms.*

ep. 809 *C* = 806 *A* = 767 *ms.* (pp. 184, 186)

5 spectatores *C A*: expectatores *ms.*/13 quaerendas *C A*: gerendas *ms.*/16 Cortesii *C A*: Cortessii *ms.*/18 calamitose *C A*: calamitosse *ms.*/19 abscessit *A ms.*: abcessit *C*/23 opiniones *C A*: oppiniones *ms.*/26 ut servi *A*: ne servi *C ms.*/ne liberi sint hi *C ms.*: non liberi autem hi *A*/27 vitia *A*: vicia *C ms.*/30 franciscos *C ms.*: franciscanos *A*/31 a re *C A*: a te *ms.*/33 haec *C ms.*: et haec *A*/34 Kalendas *C ms.*: Calendas *A*/Millesimo Quingentesimo Vigesimo *C A*: Millessimo Quingentessimo Vigessimo *ms.*

ep. 812 *C* = 809 *A* = 770 *ms.* (p. 188)

2 scloppis *corr.*: sclopis *C A ms.*/5 Cortesio *C A*: Cortessio *ms.*/7 pyratarum *C ms.*: piratarum *A*/10 Roderico *C A*: Rhoderico *ms.*/16 Caesar *C A*: Caessar *ms.*/18 Rosanum *C A*: Rossanum *ms.*/antistitem *A*: antistem *C ms.*/20 inquisitionis *C A*: inquissitionis *ms.*/22 collegae *A*: collega *C ms.*/24 Madriti *C A*: Madrito *ms.*/25 foelicem* *C ms.*: felicem *A*

ep. 814 *C* = 811 *A* = 772 *ms.* (pp. 190, 192)

3 Kalendas *corr.*: Kalendis *C*, Calendis *A ms.*/6 foelix* *C ms.*: felix *A*/13 habitatas *A*: habitate *C ms.*/14 praerogativis *C ms.*: praerogatis *A*/20 Caesar *C A*: Caessar *ms.*/22

foelicibus* *C ms.*: felicibus *A* /oceanum *C A* : occeanum ms/23 Cortesio *C A* : Cortessio *ms.*/24 Caesari *C A* : Caessari *ms.*/impraesentiarum *A* : impraessentiarum *ms.*, in praesentiarum *C*/26 Cortesius *C A* : Cortessius *ms.*/32 Aria *corr.*: Ariae *C A ms.*/33 Cortesius *C A* : Cortessius *ms.*/34 de Las Casas *C A* : de Las Cassas *ms.*/35 alias *A* : alas *C ms.*/42 curruum *A* : currium *C ms.*/44 Caesar *C A* : Caessar *ms.*/45 Caesar *C A* : Caessar *ms.*/47 Caesare *C A* : Caessare *ms.*/49 Caesarea *C A* : Caessarea *ms.*/clauso *C A* : clausso *ms.*/50 conclusio *C A* : conclussio *ms.*/51 Gillinus *corr.* (alibi): Gilius *C A ms.*/54 Gattinera *C A* : Gatinera *ms.*/Caesarem *C A* : Caessarem *ms.*/plaerosque* *C A* : plerosque *ms.*/56 autoritatem *C A* : authoritatem *ms.*/57 collisum *A* : collissum *C ms.*/Caesar *C A* : Caessar *ms.*/60 Kalendas *C*: Calendas *A ms.*/Millesimo Quingentesimo Vigesimo *C A* : Millessimo Quingentessimo Vigessimo *ms.*

Appendix II: Critical Notes to the Decades de Orbe Novo I 1-7 (collated with the Seville 1511 edition)

I 1

p. 206, 1-12 Solebat...vir] De insulis in occiduo mari felicibus auspiciis Ferdinandi et Helysabeth Hispaniarum et nostri maris insularum equa lance regum nuper inventis: quid perceperim accipio. Hoc si quidem tuis litteris tantum cupere videris ut tamen apertius omnia cognoscas a primordio rei ipsius exordiendum duxi Chrisophorus quidam Colonus ligur vir *H*/14-15 attinentibus...a quibus] attinentibus illum armarent affirmans a quibus *H*/17 destinata] assignata *H*/21-22 millesimum...coepit] millesimum a salute mundi iter institutum Colonus cepit *H*/24-25 nuncupantur...distant] nuncupantur nuper ab eis capte distant *H*/30-32 atrox...usque] atrox aestas. Has ad hec usque *H*//p. 208, 8-11 a Gallo...pedem] a gallo errante tempestatibus acto reperte forte fortuna fuerint nomine Bethancor. Pedem *H*/12-13 Lancelotum...Hispanis] lancelotum et bonaventuram patrie postmodum amore tactus hispanis *H*/15 nostris] nostris vero *H*/16-20 scilicet...gens] scilicet palmam et tenerifem Alfonsus lugo licet duriuscule: gens *H*/23 Ab his] Ex his *H*/24-25 paulisper tres] paulisper (ut ipse michi post reditum sepe numero hec avide scrutanti retulit) tres *H*/26-36 navigavit...navigatione] navigavit optatum tandem ex altiori cavea terre prospectum leti suscipiunt. Detexit navigatione *H*//p. 210 18 cum] quom *H*/22 properantes] accurrentes *H*/23-24 viderunt ... inauditam] viderunt qui applicantem inauditam *H*/27 cum] quom *H*/35 paropsidis] parapsidis *H*/37 simile nostri] simile a nostris *H*//p. 212, 2 cum] quom *H*/15-16 construunt...octoginta] construunt octoginta *H*/25-26 truculentos...vocant] truculentos illos vocant *H*/29 vexari] infestari *H*/31 pullos] puulos *H*/34 matura cum ad eorum] matura statim quom ad eorum *H*/35 intestina] intestina et *H*/epulantur...ut nos] epulantur partim sale conditos ut nos *H*//p. 214, 7 praesentiunt aliam] presentiunt nullam aliam *H*/17-18 ipsi...panem] ipsi. Panem *H*/26 panicula] mappa *H*/30-31 exuperant...est] exuperant. Est *H*//p. 216, 5-6 forte...inciderunt] forte in flumen quoddam latitudinis immense inciderunt *H*/9 Serpentes...nutriunt] Serpentes et magnitudine et numero admirabiles insule nutriunt *H*/17 de psittacis illustrissime Princeps] de psitacis illustricime princes *H*/21 cum] quom *H*/22 Aristoteles] Aristotiles *H*//p. 218, 5 reliquit] reliquias *H*/9 contactus] contactatus *H*/20-21 sperantes...commoventur] sperante ad cristianum cultum tot nationes et simplices gentes facile trahi posse iis rebus a Colono solum sed a suismet accolis (qui supra ducentos cum illo tale: tamquam dubiam provintiam fuerant agressi) auditis: commoventur *H*/26-34 imperant...pollicebatur] imperant. Is admiratus apud hispanos nuncupatur. Ex insulis preterea (ut in initio Colonus ipse iam prefectus maritimus pollicebatur) *H*//p. 220, 5-7 magnitudinem...ducentos] magnitudinem abiles ultra ducentos *H*/19 uberrimam] fertilissimam *H*/30 hac insula vela] hac vela *H*/33 Vale...1493] Vale felix *H*

I 2

p. 222, 6 quadringenta] quadraginta H: CCCC *alii in mg.*/8 quarti] tertii *H*: quart] *alii in mg.*/9 missi] destinati *H*/10 appulsa esse] applicuisse *H*/12 Praefectum marinumi prefectum maritimum *H*/14-15 scribit...dux] scribit. Quarto nonas aprilis igitur dux *H*/15-16 regii...Ab eo] regii a prefecto maritimo destinatus accessit. Ab eo *H*/18 fuerunt...recensebo] fuerunt ut tibi gratum faciam enarrata recensebo *H*/21 littoribus...in altum] littoribus actis navibus in altum *H*/24-25 propterea...insulas] propterea in caniballium insulas *H*//p. 224, 1-3 aequoris...neque] aequoris diversi arboribus vimine trunco radicibus et foliis aromaticos et suaves odores emittentibus insule referte ocurerrunt neque *H*/5 lacertos] stelliones *H*/7 quodam] quodam sublimi *H*/13 innumeros] innumeras *H*/14 singulos vicos] singulas villas *H*/15 platae tuguriis] platea *H*/23 ut...domus] ut acutam superfitiem domus *H*/26 gossampinis] bombicinis *H*/28 gossampino] bombice *H*/gossipium] bombicem *H*/29 gossipio] bombice *H*/32-33 conveniunt...ligneas] conveniunt duas in quodam loco ligneas *H*/36 didicerunt] adverterunt *H*/memoravimus] momoravimus *H*/37 gossipio] bombice *H*//p. 226, 8 dissimilia] discrepantia *H*/22 appellant...tulerunt] appellant. Tulerunt *H*//p. 228, 1 apud viros] apud eos *H*/4-5 cuneo facto] globo facto *H*/15 Madanino] Matininam *H*/25-26 creduntur ad hanc *H*/27 pervenire] accedere *H*/28 Madaninoe] Matinine *H*//p. 230, 4 aliam iterum] aliam atque aliam iterum *H*/8-9 fertilitatis accipiunt] fertilitatis ab iis quos vehebant accipiunt *H*/12-13 nomine...voluerunt] nomine insignitam fore voluerunt *H*/27 ita priusquam] ita quod priusquam *H*//p. 232, 11 facio.Ad] facio se ne ab incepto discedamus ad *H*/12 procedentes iam] procedentes ab hispanis littoribus iam *H*/14 cum] quom *H*/22 frequentiae] spistudinis *H*/31 Burichena] Burichenia *H*//p. 234, 8 rabiosis] rabiosie *H*/18 insula cui] insula quem vocant cacicum cui *H*/22-25 reliquis...Est] reliquis deinde iam optatam sed infelici eventu (quod omnes socios ibi relictos interemptos repererint) Hispaniolam a prima insula caniballium quingentas lequas distantem intra paucos dies attingunt. Est *H*/32-33 furtim deiciunt] furtim deijcientes *H*//p. 236, 7 cum] quom *H*/8 pervenissent] applicuisset *H*/10 Praefectum marinum] prefectum maritimum *H*/13 si qui] si aut qui *H*/19 plures] plures ait *H*/suo] sue *H*/24 gossampina] bombicina *H*/25-p. 235, 3 cupiebat...Altero] cupiebat.Altero *H*/10 Guaccanarillo] Guaccanerillo *H*/26-28 facinus...illa] facinus quam Cloelia romana que Tiberium ruptis vinculis porsene impium fugiens cum reliquis obsidibus virginibus enatavit aggressa est. Illa *H*//p. 240, 3-9 quaeritans...Falcatum] queritans in fauces quasdam retortas utrimque collibus erectis munitas incidit: fluvii alicuius grande hostium arbitratus portum ibi quo tutiorem aut quommodiorem nullus unquam (ut ipsi aiunt) viderit ingrediens adinvenit portum regalem proptera nominandum existimarunt falcatum *H*/18 explorant] scrutatur *H*/19 adeuntibus] applicantibus *H*/26 ut] quod *H*/34 regionis] provincie *H*//p. 242, 13-16 contenti...Fama] contenti iusserat enim: prefectus ut mihi relatum est: pena etiam preposita ne quid ulterius preterquam de locis et locorum signis curarent rem ad prefectum referunt. Fama *H*/20 nullibi] nullubi *H*/31 nullibi] nullubi *H*/32 diei...aequinoctialem] diei preterquam equinotialibus ipsi vero equinocialem *H*//p. 244, 13 diximus...non] diximus. V.nonas febr. mill. CCCCXCIIII destinavit: non *H*/29-30 Vale...1494] *om. H*

I 3

ad Ludovicum Aragonium cardinalem] incipitur ad Iulium secundum pont. max. (in decadis occeanee. Librum tertium prefatio) *H*/p. 246, 1 petis] Ioannes Ruffus britonoriensis episcopus qui apud catholicum regem tue beatitudinis vices legatus gerit indefesso spiritu die noctuque tue sanctitatis amplissimas virtutes predicans: inter ceteras litterarum cultoribus semper S.T. favisse novarumque editionum amatricem esse mihi (quem in amiciciam dignatus est admittere) sepe numero retulit. Suasitque ut occeanee decadis mee libellos (quos ipse manu habuit dispersos) colligerem: ad tuamque S. exemplar eorum mitterem: ut (si quando per otium liceat) tua S. queat animum tanta mole negotiorum promissum nova lectione reficere quibus per Christophorum colonum concivem suum regiis auspiciis tam vasta littora incognita hactenus fuisse reperta conspicet. Ubi cristiana religio que tue B. humeris inheret iam crevit in immensum: in diesque magis atque magis coalescet. Ascanii marie sfortie cardinalis tue b. vicecancellari quondam impulsu libellos primos duos conscripseram quo cadente decidit et mihi animus a scribendo: donec me (Federici regis nomine) ludovicus aragonius cardinalis tue beat. amantissimus denuo excitavit: ad quem epistolam (quae adest) conscripsi: ut qui me ad scribendum agitarent noscerentur. Hec igitur (uti apud me iacebant) tua sanctitas sibi habeat. Que de preclare gestis suis et animi constantia per commentaria adhuc apud me latentia reliquis rebus memoratu dignis que nostra tempestate in universo acciderunt conmixta (si vivere dabitur) aliquando videbit. Ad Cardi. iam petentem regis nomine ut scribam deveniamus. Petis *H*/12 marini] maritimi *H*/13 quanto] quanto celeriter *H*/15-17 discessum...singulis] discessum (qui proximus erat) ut nostri regis sororem parthenopeam reginam veterem tibi amitam: quam huc fueras commitatus: in patriam reduceres objicens: singulis *H*/18 adegisti] coegisti *H*/20 vice cancellarium scriptitare] vice cancellarium (dum fortuna fuit) scriptitare *H*/23 directae] misse *H*/24 1500] MCCCCCI *H*/25 Praefectum marinum] prefectum maritimum *H*/27 appulsum fuisse] applicuisse *H*//p. 248, 4 septingenta] octingenta *H*/6 producant ab] producant longitudinem ab *H*/7-9 praedicant...Insulae] predicant insule *H*/19-20 hortos...limitibus] ortos multi colendos limitibus *H*/29 aut sarmentis itidem] aut siccis pampinis itidem *H*/39 regionem] provintiam *H*/39-p. 250, 1 dimisit...montosa] dimisit. Est autem hec provintia montuosa *H*/3 de regionis] de provintie *H*/5-6 insulam...memoranda] insulam memoranda *H*/15 regionem provintiam *H*/24 regionem] provintiam *H*/26 regionis] province *H*/28 regionis incolae] provincie accole *H*/35 cum] quom *H*//p. 252, 12 drachmarum] dragmarum *H*/17 incolis] accolis *H*/22 incolis] accolis *H*/27 regio] provincia *H*/32 auro conmixta] auro involuta *H*/35 quum] quom *H*/gossipio] bombice *H*//p. 254, 1 regionis] provincie *H*/8-9 illum...ne] illum ut percurrere nova littora quotquot posset festinaret admonuerat ne *H*/11-12 Pontifex...Regi] Pontifex regi *H*/14-17 extra parallelum...hae] per parallelum insularum Cassiteridum que dicuntur Caput Viride. Nam he *H*/20 ab Hesperidibus] a cassiteridibus *H*/21 Portugalenses adhuc] Portugalenses *H*/22 regionem] provinciam *H*/23-24 vocitarant...vocavitque] vocitarant intra paucos dies applicuit vocavitque *H*/25 cum] quom *H*/33 latum] amplissimum *H*/34 Sancti Nicolai] Sancti Michaelis *H*/38 curvari. In] curvari. Ita ut amplissimam iam: ex cuneali et acuta primum: terra illi in dies fieret australioremque se magis reperiret. In *H*//p. 256, 6 incolasque] accolasque

H/16 incognitae reliquisse] incognite reliquisse *H*/21 cotidie] quottidie *H*/25 supra...hoc] supra ter centum hoc *H*/31-32 portum...capacem] portum ab omni procella et tempestate tutissimum omniumque navium quas maria sustinent cappacem *H*/34 immensa] immesa *H*//p. 258, 8 duodeviginti] duorum et triginta *H*/12 dentes alii evulsos] alii dentes evulsos *H*/14 qui...profugerant] qui ipsis applicantibus profugerant *H*/19-23 Colonum...incola] colonum a teneris annis inter suos educatum iuvenem iam insularium linguam callentem cuius ydioma erat istorum lingue fere simile didaco interprete qui proprius accesserat alloquitur: metu deposito accessit incola *H*/23 venirent] accederent *H*//p. 260, 1 Almirantus] prefectus *H*/3 Almiranto] prefecto *H*/7 incolae] accole *H*/10-15 invitabant...Idibus] invitabant. Idibus *H*/20 piscatorum] piscatoriam *H*/22 tacitis] taciti *H*/25 pisces alios] alios pisces *H*//p. 262, 8-9 demittunt...quattuor] demittunt. Quattuor *H*/14 Almirantus] prefectus *H*/26 laeva...ingressus] leva huius terre adiacebant ingressis *H*/27 fugere] fugiere *H*//p. 264, 6 Almirantus] prefectus *H*/9 quam celerrimo] quam celeri *H*/12 noster fugiebat] ballistarius fugiebat *H*/15 pergerent] peragrent *H*/17-18 apparuit...proficisci] apparuit per herbas profiscisci *H*/22 cum] quom *H*/25-27 silvam...Racemos] silvam (serpentibus per altas arbores passim vitibus. suapte natura productis) arboribusque aliis plurimus aromaticos fructus parturientibus consitam repererunt racemos *H*/29 cum] quom *H*/30 putruerunt] putuerunt *H*/33 cum] quom *H*/montes vela] montes qui illi in triginta milliarium prospectu apparuerunt vela *H*//p. 266, 1-3 compellarunt...intellexerat] compellarunt neque insularis ille (qui in cube initio accolarum lingua intelexerat) *H*/8 habentur] abraduntur *H*/13 specularis] specularia *H*/14-20 Nec...littora] Nec an incolarum essent ignes ad necessitatem parati an (uti suspectis bellorum temporibus fieri solet) per eos fumos signa vicinis darent ut se in tutum reciperent aut ut in unum convenirent si quid nostri contra eos moliri tentarent aut forte (quod magis consonum videtur) ut tanquam ad rem mirandam nostra navigia inspecturi concurrerent bene constitit. Littora *H*/21-22 insulis implicitum] insulis coagulatum *H*/31 albidarum aquarum] albidarum ac spissarum aquarum *H*/33 cum] quom *H*//p. 268, 2 quos] quas *H*/4 cum] quom *H*/16 terras] provincias *H*/19-20 itinera...scias] itinera sibi (quom e corpore prosiliunt) animas habere duo scias *H*/21 sunt] sint *H*/29 regionum] provinciarum *H*/30 cum] quom *H*/33 indigenas debellaret] indigenas comprimeret *H*//p. 270, 2 cum] quom *H*/19-20 delectatur...Inde] delectatur. Inde *H*/35-36 De quibus...Vale] De quibus pauca narrare (quod non erit absurdum audire) decrevi sed alio tempore alioque libro coligenda satius duco. Vale *H*

I 4

p. 272, 1 arbitratur Indico] arbitratur predicatque indico *H*/Praefectus marinus] prefectus maritimus *H*/2 Boilum et Petrum] Boilum Petrum *H*/4 regionis] provincie *H*/corrupto animo] corrupto in se animo *H*/5 quid horum] quid de se horum *H*/7 alios eorum loco qui] alios qui eorum loco qui *H*/9 cum] quom *H*/10 possent redire] possent provideret redire *H*/14 cum] quom *H*/conspicerent] conpspicerent *H*/18 fuerat...indomita] fuerat fere omnia indomita *H*/23 quotquot...incolae] quotquot pallantes incole *H*/24 sacra offerentes deo] sacra diis offerentes *H*/33 regionis] provincie *H*//p. 274, 6 mittuntur qui] destinantur qui *H*/7 servire] inservire *H*/11 regionem] provinciam *H*/31 ut quinquaginta] ut plusquam quinquaginta *H*/33 cum] quom *H*/35 insulares commeatus] insularia alimenta *H*//p. 276, 3 regione] provincia *H*/5 regio] provincia *H*/8 regiones] provincias *H*/12 nostris...quaedam] nostris alimenta quedam *H*/17 scaturientium...arcem]

scaturientium ornato arcem *H*/21 Subtristes an] Subtristes tamen quottidie an *H*/31 ut]
quod *H*/33 librarum] librarium *H*/36 eductum] evulsum *H*//p. 278, 9 vulgarem] mediocrem *H*/11-12 mercatores...appellant] mercatores itali verzinum appellant *H*/15 gossipio]
bombice *H*/23-24 potuisse...Hispani] potuisse citius insulares vinci aut domari eorumque
vires frangi ad imperium insule libere capessendum refert hispani *H*/34 regionum]
provinciarum *H*//p. 280, 4 regionis] provinciae *H*/5 ille statueret] ille iniungeret *H*/9
vero terras] vero provincias *H*/gossipium] bombix *H*/23-25 diversi...Ad Caunaboam]
diversi. Ad Caunaboam *H*/27-28 liberaret animo] eximeret animo *H*/29 regionem]
provinciam *H*/32 die grassationis] die insultibus *H*/34 regione] provincia *H*/36 suppete-
rent] sufficerent *H*//p. 282, 1 noverint] moverint *H*/regionem] provinciam *H*/6 ignarus
ad] ignarus applicans ad *H*/7 cuique] unicuique *H*/9 opponit] apponit *H*/14 acie confli-
gere] acie (quom omnes eo ordine apropinquare conspicerent) confligere *II*/24 regio]
provincia *H*/29-30 exortum...ad] exortum qui quascumque maximas arbores offendebat
radicitus everteret predicant. Is turbo quom ad *H*/pervenisset] applicuisset *H*/34 - p.
284, 2 plusquam...neque] plusquam lacerti mensura fatentur. Insularibus hec stupentibus
murmurantibus intra se gentem hanc flagitiosam facinorosam violentiam que auream
eorum quietem otiumque placidissimum sua avaricia et cupiditate perturbarat hec portenta tulisse. neque enim *H*/4-5 insulam...neque] insulam ab aerea plaga demissum
hactenus fuisse neque *H*/9 Caunaboam repetamus] Ad caunaboam redeamus *H*/10 cum]
quom *H*/16 manu...quas] manu eas aurifodinas quas *H*/22 diiudicare...Metallarii] dijudi-
care. Metallarij *H*/26 auri drachmas singulis] auri pondo singulis *H*/27 Adelantatus]
antelatus *H*/30 venturus alacer] venturus et antea constituerat alacer *H*

I 5

p. 286, 1 adelantatus] atelatus *H*/3-4 ferebatur calones] ferebatur (fiunt nam in
Hispania muri fere omnes ex materie terrea calce tamen admixta calones *H*/4 muratores
inter] muratores ipsius inter *H*/9 habuit permutatione] habuit per permutationem *H*/19
cum excariis rebus] cum alimentis *H*/21 viritim...dividuntur viritum luxta ex Hispania
constitutionem latam dividuntur *H*/22 vecta esse] applicuisse *H*/28 ditionariis] accolis
H/30-31 mittit...arcemque] mittit habitacula vero post explorata diligentius meridionalia
littora transportat arcemque *H*/33 appulsus est] applicuit *H*/34-288, 1 refertissimus...utrinque] refertissimus per cuius decursum terdecim millia passuum ad duodecimum usque lapidem ad arcem auream navigia possunt conscendere in portum amenissi-
mis utrinque *H*/4 onustos in caput] onustos usque in caput *H*/12 milliaria...Naibam]
milliaria viginti supra centum in fluvium Naibam *H*/16-17 ad regulorum...per diversa]
ad regulorum provincias quorum nemora meridionali ad occidentis angulum insule lateri
adiacentia ex coccineis arboribus constant per diversa *H*/21 adelantatus] antelatus *H*/26
regia...sita] regia insule calcam occidentalem versus sita *H*/27 vocatur] vocitatur *H*/32
adelantatus inquit] antelatus autem inquit *H*/33 marino] maritimo *H*//p. 290, 1 adelan-
tatus] antelatus *H*/2 gossampii] bombicis *H*/3 regionem] provinciam *H*/11-12 ad navium...dicunt] ad navium amplustria contexenda esse dicunt *H*/12 gossampii...tributa]
bombicis secundum telluris varie naturam tributa *H*/13 veniunt] applicant *H*/17 digna]
digna acta fuisse *H*/appropinquantibus...foeminae] appropinquantibus rege et antelato
primum triginta femine *H*/20 quibusdam...corruptae] quibusdam bombicinis tanquam
corrupte *H*/28 adelantato] antelato *H*/29 coenam...nocte] cenam invenientes longo itinere
et vigiliis vires perditas revocant nocte *H*/30-31 superveniente...hospitia] superveniente

secundum cuisuque statum ad hospitia *H*/32 pro eorum consuetudine] iuxta eorum consuetudine *H*//p. 292, 13 caperet...non modo] caperet ignarus quom non modo *H*/16 per regiones] per provincias *H*/20 condidit a Sperancia] condidit Sperancia *H*/27 incolarum] accolarum *H*/29 ca[it est regni] caput est provincie *H*/33 cum] quom *H*/34 finium] provinciae *H*/35 animis...defectioni] animis propter eorum vi et rapinas vivere studereque defectioni *H*//p. 294, 2 cum] quom *H*/4 cum quindecim] quindecim *H*/5 adelantatus] antelatus *H*/9 mittuntur] destinantur *H*/13 adelantatus] antelatus *H*/20-22 potuisset...intonuit] potuisset reliquos simul et Guarionexium dimisit aderat uti arbitrantur quinque millium hominum multitudo quod supplices omnes pro suorum regum liberatione inermes confluxerant intonuit *H*/23 adelantatus] antelatus *H*/25 ne...molirentur] ne quid tale molirentur *H*/26-27 habuit...deliquentes] habuit copiosissimam de nostrorum potentia miseria in delinquentes *H*/32 regio] provincia *H*/34 discessu] digressu *H*/36 adelantatus] antelatus *H*//p. 296, 2 partis] provincie *H*/3 adelantatum] antelatum *H*/gossampium] bombicem *H*/4 incolis] accolis *H*/5 adelantatus] antelatus *H*/pergit honorifice] pergit applicat honorifice *H*/10-11 persuaserat...duos] persuaserat. Duos *H*/17 inter eorum edulia *H*/20 horrorem non modo] horrorem quendam non modo *H*/22 adelantatus] antelatus *H*/26 helluones] ganeones *H*/31 a iugulo ad inguina] a iugulo usque ad uterum et inguina *H*//p. 298, 5 quum] quom *H*/gossipio] bombice *H*/6 adelantatus] antelatus *H*/8 regiones] provincias *H*/10-11 portaretur...imperent] portaretur volantes ad Hisabellam nucios destinat qui adduci (procul habita omni mora) peractam caravellam de duabus quas inceptas iam diu fuisse supra memoravimus suo nomine imperent *H*/15-16 mulier...ubi] mulier uxor quondam Caunaboe de qua supra memoravimus ubi *H*/16-18 suum...sex] suum applicuisse cognovit fratri persuadet ut ambo cum antelato ad illam videndam profiscatur. Antelato diu renuente et ne laborem illum summant persuadente pergunt tamen sex *H*/28 Hispaniolae] Hispane *H*/35 adelantato] antelato *H*//p. 300, 1 gossampi] bombicis *H*/2 cum pervenissent] quom applicuissent *H*/3 adelantatus] antelatus *H*/6-7 voluit...vehi] voluit mulier cum antelato proficisci *H*/10 adelantatum] antelatum *H*/11-12 cum...fistulae] quom autem proprius accederent fistule *H*/19-20 tum...remis] tum vero quom sine remis *H*/21 per aequor] equor *H*/22 cum] quom *H*/25 navi pane] navi insulari pane *H*/32 adelantatum] antelatum *H*//p. 302, 1 ditionariis] accolis *H*/10 cum] quom *H*/17 defendatque] defendat *H*/20 adelantatus] antelatus *H*/32 almierantus] prefectus *H*//p. 304, 1 appulsa sunt] appulerunt *H*/11 adelantatus] antelatus *H*

I 6

p. 306, 11 reliquis...vehentibus] reliquis quom prius duas misisset alimenta vehentibus *H*/12 caravelis australis] caravellis de quibus alias australis *H*/16 mediae Hesperides] medie Cassiterides *H*/21 labe] elephantia *H*/inde...aer] inde igitur quom esset ibi aer *H*/25 ut fere] quod fere *H*//p. 308, 3 ardoribus] torroribus *H*/10 cum] quom *H*/12 adeunt] accedunt *H*/23 invenerunt] adverterunt *H*/25 a longe...prospiciunt] a longe ab euro venientem prospiciunt *H*/29 gossampina] bombicina *H*/35 ea navigatione...affirmat] ea navigatione et malachiis pertinaciter prefectus affirmat *H*/36 incolis] accolis *H*//p. 310, 3-8 non video...tintinnabula] non video. Iuvenes ut aliceret prefectus specula vasa enea tersa lucida tintinabula *H*/19-20 e converso paratis sagittis] e converso ballistis armatis *H*/22 adhaeserunt] applicuerunt *H*/31 decidenti cederet] decidenti (quom arbores secum et ingentia fara rotando trahit) cederet *H*//p. 312, 2-4 defluxus ruebat...ex faucibus] defluxus accedebat ex faucibus *H*/17-18 casas nullas...ruricolae] casas nullas. Id illi quod nostris nos accidere sepe numero coniectati sunt nam ruricole *H*/21 cum] quom *H*/22 appulsam esse] appulisse *H*/30 portenderet omnes recensent] portendere polliceretur omnes recenseret *H*/32 surgere] assurgere *H*/33-34 odores afflari] odores quibus nostrorum animi recreabantur afflari *H*/36 propius...cacichi] propius accedentibus eius provintie cacichi *H*//p. 314, 2 offerendo] offerentes *H*/7 maiora] maiora sibi *H*/14 accomodatius] accomodatius (uti aiebat) *H*/18 adeuntes] adentes *H*/29 uvis sed] uvis (neque enim vites habent) sed *H*//p. 316, 1 gossampino] bombicino *H*/17 navem si vis] navem quom vis *H*/21-24 Cumana...Curiana] om. *H*/31 herbidum ingressus est] herbidum (quamvis in defluentis amnis similitudinem aqua decurreret) ingressus est *H*/31-32 semen...aemulbatur] semen lentisci semen (ut aiunt) emulabatur *H*//p. 318, 9 possit] posset *H*/15 quum] quom *H*/19 culmine] om. *H*/20 memoravimus] memoravimus culmine *H*/24 quum] quom *H*/30-31 postmodum...continentem] postmodum terram ipsam accuratius utilitatis causa investigarunt permensi sunt continentem *H*//p. 320, 4-5 visendorum militum] visendarum gentium *H*/6 tetendit] applicuit *H*

I 7

p. 322, 9-10 punireque...Illi] punireque unumquenque secundum comissa queat. Illi *H*/20 e contrario quum] e contra quom *H*/23 stupratores] strupatores *H*/30 insulam] provinciam *H*//p. 324, 5 Adelantatum] Antelatum *H*/8 cum] quom *H*/Adelantatus] antelatus *H*/11 exploratores hostium] exploratores *H*/14 fluvium delitescere] fluvium expectare *H*/15-16 incautos...vadum] incautos adoriantur fassus est delitescere Antelatus igitur monitus quom iuxta loci et temporis exigentiam acies suas instruxisset per fluminis profluentis ripam vadum *H*/17-18 ascendit...emissis] ascendit. Quom autem apertiorem latioremque fluminis alveum comperisset locumque ob sparsas per planiciem fluminis aquas vadosum emissis *H*/20-21 prodeunt...Nigro] prodeunt enim omnes veluti maroniani agatirsi picti omnes et aspersi veluti panthere. Nigro *H*/23 ad genua usque] usque ad genua *H*/25 transitum] trasitum *H*/28 Adelantatus] Antelatus *H*//p. 326, 3 quum] quom *H*/4 silvis moveri] silvis bullire *H*/9 duos...a] duos quom fugerent assecuntur a *H*/Maiobanexium] maiobonexium *H*/12 Adelantatus] antelatus *H*/13 donec regionem diligentius] donec terrae natura diligentius *H*/17 Adelantatum] antelatum *H*/18 Adelantato] antelato *H*/21 insequuntur] insecuntur *H*/23 Maiobanexium] maiobanexium *H*/24 mittit] destinat *H*/incolis] accolis *H*/26-28 sed...propterea] sed ut guarionexius qui ad te confugit tibique ut arma in maximum tuorum incommodum sumeres persuasit commissorum penas deprehensus luat efflagitat propterea *H*/29 monetque] monet *H*/30 Praefectus marinus] prefectus maritimus *H*//p. 328, 5 Adelantatus] antelatus *H*/6 Maiobanexioque propior] Mariobanexioque propinquior *H*/8 intimis...quocum] intimis aliquem mittat quocum *H*/10 rex ire imperat] rex destinat *H*/Adelantatus] antelatus *H*/13 incolas] accolas *H*/14 Maiobanexius] maiobaunexius *H*/17 Maiobanexius] Maiobaunexius *H*/19 dona...multa] dona quom ad eum accederet multa *H*/20 tripudiareque] trepudiareque *H*/28 Adelantatum] antelatum *H*/29 primus] primas *H*/Adelantati] antelati *H*/30 cum fida custodia] cum ingenti custodia *H*/32 Adelantato] antelato *H*/33 Adelantatus] antelatus *H*//p. 330, 3 constituit. Vadit] constituit. Accedit *H*/8 Cum] quom *H*/9 Adelantati] antelati *H*/11-13 veniam...recedunt] veniam multi et ut redire ad conceptionem liceat ubi plurimi ex eis predia insulari more habebant cultissima petunt. Indulgetur recedunt *H*/13 Adelantato] antelato *H*/21 Adelantatus] antelatus *H*/22 quaeritare si] queritare ut si *H*/23-24 quidam...quos] quidam ipsius quos *H*//p. 332,

1 regionis] provincie *H*/4 comitabatur. Eam] comitabatur quam *H*/4-5 natura...creavit]
natura creavit *H*/5 vir ipsius] vir eius *H*/10 incolis] accolis *H*/11 incolarum] accolarum
H/13 adiit] accedit *H*/16 ad clementiae] ad miserie *H*/21 cum] quom *H*/29-30 vinctos
adductos esse didicerunt] victos applicuisse didicerunt *H*/34 Adelantatum] antelatum *H*//p.
334, 3 Adelantatus] antelatus *H*

Appendix III: Critical Notes to the *Decades de Orbe Novo* I 1-7; III 4

I 1

p. 206 Sfortiam C^1 C^2: Sphorciam *B P*//p. 206, 4 huiuscemodi C^1 C^2 *B*: huiusmodi
P/9 autoribus C^1 C^2 *B*: authoribus *P*/litteris C^1 *B P*: literis C^2/10 cupere C^2 *B P*: te
cupere C^1/videris C^1 *B P*: ostendis C^2/initio rei C^2 *B*: initio C^1 *P*/12 quidam C^1 *B P*:
om. C^2/ligur C^2 *B P*: lygur C^1/Helisabethae C^1 C^2 *B*: Elizabethe *P*/14 attinentibus C^1 C^2
B: attingentibus *P*/15 religio et margaritarum C^2 *B P*: religio margaritarum C^1/16
aromatum atque C^1 *B P*: aromatumque C^2/18 caveatum C^1 *B P*: om. C^2/duo mercatoria
levia C^1 C^2 *B*: duo levia mercatoria *P*/sine caveis C^1 *B P*: om. C^2/26 lequas C^1 *B P*:
leucas C^2/27 lequas C^2 *B P*: lequas: leucas C^2/quattuor C^1 *B*: quatuor C^2 *P*/29 urget
incolas C^1 *B P*: urget inaestas C^2/30 aestas. Sunt C^1 *B P*: aestas eo quod extra omne
clima Europae ad meridiem sitae sint. Sunt C^2/31 appellant Canarias C^1 *B P*: appellant
eas puto Hesperidas esse Meduseas Canarias C^2//32 - p. 208, 1 eo quod...meridiem C^1
B P: om. C^2/9 Betanchor C^1 *B P*: Bethancor C^2/Catherinae C^2 *B*: Caterinae C^1, Catharinae
P/11 Betanchor C^1 *B P*: Bethancor C^2/12 Lancelotum C^1 C^2 *B*: Lancelotam *P*/13 heres
C^1 C^2 *B*: haeres *P*/17 Tenerifen Alphonsus C^1: Teneriphen Alfonsus C^2 *B P*/24 secutus
C^1 *B P*: sequutus C^2/laevam *P*: levam C^1 C^2 *P*/26 primum secreto C^1 *B P*: primum
tacite C^2/27 apertus mox C^1 *B P*: mox apertis C^2/29 ligure C^2: lygure C^1 *B P*/33
depascebat C^1 C^2: deposcebat *B P*/34 si C^1 C^2 *B*: et si *P*//p. 210, 1 vocitavit C^1 *B P*:
vocavit C^2/8 lequas C^1 *B P*: leucas C^2/14 Ophiram C^1 C^2 *B*: Ophyram *P*/20 planities *P*:
planicies C^1 C^2 *B*/25 gallicis C^1 C^2 *B*: galicis *P*/26 insecuti C^1 *B P*: insequuti C^2/30
quom C^1: quam C^2, quum *B P*/36 tintinnabulum *B*: tintinabulum C^1 C^2 *P*//p. 212, 12
lintribus C^1 *B P*: linthribus C^2/16 esse C^1 C^2 *P*: esse esse *B*/plerasque *B P*: plaerasque
C^1 C^2/25 rettulerunt *corr.*: retulerunt C^1 C^2 *B P*/31 gallinaceos C^2 *B P*: galinaceos C^1//p.
214, 2 nefas C^2 *B P*: nephas C^1/4 gallinas C^2 *B P*: galinas C^1/11 indigenae C^2 *B P*:
indiginae C^1/22 lethaliorem C^1 *P*: letaliorem *B*, loethaliorem C^2/illico C^1 C^2 *P*: ilico
B/26 spitama C^1 C^2 *B*: spithama *P*/29 maturuerunt C^1 *B P*: matuerrunt C^2//p. 216,
3 pillulas C^1 C^2 *B*: pilulas *P*/10 silvestres C^1 C^2: sylvestres *B P*/17 recitasse quoniam C^1
C^2 *B*: recitasse quamvis *P*/18 Christophori C^2 *B P*: Christofori C^1/sphaerae *B*: spherae
C^1 C^2 *P*/22 libri C^1 C^2 *P*: libi *B*/25 gossampii *corr.*: gosampii C^1 C^2 *B P*/29 cinnamomi
corr.: cinamomi C^1 *B P*, cynamomi C^2/30 zingiberim *B P*: zingiverim C^1 C^2/medulla C^2
B P: medula C^1//p. 218, 2 zephyris...ver C^1 *B P*: zephyris propter ver C^2/3 constituens
C^1 *B P*: constituit C^2/7 amicitiae C^2 *B P*: amiciciae C^1/12 abducens C^1 *B P* abduxit
C^2/13 litteris C^1: literis C^2 *B P*/16 reliquave C^1 C^2: reliquaque *B P*/24 supremique *B P*:
supremi C^1 C^2//p. 220, 12 hordeum C^1 C^2 *P*: ordeum *B*/16 duriciei C^2: duricei C^1,
duritiei *B P*/19 sidera C^1 *B P*: sydera C^2/23 autoritate C^2 *B*: auctoritate C^1, authorite
P/24 aggressi *B P*: agressi C^1 C^2/25 tertii scripsi: III C^1 C^2 *P*: IIII *B*/26 Fortunatas C^1
C^2: Fortunatas insulas *B P*/Kalendis C^1 C^2: Calend. *B P*/30 cadente C^1 *B P*: cadene
C^2/31 coepit C^2 *B P*: accepit C^1/33 felix C^1 *B P*: faelix C^2/34 Idibus *P*: Idus C^1 C^2 *B*

p. 222 Sfortiam *corr.*: Sphorciam C^1 B P, om. C^2//p. 222, 6 quadringenta C^1 C^2: quadraginta B P/9 rettulerunt *corr.*: retulerunt C^1 C^2 B P/10 appulsa P: appulsas C^1 C^2 B/22 attingerent P: atingerent C^1 C^2 B/23 laevam P: levam C^1 C^2 B/26 noticia C^1 C^2: notitia B P/27 quod C^1 C^2 B: quo P/31 lequas C^1 B P: leucas C^2//p. 224, 1 a puppi B: appupi C^1, a pupi C^2 P/4 ulla C^2 B P: ula C^1/16 illorum C^1 B P: illlorum C^2/30 appellat C^1 B P: appellant C^2/37 numen C^1 B P: numem C^2/gossipio B P: gosipio C^1 C^2//p. 226, 16 Quaeritando *corr.*: quaesitando C^1 C^2 B P/27 saepenumero C^2 B P: sepenumero C^1/29 glaucae C^2 B P: glauce C^1/32 delicias B P: delitias C^1 C^2/36 illae C^2 B P: ille C^1//p. 228, 6 pedem C^2 B P: pede C^1/8 lintribus P: linthribus C^1 C^2 B/9 anchoras C^1 C^2 B: ancoras P/11 permotus C^1 C^2 P: praemotus B/12 laevaque B P: levaque C^1 C^2/postergabat C^2 B P: post tergabat C^1/15 Madanino C^1 C^2 B: Madannina P/19 rettulit *corr.*: retulit C^1 C^2 B P/28 Madaninoe C^1: Madanino C^2 B, Madaninae P/34 Canibales C^2 B P: Caniballes C^1//p. 230, 13 anchoras C^1 C^2 B: ancoras P/15 quattuor C^1 C^2: quatuor B P/20 Canibales C^2 B P: Caniballes C^1/Guadalupeam C^2 B P: quadalupeam C^1/21 silvas C^1 C^2: sylvas B P/31 adverterant C^1 B P: animadverterant C^2/32 inter eos C^1 C^2 B: inter reos P//p. 232, 3 coopertum C^1 B P: coopertur C^2/strenue C^2 B P: strenne C^1/6 libyci B P: libici C^1, lybici C^2/8 horrore C^2 B P: horore C^1/10 Methymnae P: Methimanae B, Methimane C^1 C^2/13 Africum *corr.*: Aphricum C^1 C^2 B P/15 insulis C^1 B P: in insulis C^2/23 illiderentur C^1 C^2 B: illuderentur P/32 Canibalibus B P canniballibus C^1, cannibalibus C^2//p. 234, 2 Canibalibus B P: canniballibus C^1, cannibalibus C^2/3 inimicitias B P: inimicicias C^1 C^2/4 Canibalium B P: canniballium C^1, cannibalium C^2/5 Canibales B P: canniballes C^1, cannibales C^2/9 interpretes C^2 B P: interpraetes C^1/15 planities P: planicies C^1 C^2 B/16 Canibalium B P: canniballium C^2/21 Canibalibus B P: canniballibus C^1, cannibalibus C^2/Canibalium B P: canniballium C^1, cannibalium C^2/24 infoelici C^1 C^2: infelici B P/35 interpretes B P: interpraetes C^1 C^2/36 hos non B: hos C^1 C^2 P//p. 236, 2 amicitia B P: amicicia C^1 C^2/5 eventum C^1 C^2 B: adventum P/6 interpretes C^2 B P: interpraetes C^1/12 ballistas *corr.*: balistas C^1 C^2 B P/18 rettulerunt C^1 C^2: retulerunt B P/19 sit C^1 B P: sint C^2/22 supellectilia B P: suppellectilia C^1 C^2/combussisse C^2 B P: combusisse C^1/24 rettulit C^1 C^2: retulit B P/29 tyrannos C^2 B P: tirannos C^1/34 solliciti C^1: soliciti C^2 B P//p. 238, 7 rettulit *corr.*: retulit C^1 C^2 B P/valitudine C^1: valetudine C^2 B P/9 consilio C^1 C^2 B: concilio P/14 Canibalibus B P: canniballibus C^1, cannibalibus C^2/Catherinam C^1 C^2: Catharinam B P/17 aspectu C^1 C^2 B: adspectu P/23 Catherina C^1 C^2: Catharina B P/26 aggressa C^2 B P: agressa C^1/33 Catherinam C^1 C^2: Catharinam B P/quattuor C^1 C^2: quatuor B P//p. 240, 6 utrinque C^1 C^2: quinque B P/10 laevam C^1 B P: levam C^2/22 fundalibus *corr.*: fudalibus C^1 C^2 B P/23 Canibales C^2 B P: canniballes C^1/26 amicitiam C^2 B P: amiciciam C^1/30 erat C^1 B P: erant C^2/32 harundineis C^1 C^2 B: arundineis P/37 cacico C^2 B P: cacicco C^1//p. 242, 4 quattuor C^1 C^2: quatuor B P/7 colligebant C^1 C^2 B: collegabant P/8 profunditate C^1 B P: profunditatem C^2/9 dextra C^1 B P: dextera C^2/15 praeposita C^1 C^2 B: proposita P/21 illorum omnium fluminum C^1 C^2 B: illorum fluminum omnium P/24 rettulit *corr.*: retulit C^1 C^2 B P/sphaerae B P: spherae C^1 C^2/34 litterarum C^1: literarum C^2 B P//p. 244, 9 terdecim C^1 C^2 B: tredecim P/14 internicione C^1 B P: internitione C^2/16 syrophoenicibus C^2 B: syrophenicibus C^1 P/18 medulla C^2 B P: medula C^1/19 cinnami C^1 B P: cynnami C^2/autumant C^1 B P: autumnat C^2/30 Ex...1494 C^1 B P: om. C^2/Kalendas *corr.*: Calendas C^1 B P

p. 246, I Phoebaeos *C¹ C² B*: Phoebeos *P*/3 Helisabeth *C¹ C² B*: Elisabeth *P*/5 Federici *C¹ C²*: Foederici, *B*, Frederici *P*/6 litteras *C¹*: literas *C² B P*/15 cotidie *C¹ B*: quotidie *C² P*/19 infoelicem *C¹ C²*: infelicem *B P*/20 Sfortiam *C¹ C² B*: Sphorciam *P*/21 incoeperam *C¹ C² B*: inceperam *P*/22 Federici *C¹ C²*: Foederici *B*, Frederici *P*/23 litterae *C¹*: literae *C² B P*/24 Mai anno 1500 *P*: Mai MDXXIII *C² B*, Mai *C¹*/25 percurrisse *C¹ C² P*: praecurrisse *B*/26 quarto *C¹ B P*: om. *C²*//p. 248, 13 planities *P*: planicies *C¹ C² B*/15 viginti *C¹ C² B*: viginiti *P*/planitiem *P*: planiciem *C¹ C² B*/20 holerum *C¹ C²*: olerum *B P*/25 hortensia *C¹ C² B*: hortentia *P*/36 rettulerunt *corr.*: retulerunt *C¹ C² B P*//p. 250, 4 quattuor *C¹*: quatuor *C² B P*/6 quattuor *C¹* quatuor *C² B P*/16 planitiem *P*: planiciem *C¹ C² B*/planitiei *P*: planiciei *C¹ C² B*/21 Cibavi *C¹ C² B*: Cibavae *P*/29 cotidie *C¹ B P*: quotidie *C²*/33 spacium *C¹ C² B*: spatium *P*//p. 252, 1 quattuor *C¹*: quatuor *C² B P*/3 dietam *C¹ C²*: diaetam *B P*/6 magnifacere *C¹ B P*: magnifare *C²*/10 Hamadriadem *C¹ C² B*: Hamadryadem *P*/13 collegerant *C¹ C² B*: collegerunt *P*/18 rettulit *corr.*: retulit *C¹ C² B P*/25 silvis *C¹ C²*: sylvis *B P*/29 scindatur *C¹ C²*: secetur *B P*/30 quattuor *C¹*: quatuor *C² B P*//p. 254, 2 Cibavi *C¹ C² B*: Cibavae *P*/Kalendis *C¹ C² B*: Calend. *P*/7 septuagesimum *C² B P*: septuagessimum *C¹*/Regum coni.: regii *C¹ C² B P*/8 admonuerant *C¹ C²*: admonuerat *B P*/ut *C¹ B P*: om. *C²*/9 dicioni *C¹ P*: ditioni *C² B*/10 Portugaliae *C¹ C²*: Portugalliae *B P*/16 lequas *C¹ B P* leucas *C²*: Portugalliae *B P*/19 Africae *C¹ B P*: Affricae *C²*/21 Portugalenses *C¹ C²*: Portugallenses *B P*/23 vocitarant *C¹ C² B*: vocitarat *P*/26 Instat *C¹ C²*: constat *B P*/34 Sancti Nicolai *C² B P*: Sancti Michaelis *C¹*/35 lequas *C¹ B P*: leucas *C²*//p. 256, 11 amicitiam *C² B P*: amiciciam *C¹*/Iamaica *B P*: Iamayca *C¹ C²*/13 Chersoneso *corr.*: Chersonesso *C¹ C² B P*/19 Chersonessum *corr.*: Chersonessum *C¹ C² B P*/lequas *C¹ B P*: leucas *C²*/27 laevam *C¹ B P*: levam *C²*/28 passim *C¹ B P*: passuum *C²*/35 casulas *C² B P*: causulas *C¹*//p. 258, 6 Aegyptiis *C² B P*: egyptiis *C¹*/crocodillis *C¹ C²*: crocodilis *B P*/7 crocodillorum *C¹ C²*: crocodilorum *B P*/8 duodeviginti *C¹ B P*: duorum et triginta *C¹*/9 maiores *C¹ C² B*: moiores *P*/12 astricta *C¹ C² B*: adstricta *P*/22 propius *C¹ B P*: proprius *C²*/25 amicitiam ineunt *C² B P*: amiciciam iniunt *C¹*/35 amicitiam *C² B P*: amiciciam *C¹*//p. 260, 3 Almiranto *C² B P*: almirato *C¹*/4 montosa *C¹ B P*: montuosa *C²*/14 aequante *C²*: aequate *C¹*, aequare *B P*/15 laevam ad austrum *B P*: levam ad astrum *C¹ C²*/24 aequora *C¹ B P*: equora *C²*/25 venatorio *C¹ C² B*: venatario *P*/26 grandiori *C¹ B P*: parvae *C²*/32 quom *C¹*: quum *C² B P*/33 conchile *C¹ C²*: conchyle *B P*//p. 262, 9 appellant *C² B P*: appallant *C¹*/quattuor *C¹*: quatuor *C² B P*/11 illautus *C¹ C² B*: illotus *P*/14 Almirantus *C² B P*: almiratus *C¹*/15 cacicum *corr.*: cazicum *C¹ C¹ C² B P*/16 cacicum *corr.*: cazicum *C¹ C² B P*/19 cacichi *corr.*: cazici *C¹ C² B P*/26 laeva *B P*/26 leva *C¹ C²*/adhaerebant *C¹ C² B*: ahdaerebant *P*/28 quattuor *C¹*: quatuor *C² B P*/29 haedos *corr.*: hedos *C¹*, aedos *C²*, hoedos *B P*/33 verrerent *C¹ C²*: verreret *B P*/34 milliaria *C¹ B P*: miliaria *C²*/35 quom *C¹ P*: quum *C² B*/36 milliare *C¹ B P*: miliare *C²*/37 lignandique *C² B P*: lignadique *C¹*//p. 264, 3 silvam *C¹ C²* sylvam *B P*/6 Almirantus *C² B P*: almiratus *C¹*/14 milliaria *C² B P*: miliaria *C¹*/16 planitiem *P*: planiciem *C¹ C² B*/17 unquam *C¹ C² B*: usquam *P*/19 milliare *C¹ B P*: miliare *C¹*/25 silvam *C¹ C²*: sylvam *B P*/32 rettulerunt *corr.*: retulerunt *C¹ B P*, tulerunt *C²*/36 populatissimam *C¹ C²*: populosissimam *B P*//p. 266, 6 coenosa *C²*: caenosa *C¹ B P*/8 conchilia *C¹ C²*: conchylia *B P*/12 millia *C¹ B P*: milia *C²*/21 Africum *C¹ B P*: Affricum *C²*/30 detardarent *C² B P*: detarderent *C¹*/34 posito *C¹ B P*: possito *C²*//p. 268, 4 ex *B P*: om. *C¹ C²*/12 assistit *C²*: asistit *C¹*, adsistit *B P*/28 praemiis *C¹*

B P: premiis *C²*//p. 270, 9 obortis *C¹ C² B*: abortis *P*/15 Aetas *C² B P*: etas *C¹*/16 sepibus *C¹ C²*: saepibus *B P*/sepiunt *C¹ C²*: saepiunt *B P*/21 Iamaicam *P*: Iamaycam *C¹ C² B*/24 laevam *B P*: levam *C¹ C²*/meridionale *C² B P*: meredionale *C²*/26 Kalendas *C¹ C² B*: Calend. *P*/30 valitudo *C¹ C²*: valetudo *B P*/33 valitudinem *C¹ C²*: valetudinem *B P*

I 4

p. 272 ad cardinalem...nepotem *C¹ B P*: om. *C²*//p. 272, 9 huiuscemodi *C¹ C² B*: huiusmodi *P*/18 secuta *C¹ B P*: sequuta *C²*/20 Insularum *C¹ C² B*: insularium *P*/24 rabide *C¹ C² B*: rapide *P*/25 interfecerant *C²*: interficerant *C¹ B P*/28 superiore libro *C¹ B*: superiori libro *P*, superiore capite *C²*/29 amicitiam *C² B P*: amiciciam *C¹*//p. 274, 2 obsessum *C² B P*: obsesum *C¹*/11 amicitiam *C² B P*: amiciciam *C¹*/17 obtruncasset *C² B P*: obtrucasset *C¹*/25 blanditiis *C² B P*: blandiciis *C¹*/31 millia *C¹*: milia *C² B P*/35 commeatus *C² B P*: comeatus *C¹*//p. 276, 2 libro *C¹ B P*: capite *C²*/9 fassus *C¹ B P*: falsus *C²*/12 premebatur *C¹ B P*: praemebatur *C²*/16 huius *C¹ C² P*: huius huius *B*/17 Cibavi *C¹ C² B*: cibavae *P*/22 sciscitabantur *C² B P*: sciscitabatur *C¹*/24 tofi *C¹ C² B*: tophi *P*/30 huiuscemodi *C¹ B P*: huiusmodi *C²*/corinthiaco constari *C¹ C²*: corinthia constari *B P*/32 laevorsum *B P*: levorsum *C¹ C²*/33 tricentarum *C¹ C² B*: trecentarum *P*//p. 278, 3 lapidibus *C¹ C² B*: lipidibus *P*/10 silvas *C¹ C²*: sylvas *B P*/14 Hispalim *C¹ C² B*: hispani *P*/26 obiices *C¹ C² B*: obices *P*//p. 280, 2 impollutum *C¹ C² B*: impolutum *P*/10 oriantur *C¹ C²*: oriuntur *B P*/15 Plerique *B P*: plaerique *C¹ C²*/24 agrestique *C¹ B P*: aggrestique *C²*/25 Caunaboam *B P*: Caunoboam *C²*, Canoboam *C¹*/27 quomodo *B P*: quum *C¹ C²*/29 dicionem *corr.*: ditionem *C¹ C² B P*/praesidia *C² B P*: presidia *C¹*/32 quoto die grassationis *C¹ C²*: quotidie grassatione *B P*//p. 282, 3 sagittis *C¹ C² B*: sagitis *P*/17 commodior *C² B P*: cummodior *C¹*/28 sidera *C¹ B P*: sydera *C²*/30 tipho *C¹ C² B*: typho *P*/31 anchoris *C¹ C² B*: ancoris *P*//p. 284, 1 τυφωνες *scripsi*: tiphones *C¹ C² B*, typhones *P*/7 immo *C¹ C² P*: imo *B*/8 planitiem *P*: planiciem *C¹ C² B*/16 lequas *C¹ B P*: leucas *C²*/17 sexaginta *P*/18 effossos *C¹ B P*: effosos *C²*/21 per sinum persicum *B P*: persinum per siccum *C¹ C²*/24 millia *C¹ B P*: milia *C²*/25 mercennarius *C¹* mercenarius *C² B P*/28 litteras *C¹*: literas *C² B P*/29 peractae *C² B P*: peracte *C¹*/31 fratri *C² B P*: frarri *C¹*

I 5

p. 286 Aragonium *C² B P*: Aragonum *C¹*//p. 286, 1 Bartholomaeus *corr.*: Bartholomeus *C¹ C² B P*/7 milliare *C¹ B P*: miliare *C²*/15 Manicautexius *C¹ C² B*: Manicauexius *P*/19 exegit *C¹ C² B*: exigit *P*/20 vaccinisque *B P*: vacinisque *C¹ C²*/caravelae *B P*: caravellae *C¹ C²*/33 appulsus *P*: apulsus *C¹ C² B*//288, 1 amoenis *C² B*: amenis *C¹ P*/6 vailtudinarios *C¹*: valetudinarios *C² B P*/7 inceperant *C¹ B P*: incoeperant *C²*/caravelas *B P*: caravellas *C¹ C²*/12 lequas *C¹ B P*: leucas *C²*/milliaria *C¹ B P*: miliaria *C²*/17 laevorsum *C¹ B P*: levorsum *C²*/18 silvas *C¹ C²*: sylvas *B P*/19 preciosae *C² B*: preciose *C¹ P*/24 Naibenses *C¹ C² B*: Naibanses *P*/27 vocatur *C² P*: vocat *C²*, om. *B*/lequas *C¹ B P*: leucas *C²*//p. 290, 3 cannabi *corr.*: canabi *C¹ C² B P*/8 lequas *C¹ B P*: leucas *C²*/10 dioeceses *C²*: dioceses *C¹ B P*/cannabi *corr.*: canabi *C¹ C² B P*/11 lino *P*: ligno *C¹ C² B*/12 aliis aliis *C² P*: alii alii *C¹ B*/15 Beechium Anacauchea *corr.*: Beechium

475

Anachaucoam C^1 C^2, Beuchium Anacauchoam B, Beuchium Anachaucoam P/20 femoralibus C^1 B P: foemoralibus C^2/35 planitiem P: planiciem C^1 C^2 B/p. 292, 1 troicus C^2 B: toicus C^1 P/harundineus C^1 B: arundineus P, harundienus C^2/4 illae $corr.$: ille C^1 C^2 B P/6 quattuor C^1 B: quatuor C^2 P/10 valitudinarios C^1: valetudinarios C^2 B P/11 incepta C^1 B P: incoepta C^2/16 valitudinarios C^1: valetudinarios C^2 B P/21 Catherinam C^1 C^2: Catharinam B P/Catherina C^1 C^2: Catharina B P/22 milliaria C^1 B P: miliaria C^2/14 planitie P: planicie C^1 C^2 B/27 millia C^1 B P: milia C^2/37 provinciae C^1 C^2: regionis B P//p. 294, 6 reliquisve C^1 C^2: reliquisque B P/11 congressi C^1 C^2 P: ingressi B/14 cepitque B P: coepitque C^1 C^2/15 quattuordecim C^1: quatuordecim C^2 B P/17 reliquosve C^1 C^2: reliquosque B P/21 millium C^1 B P: milium C^2/23 sidera C^1 B P: sydera C^2/27 sedent C^1 C^2 B: sedant P/28 astruant C^1 C^2 B: adstruant P/32 solliciti $corr.$: soliciti C^1 C^2 B P/35 incedebant C^2 B: incidebant C^1 P//;. 296, 1 Beechius Anacauchea $corr.$: Beechiusan Acauchea C^1 C^2, Beechius Anacauchoa B P/11 Anacaona B P: Anaccaona C^1 C^2/12 Beechii Anacaucheae $corr.$: Bechii Aunachauchoae C^1 C^2 P, Beuchii Anacauchoae B/13 benivolentiam C^1 B P: benevolentiam C^2/18 crocodillisque C^1 C^2 P: crocodilisque B/simillimos C^1 C^2: similimos B P/29 quam uno C^1 B P: quam C^2//p. 298, 3 si C^1 B P: sic C^2/9 ad regiamque C^1 C^2 B: ad regiamve P/Beechii Anacaucheae $corr.$: Beuchii Anachaucheae C^1, Beuchii Anacaucheae C^2, Beuchii Anacauchoae B P/11 caravelam $corr.$: caravellam C^1 C^2 B P/12 se C^1 B P: ad se C^2/14 Beechii Anacaucheae $corr.$: Beuchii Anachaucheae C^1, Beuchii Anacaucheae C^2, Beuchii Anacauchoae B P/16 Caunaboae B P: Caunaboe C^1 C^2/18 millia C^1 B P: milia C^2/22 attinentia C^1 C^2 B: attinentes P/24 Ioannis C^2: Io. C^1 P, Ioannes B/25 Baptista C^1 C^2 B: Babtista P/26 quidquid C^1 B P: quicquid C^2/31 caelant C^2 B: celant C^1 P/34 sedilibus B: sedibus C^1 C^2 P/35 quattuordecim C^1: quatuordecim C^2 B P/36 quattuor C^1: quatuor C^2 B P//p. 300, 1 neti C^1 B P: necti C^2/12 pulsantur C^1 B P: pulsant C^2/14 puppim B: pupim C^1 C^2, puppi P/18 antennis B P: antenis C^1 C^2/23 laevam C^1 B P: levam C^2/26 Beechium Anacaucheam C^1 C^2: Beuchium Anacauchoam B P/29 Roldanum C^2 P: Rodalnum C^1 B/33 Roldani C^2 P: Rodalni C^1 B/p. 302, 1 ditionarii C^2 B P: dictionariis C^1/2 lequas B P: leuquas C^1, leucas C^2/4 Ciguavos $corr.$: Ciguaios C^1 C^2 B P/5 Maiobanexium B P: Maiobannexium C^1 C^2/8 pulchra C^2: pulcra C^1 B P/planities P: planicies C^1 C^2 B/11 planitiem P: planiciem C^1 C^2 B/14 rettulitque $corr.$: retulitque C^1 C^2 B P/17 facinorosorum C^2 B P: facinorosum C^1/18 Maiobanexius B P: Maiobannexius C^1 C^2/21 insularium C^1 C^2: insularum B P/milliare B P: miliare C^1 C^2/duodecimum C^1 B P: duodecim C^2/26 infoelicem C^1 C^2 P: infelicem B/30 secutique C^1 B P: sequutique C^2//p. 304, 1 Ximenez C^1 P: Ximenex C^2, Ximenus B/10 subornaverant C^1 C^2 B: subornaverunt P/17 libri C^1 B P: capituli C^2

I 6

p. 306 ad...nepotem C^1: ad eundem cardinalem Ludovicum Aragonium B P, om. C^2//p. 306, 4 piratas C^1 B P: pyratas C^2/6 laevorsum B: levorsum C^1 C^2 P/7 occurrit C^1 C^2 P: incurrit B/12 caravelis B P: caravellis C^1 C^2/13 aequinoctialem C^1 C^2 B: equinoctialem P/14 reperiret C^1 C^2: reperirent B P/16 terdecim C^1 C^2: tredecim B P/19 Portugalenses C^1 C^2 B: Portugallenses P/21 mundantur C^1 C^2 B: mundatur P/22 africum C^1 (alibi): apricum C^1 B P, affricum C^2/23 malachiis C^1 C^2 P: malaciis B/25 crepebant C^1 C^2 B: crepabant P/27 rettulit $corr.$: retulit C^1 C^2 B P/30 actis C^1 C^2 P: actus B/32 flatu C^1 B P: flactu C^2/secutus C^1 B P: sequutus P/33 paralleli P: paralelli

C^1 C^2 B//p. 308, 1 se C^1 C^2 B: *om.* P/3 malachiis C^1 C^2 P: malaciis B/6 Kalendas C^2: Calendas C^1 B P/7 prae C^2: pre C^1 B P/12 attigerunt C^1 C^2 B: attigerant P/21 Puntam C^2: Putam C^1 B P/Arenalis C^1 C^2 B: Arenalem P/26 quattuor C^1: quatuor C^2 B P/29 scissis C^1 B P: scisis C^2/31 paralleli P: paralelli C^1 C^2 B/32 convallium C^1 B P: convalium C^2/34 parallelis P: paralellis C^1 C^2 B//p. 310, 8 tintinnabula B P: tintinabula C^1 C^2/21 adeunt C^1 B P: addeunt C^1/23 puppi B P: pupi C^1 C^2/28 advolarunt C^1 C^2: avolarunt B P/p. 312, 3 ori C^1 C^2 B: ori Draconis P/6 sinum ipsum C^1 C^2: sinum B P/9 percunctanti C^1 C^2 B: percontanti P/rettulerunt *corr.*: retulerunt C^1 C^2 B P/10 lequas C^1 B P: leucas C^2/11 quattuor C^1 C^2 P: quatuor B/17 rettulerunt *corr.*: retulerunt C^1 C^2 B P/26 quattuor C^1 P: quatuor C^2 B/hominibus C^1 B P: homnibus C^2/36 cacichi C^1 C^2: cacici B P//p. 314, 4 confluunt C^1 C^2 B: canfluunt P/10 immo C^1 C^2 P: imo B/21 grandaevus C^2: grandevus C^1 B P/23 sphaericam *corr.*: sphericam C^1 C^2 B P//p. 316, 2 caetera B P: caeteri C^1 C^2/8 silvestribus C^1 C^2: sylvestribus B P/15 pelagi C^2 B P: pellagi C^1/22 regiunculae C^1 C^2 B: regiumculae P/milliarium C^1 B P: miliarium C^2/23 lequas C^1 B P: leucas C^2/28 lequarum C^1 B P: leucarum C^2/p. 318, 9 crepusculo C^1 C^2 P: corpusculo B/14 sphaericum B: sphericum C^1 C^2 P/17 appensi C^1 C^2 B: apensi P/regionem C^1 B P: regonem C^2//p. 320, 6 nonagesimi C^1 C^2 P: nonagesimi anni B/8 absinthii C^2: absinthi C^1 B P/omnia C^1 C^2 P: omnibus B

I 7

p. 322 ad eundem cardinalem Ludovicum Aragonium B P, *sed om.* C^1 C^2//p. 322, 6 incoepit C^2: incaepit C^1, incepit B P/17 versare B P vesare C^1 C^2//p. 324, 6 millibus B: milibus C^1 C^2 P/7 inimicitias B P: inimicicias C^1 C^2/9 planitiem P: planiciem C^1 C^2 B/10 Ciguavorum P: Ciguaiorum C^1 C^2 B/18 planitie P: planicie C^1 C^2 B/19 silvis C^1 C^2: sylvis B P/23 summo C^2 B P: sumo C^1/26 telorum C^1 B P: tellorum C^2/31 silvas C^1 C^2: sylvas B P//p. 326, 1 silvis C^1 C^2: sylvas B P/2 longae hastae C^2 B P: longe haste C^1/4 silvis C^1 C^2: sylvis B P/9 castra metatus C^2 B P: castramentatus C^1/16 silvis C^1 C^2: sylvis B P/19 silvis C^1 C^2: sylvis B P/20 plerosque B P: plaerosque C^1 C^2/22 silvas C^1 C^2: sylvas B P/25 amicitiam B P: amiciciam C^1 C^2/28 sumeres C^2 B P: summeres C^1/deprehensus C^1 C^2 B: depraehensis P//p. 328, 2 esse iudico C^1 B P: esse se iudicare C^2/4 amicitiam B P: amiciciam C^1 C^2/27 quoat C^1 B P: quoad C^2/28 immo C^1 C^2: imo B P/32 Ciguavensibus *corr.*: Ciguaiensibus C^1 C^2 B P//p. 330, 6 alia C^1 C^2: alii B P/10 agebatur B: agebat C^1 C^2, gebatur P/19 coenosae C^1 C^2 P: caenosae B/28 ciguavo P: ciguaio C^1 C^2 B//p. 332, 5 quom C^1: quum C^2, cum B P/8 dicioni C^1: ditioni C^2 B P/9 obiice C^1 C^2: obice B/redderet B P: rederet C^1 C^2/12 solum ducens C^1 C^2: secum ducens B P/15 Ciguavos *corr.*: ciguaios C^1 C^2 B P/16 clementiae C^1 B P: claementiae C^2/29 adductos B P: aductos C^1 C^2/31 tulisse B P: tullisse C^1 C^2/33 characteribus P: caracteribus C^1/litteras C^1: literas C^2 B P//p. 334, 1 pararet C^2 B P: pareret C^1/2 tutaretur C^1 B P: tutarentur C^2/3 armatos C^1 C^2 B: armato P/4 apprehendit C^2 B: appraehendit C^1 P

III 4

p. 336, 2 parumper C^1 C^2 B: paruper P/3 et C^1 B P: *om.* C^2/7 quattuor C^1 B: quatuor C^2 P/9 praehendit C^1 C^2: prehendit B P/10 appulsus C^2 P: apulsus C^1 B/27 quod nec C^1 C^2: ut nec B P/28 potentiam C^1 B P: pontentiam C^2/31 tintinnabula B P: tintinabula C^1 C^2//p. 338, 1 genere quodam B P: generi cuidam C^1 C^2/3 gossampina B P: gosampina C^1 C^2/4 intexta C^2: intesta C^1 B P/5 praehenderunt C^1 C^2 P: prehenderunt B/7 benivolos C^1 C^2 B: benevolos P/14 obstipo B P: obstippo C^1 C^2/18 tractu C^1 B P: tractatu C^2/21 postferendam C^2 B P: postferandam C^1/24 ilicetis B P: illicetis C^1, illignetis C^2/25 septem C^1 B P: septam C^2/26 dactiliferae C^1 C^2: dactyliferae B P/27 labruschis C^1 C^2: labruscis B P/32 mirabolanos C^1 C^2 P: myrobalanos B/33 checubos C^1 C^2: chebulos B P/34 ages B P: aies C^1 C^2/batatas C^1 C^2: battatas B P/35 tigres C^1 C^2 P: tigrides B//p. 340, 7 Agathyrsos B: Agatirsos C^1 C^2 P/inficiunt C^1 C^2 P: infiunt B/8 plerique B: plaerique C^1 C^2 P/9 appetitu B: a petitu C^1 C^2 P/10 defluebant C^1 C^2: fluebant B P/14 Kalendas corr.: Calendas C^1 C^2 B P/15 lequas C^1 B P: leucas C^2/ostium B: hostium C^1 C^2 P/18 fuisse vim C^1 C^2: vim fuisse B P/19 lequas C^1 B P: leucas C^2/23 lequarum C^1 B P: leucarum C^1/26 femore B: foemore C^1 C^2 P/27 plerisque B: plaerisque C^1 C^2 P/crocodillorum C^1 C^2 P: crocodilorum B/29 dedit coni.: dedi C^1 C^2 B P/30 fultam C^2 P: fultum C^1 B/squalidis C^1 C^2 B: squallidis P/33 cacicum B P: cacichum C^1 C^2/34 saccus C^1 C^2 B: sacchus P/36 cupram C^1 B P: capram C^2/37 chiuys C^1 C^2: chyuis B P//p. 342, 2 quattuor C^1 P: quatuor C^1 P/4 quattuor C^1 P: quatuor C^2 B/lequas C^1 B P: leucas C^2/5 terdecim C^1 C^2 B: tredecim P/6 praehendit C^1 C^2 P: prehendit B/praeditas C^2 B: preditas C^1 P/7 aemulantium B: emulantium C^1 C^2 P/8 lequas C^1 B P: leucas C^2/9 lequarum C^1 B P: leucarum C^1/spacio C^1 C^2 P: spatio B/16 valitudinem C^1 C^2: valetudinem B P/18 Mirabolanus C^1 C^2: Myrobalanus B P/23 commercia corr.: comertia C^1 B P, commertia C^2/25 benivolentiam C^1 C^2 P: benevolentiam B/28 suspicati quod C^1 C^2: suspicat quod B P//p. 344, 9 refluxu C^2 B P: reflexu C^1/11 quae C^1 B P: quam C^2/18 cercopitheco B P: cercopiteco C^1 C^2/suspensus C^1 B P: suspenssus C^2/sese C^1 C^2 P: se B/22 cercopithecus B P: cercopitecus C^1 C^2/23 cercopitheco B P: cercopiteco C^1 C^2/24 cepitque corr.: coepitque C^1 C^2 B P/28 cercopitheco B P: cercopiteco C^1 C^2/29 cercopithecus B P: cercopitecus C^1 C^2/31 cercopithecus P: cercopitecus C^1 C^2 B/34 silvaeque C^1 C^2: sylvaeque B P/35 lequas C^1 B P: leucas C^2//p. 346, 1 lequas C^1 B P: leucas C^2/2 quattuor C^1 B: quatuor C^2 P/20 commercia B: comertia C^1 P, commertia C^2/27 lequas C^1 B P: leucas C^2/29 expuentes C^2: espuentes C^1 B P/33 commercium corr.: commertium C^1 C^2 B P//p. 348, 1 ballistae, corr.: balistae C^1 C^2 B P/2 commerciantur corr.: commertiantur C^2, comertiantur C^1 B P/4 conchilia C^1 C^2 P: conchylia B/7 Durubba C^1 C^2: Duribba B P/9 Embigar C^1 C^2 B: Embigaar P/12 lequarum C^1 B P: leucarum C^2/lequas C^1 B P: leucas C^2/13 Nicuesae C^1 B P: Nicuessae C^2/discursu C^1 B P: discurssu C^2/15 lequas C^1 B P: leucas C^2/22 tegunt C^1 B P: teguntur C^2/25 crocodillis C^1 C^2 P: crocodilis B/28 crocodillo C^2: crocodilo C^1 B P/rettulerunt C^1: retulerunt C^2 B P/31 aquarum C^1 B P: aquatum C^2//p. 350, 1 anchoris C^1 C^2 B: ancoris P/6 lequas C^1 B P: leucas C^2/10 Bartholomaeum P: Bartholomeum C^1 C^2 B/15 quidam C^1 C^2 P: om. B/20 dicionis C^1 B P: ditionis C^2/23 ditiorem B P: ditius C^1 C^2/30 coeperant B: cpaeerant C^1 P, ceperant C^2//p. 352, 4 benigne C^1 B P: begnine C^2/11 praehendere C^1 C^2 P: prehendere B/12 viribus B P: ubi C^1 C^2/14 appulsi C^2: apulsi C^1 B P/23 coniectetur C^1 C^2 P: coniectet B/25 cuna C^1 C^2: cunis B P/29 mare C^1 C^2 P: mari B/32 lequas C^1 B P: leucas C^2//p. 354, 7 lequarum C^1 B P: leucarum C^2/Cerabaroo C^1 C^2: Cerabaro B P/27 Adriatico B P: Adriaco C^1 C^2/28 Portugalenses C^1 C^2 P: Portugallenses B/29 ac C^1 C^2 B: ad P/33 in C^1 B P: i C^2/34 Apennini B: Apenini C^1 C^2 P/variis C^1 B P: varii C^2//p. 356, 5 ea primus C^1 C^2 B: ea omnium primus P/9 occidentem C^1 C^2: occidentem usque B P/10 corporis C^1 C^2 B: corporis quemadmodum P/14 Graeciam C^2: Graetiam C^1 B P/16 Meotide C^1 C^2

P: Maeotide *B*/28 hunc *B P*: hoc *C¹ C²*/30 Nunez *C¹ B P*: Nunnez *C²*/33 aditibus *C¹ B P*: additibus *C²*/34 intervallis *C²*: intevallis *C¹ B P*//p. 358, 4 angustis *P*: angustiis *C¹ C² B*/12 appellant *C¹ C² B*: ap appellant *P*/13 ostia *B*: hostia *C¹ C² P*/15 lamas *B*: lammas *C¹ C² P*/16 cenagales *C²* cenegales *C¹ B P*/24 balbutiunt *C¹ C²*: pueriliter sentiunt *B P*/28 crocodillorum *C¹ C²*: crocodilorum *B P*/34 sint *C¹ B P*: sin *C²*/35 esse eos *C¹ C² P*: eos esse *B*//p. 360, 1 praedicant *C¹ B P*: predicat *C²*/auro *C¹ C² B*: auri *P*/3 asportent *C¹ C² B*: absportent *P*/13 pulchre *corr.*: pulcre *C¹ C² B P*/16 Cumananus *C¹ C² B*: Cumanus *P*/19 topazios *B*: topacios *C¹ P*, topatios *C²*/21 annulatos *C¹ B P*: annullatos *C²*/23 quando *C² B P*: quado *C²*/27 suffumigationes *C¹ B P*: suffumigatoines *C²*/p. 362, I Aria *corr.*: Ariae *C¹ C² B P*/2 plerique *corr.*: plaerique *C¹ C²*, quidam *B P*/pullulant *C²*: pululant *C¹ B P*/3 cotidie *C²*: cottidie *C¹ B P*

BIBLIOGRAPHY

Compiled by
SIMONETTA CONTI

Since the body of studies concerning Peter Martyr d'Anghiera and his work is very large, and much scholarship, by both Italian and foreign authors, has been devoted to him, the reader is directed to the following volumes for more complete bibliography:

— *Pietro Martire d'Anghiera nella storia e nella cultura.* Secondo Convegno Internazionale di Studi Americanistici (Genova-Arona, 16-19 October 1978). Genoa: AISA, 1980.

— The bibliographic appendix compiled by J.H. Sinclair in the 1944 edition of the *Decades* by J. Asensio Torres (1st ed. 1892), which includes editions and translations since 1504.

As for the works of Peter Martyr and studies of them, other than those cited in the appendices, we list a few recent and easily available editions and some of the more important criticism.

GAFFAREL, P. ed. "Première décade du *De Orbe novo* de Pierre Martyr d'Anghiera." *Revue de Géographie* 30 (Paris: 1892): 444-53; 31 (1892): 49-54, 121-26, 205-18, 298-304, 376-80, 446-50; 32 (1893): 56-63, 131-36, 212-15, 296-301, 379-82, 464-67; 33 (1893): 62-67. The same edition is available in an off-print, Paris: Juin, 1893.

GAFFAREL, P. and F. LOUVOT. "Lettres de Pierre Martyr Anghiera, relative aux découvertes maritimes des Espagnols et de Portugais." *Revue de Géographie* 20 (Paris, 1884): 458-66; (1885): 59-64, 143-48, 207-214, 302-8, 385-91, 464-69; (1886): 65-70.

GAFFAREL P., trans. *Décades,* by Peter Martyr [French translation]. Paris: Leroux, 1907 [755 pages].

Mc NUTT, F.A., ed. *De Orbe Novo,* by Peter Martyr. New York: Putnam and Sons, 1912.

CELOTTI, T., trans. *Il Nuovo Mondo* by Peter Martyr [Italian translation]. Milan: Alpes, 1930 [338 pages]. Republished Milan: Ist. Ed. It., 1958 [271 pages].

PETER MARTYR of Anghiera. *Décadas del Nuevo Mundo* [adapted from the Asensio edition of 1892]. Buenos Aires: Bajel, 1944.

LÓPEZ DE TORO, J., ed. *Epistolario,* by Peter Martyr. 4 vols. Documentos inéditos para la Historia de España. Madrid: Impr. Gongora, 1955-57.

O'GORMAN, E., ed. *Décades del Nuevo Mundo,* by Peter Martyr. Mexico: Porrúa, 1964.

KLINGELHÖFER, H., trans. *Acht Dekaden über die neue Welt,* by Peter Martyr [German translation]. 2 vols. Darmstadt: 1972-73.

GIL, J. and C. VARELA. *Cartas de particulares a Colón y Relaciones coetáneas,* by Peter Martyr. Madrid: Alianza Editorial, 1984.

AGOSTO, A. "I documenti riguardanti la Spagna dei tempi di Pietro Martire d'Anghiera nell'Archivio di Stato di Genova." In *Pietro Martire d'Anghiera nella storia e nella cultura.* 447-52.

ALEGRÍA, R.E. "Pedro Martir de Anglería y otros." Revista Española de antropología americana (Madrid: 1978): 171-79.

Mc ALISTER, L.N. *Dalla scoperta alla conquista. Spagna e Portogallo nel Nuovo Mondo.* Bologna: Il Mulino, 1986.

ARMILLAS VICENTE, J.A. "Aragón visto por un humanista: Pedro Martir de Anglería." *Estudios* (Madrid: 1974): 25-39.

ASENSIO TORRES, J. *Fuentes históricas sobre Colón y América.* 4 vols. Madrid: Impr. F. Sales, 1892.

BALLESTEROS GAIBROIS, M. *La nouvedad indiana.* Madrid: Alhambra, 1987.

BERNAIS, J. *Petrus Martyr Anglerius und sein Opus epistolarum.* Strasburg: 1891.

BOSCOLO, A. "Pietro Martire d'Anghiera Consigliere delle Indie e Abate di Giamaica." In *Pietro Martire d'Anghiera nella storia e nella cultura.* 143-47.

BOSIO, B. "L'impresa militare di Carlo VIII in Italia secondo l'epistolario di Pietro Martire d'Anghiera ed altri autori." In *Pietro Martire d'Anghiera nella storia e nella cultura.* 343-446.

BRANDI, K. *Carlo V.* Turin: Einaudi, 1961.

CANTÙ, F. "Ideologia e storiografia in Pietro Martire d'Anghiera: rapporti fra vecchio e nuovo mondo." In *Pietro Martire d'Anghiera nella storia e nella cultura.* 225-39.

CASTELLANO, F. "Accuse di falso a Pietro Martire d'Anghiera." In *Pietro Martire d'Anghiera nella storia e nella cultura.* 541-48.

CASTILLO MATHIEU, N. "El periodista de la conquista." *Boletín cultural y bibliográfico* 16.6 (Bogotá: 1979): 64-71.

CIAMPI, I. "Le fonti storiche del Rinascimento: Pietro Martire d'Anghiera." *Nuova Antologia* 30 (Florence: 1875).

CRO, S. "La utopía cristiano-social en el Nuevo Mundo (Pedro Martir, Las Casas, Vasco de Quiroga, los Jesuitas en Paraguay)." *Annales de Literatura Hispano-americana* 6.7 (1978): 87-129.

DAMONTE, M. "Pietro Martire d'Anghiera e l'umanesimo spagnolo." In *Pietro Martire d'Anghiera nella storia e nella cultura.* 175-86.

DELLA CORTE, F. "I Carmina di Pietro Martire." In *Pietro Martire d'Anghiera nella storia e nella cultura.* 183-94.

DELLA CORTE, F. "Pietro Martire d'Anghiera e il Cantalicio *preceptores publici* a Rieti." In *Letteratura e Filologia, Studi in onore di C.F. Goffis.* Foggia: 1985.

DELLA CORTE, F. "Un poeta alla Corte d'Isabella." *Columbeis II* (Genoa: 1987): 231-41.

FERRO, G. "Interessi geografici nell'opera di Pietro Martire d'Anghiera." *Bollettino della Società Geografica Italiana* (Rome: 1981): 329-40.

FOSSATI RAITERI, S. "Una fonte di informazione di Pietro Martire: gli ambasciatori alla corte di Spagna." In *Pietro Martire d'Anghiera nella storia e nella cultura.* 469-78.

FUETER, E. *Storia della storiografia moderna*. Milan and Naples: Ricciardi, 1975.

GAZZERO RIGHI, M.L. "L'Opus epistolarum di Pietro Martire d'Anghiera visto alla luce della critica tedesca della fine del XIX secolo." In *Pietro Martire d'Anghiera nella storia e nella cultura*. 261-85.

GERBI, A. *La natura delle Indie Nove. Da Cristoforo Colombo a Gonzalo Fernández de Oviedo*. Milan and Naples: Ricciardi, 1975.

GERIGK, J. *Das Opus epistolarum des Petrus Martyr, ein Beitrag zur Kritik der Quellen des ausgehenden 15. und beginnenden 16. Jahrhunderts*. Braunsberg: Druck der Ermlaendischen Zeitungs, und Verlagsdruckerei, 1881.

GIL, J. "Los humanistas españoles ante el Descubrimiento." *Humanismo y Descubrimiento* (Granada: 1982).

GIL, J. "Pedro Martir de Anglería intéprete de la cosmografía colombina." *Annuario de Estudios Americanos* 39 (Seville: 1982): 487-502.

GIUNTA, F. "Pietro Martire d'Anghiera e le guerre d'Italia." In Pietro Martire d'Anghiera nella storia e nella cultura. 295-319.

HARRISSE, H. *Bibliotheca Americana Vetustissima. A Description of Works Relating to America between the Years 1492 and 1551*. 2 vols. New York: Philes, 1866.

HEIDENHEIMER, H. *Petrus Martyr Alerius und sein Opus epistolarum. Ein Beitrag zur Quellenkunde des Zeitalters der Renaissance und der Reformation*. Berlin.

HUMBOLDT, H. v. *Kritische Untersuchungen ber die historische Entwicklung der geographischen Kenntnisse von der neuen Welt und die Fortchritte der nautischen Astronomie in dem 15. und 16. Jahrhundert*. Berlin: 1863.

LUNARDI, E. "Contributi alla biografia di Pietro Martire d'Anghiera." In *Pietro Martire d'Anghiera nella storia e nella cultura*. 3-62.

LUNARDI, E. "Dal latino di Pietro Martire alcune precisazioni sulle vicende colombiane." *Colombeis II* (Genoa: 1987): 243-59.

LUNARDI, E. "La rivelazione del Mondo Nuovo è in Pietro Martire d'Anghiera." In *Atti del III Convegno Internazionale di Studi Colombiani*. 483-96. Genoa: 1979.

LUNARDI, E. "Pietro Martire d'Anghiera: il primo americanista nella storia e nella cultura del suo tempo." *Terra ameriga* no. 37-40 (Genoa: 1976): 9-20.

MAGIONCALDA, E. "Notizie sulla *cucina indigena* al tempo della scoperta (Pietro Martire, Dec. I, 1-7; III, 4)." *Columbeis II* (Genoa: 1987): 261-266.

MARIEJOL, H. *Un lettré italien à la cour d'Espagne (1488-1526). Pierre Martyr d'Anghiera, sa vie et ses oeuvres*. Paris: Hachette et Cie, 1887.

MAYNARD, T. "Peter Martyr of Anghiera, Humanist and Historian." *Catholic Historical Review* 16 (New York: 1930-31): 435-448.

MAZZACANE, R. "Mare clausum: Pietro Martire d'Anghiera e l'accenno alla partizione dell'oceano (Dec. I, 3; II, 8)." *Columbeis II* (Genoa: 1987): 267-75.

MENÉNDEZ PELAYO, M. *Historia de las ideas estéticas*, vol. 7. Madrid: 1927.

MENÉNDEZ PELAYO, M. "Los historiadores de Colón." In *Obras completas*, vol. 8. Madrid: CSIC, 1942.

MESEGUER FERNÁNDEZ, J. "El arzobispo Cisneros y la Iglesia misionera en América (1500-1512)." *Archivio Ibero-Americano* 45 (Madrid: 1985).

MESSEDAGLIA, L. "Pietro Martire d'Anghiera e le sue notizie sul mais e su altri prodotti naturali d'America." In *Atti de R. Istituto Veneto di Scienze Lettere e Arti*, vol. 90. 293-346. Padua: 1930.

O'GORMAN, E. *Cuatro historiadores de Indias, siglo XVI. Pedro Martir de Anglería, Gonzalo Fernández de Oviedo y Valdes, Fray B. de las Casas, Joseph de Acosta*. Mexico: Secretaría de Educación Pública, 1972.

DE LAS N. OLMEDILLAS GÓMEZ, M. *Pedro Martir de Anglería y su ideologia exoticista. Exoticismo americanista*. Madrid: Facultad de Filosofia y Letras, 1961.

DE LAS N. OLMEDILLAS GÓMEZ, M. *Pedro Martir de Anglería*. Madrid: 1974.

PENNESI, G. "Pietro Martire d'Anghiera e le sue relazioni sulle scoperte oceaniche." In *Raccolta Colombiana*, pt. 5, vol. 2. 7-109. Rome: 1894.

PÉREZ EMBID, F. "Pedro Martir de Anglería, historiador del descubrimiento de América." *Anuario de Estudios Americanos* 32 (Seville: 1975): 205-15.

PONTE, G. "Pietro Martire d'Anghiera scrittore." *La Rassegna della Letteratura Italiana* 73 (Rome: 1979): 5-27.

PRESCOTT, W.H. *History of the conquest of Mexico, with a Preliminary View of the Ancient Mexican Civilization, and the Life of the Conqueror, Hernando Cortés*. London: 1857.

RAMOS PÉREZ, D. "El inicio de la historiografía americanista y el lugar donde se llevó a cabo: la datación del comienzo de las décadas de Pedro Martir de Anglería." In *Scritti in onore del Prof. P. E. Taviani*, vol. 3. 267-285. Genoa: ECIG, 1986.

RIBER, L. *El humanista Pedro Martir de Anglería*. Barcelona: Barna, 1964.

RICO, F. "Il nuovo mondo di Nebrija e Colombo. Note sulla geografia umanistica in Spagna e sul contesto intelletuale della scoperta dell'America." In *Vestigia. Studi in onore di G. Billanovich*, vol. 2. 576-606. Rome: 1984.

ROMEO, R. *Le scoperte americane nella coscienza italiana del Cinquecento*. Milan and Naples: Ricciardi, 1954.

SALAS, A.M. *Tres cronistas de Indias. Pedro Martir, Oviedo, Las Casas*. Mexico: 1959.

SANTI BARBERINI, E. "Un particolare aspetto del contributo di Pietro Martire d'Anghiera attraverso le sue opere, alla conoscenza del *Mondo Nuovo*." In *Pietro Martire d'Anghiera nella storia e nella cultura*. 195-218.

SCHUMAECHER, H.A. *Petrus Martyr, der Geschichtsschreiber des Weltmeeres. Eine Studie*. New York: E. Steiger, 1879.

SINCLAIR, H. "Bibliografía de Pedro Martir de Anglería." *Revista Chilena de historia y geografía* 68 (Santiago, Chile: 1931): 186-219.

SKELTON, R. and G.B. PARKS, ed. *P. Martire d'Anghiera. Summario de la generale historia de le Indie Occidentali*, vol. 3. 37-61. Amsterdam: Theatrum Orbis Terrarum, 1967.

SORANZO, G. "Pietro Martire d'Anghiera, *laudator* di Re Ferdinando e di Isabella, nel suo Epistolario." In *Fernando el Católico. Pensamiento politico, politica internacional y religiosa*. 88ff. V Congreso Historico de la Corona de Aragón. Zaragoza: 1955.

TAVIANI, P.E. *Cristoforo Colombo. La Genesi della grande scoperta*. 2 vols. Novara: Istituto Geografico De Agostini, 1980.

TAVIANI, P.E. *I viaggi di Colombo. La grande scoperta*. 2 vols. Novara: Istituto Geografico De Agostini, 1984.

THACHER, J.B. *Christopher Columbus. His Life, His Work, His Remains*, vol. 1. 3-110. New York: 1903.

VARELA, C. *Cristóbal Colón. Textos y documentos completos*. Madrid: Alianza Editorial, 1982.

WAGNER, R. "Peter Martyr and His Works." *Proceedings of the American Antiquarian Society* 56 (Worchester, MA: 1946): 239-88.

INDICES

INDEX OF NAMES

CEMACO: 25, 111

CEMPOAL: 205

CENET, MARCHESA of, *see* Mendoza, Mencia of

CERES: 61

CHARLES, prince (then Emperor Charles V): 26-32, 123, 131, 161, 389-91, 393, 395, 401-4, 420, 431, 433, 440

CHARLES VIII [king of France]: 19-21, 35, 41, 43, 45, 49, 51, 71, 77

CISNEROS, FRANCISCO JIMENEZ DE [archbishop of Toledo]: 10, 21, 69, 384, 418, 439

CLEMENT VIII, pope: 439

CODRO: 187

CLOELIA: 242-3

COLMENARES, ENRIQUE DE: 26, 123

COLOMBO, BARTHOLOMEW: 201, 203, 223, 289, 291, 353, 411, 427, 437, 442, 444, 446-7

COLOMBO, CHRISTOPHER: *see* Columbus

COLOMBO, DIEGO: 263, 267, 273, 277

COLOMBO, FERNANDO: 427

COLUMBUS, CHRISTOPHER: 5-7, 9, 11, 14, 19-24, 35, 37, 39, 41, 43, 47, 49, 51, 53, 55, 61, 71-2, 79, 83, 105, 201-5, 211, 221, 223, 251, 253, 277, 283, 311, 339, 341, 351, 353, 355, 357, 379, 381, 383, 392, 395, 397, 399-401, 407-8, 410-15, 421-30, 434-5, 437-9, 441-7

COMOGRO: 204

CÓRDOBA, bishop of, *see* Manrique, Alonso

CORSI, GIOVANNI: 26, 125

CORTÉS, HERNÁN: 27, 29-32, 137, 153, 161, 165, 173, 183, 187, 193, 205-7, 431-2, 434, 440

COSA, JUAN DE LA, *see* Juan de la Cosa

COUNT of BENEVENTO: 155

COUNT of CABRA, *see* Fernández de Córdoba

COUNT of POTENZA: 31, 181

COUNT of SALVATIERRA: 159

COUNT of TENDILLA, *see* López de Mendoza

COUNT of VERBANO, *see* Borromeo, Giovanni

CRASSUS: 187

CROY, GUILLAUME de [Lord of Chèvre (Chièvres)]: 26-7, 30, 127, 133, 175, 390-1, 418, 431

CUENCA, bishop of: 193

CUEVA, ALFONSO DE LA, duke of Albuquerque: 28, 149

CUNEO, MICHELE DA: 427

DABAIDA [after which the San Juan river is named]: 361

DAL VERDE, SIMONE: 427

DAMONTE, M.: 14

DEMETER: 60

DUKE OF VISEU, *see* Emanuel of Portugal

EGIDIO: 30, 173, 183, 193, 206, 434

EGUÍA, M. de: 9-12, 439

ELEONOR of HAPSBURG [queen of Portugal], *see* Hapsburg

ELISIO, GIOVANNI BATTISTA: 303

EMANUELE, king of Portugal [Duke of Viseu]: 21, 23, 26-7, 29, 32, 59, 67, 161

ENCISO, *see* Fernández de Enciso, Martín

ESTE, IPPOLITO I, cardinal of Esztergom: 24, 109

FADRIQUE, don [Professor, University of Salamanca]: 376

FAJARDO (Fagiardo) ELEONORA: 380

FAJARDO (Fagiardo) PEDRO, marquis: 24, 101, 127, 129, 133, 135, 137, 141, 157, 380, 396, 431

FALEIRO, RUY: 27, 131

FEDERICO, king of Naples, *see* Aragon, Federico:

FERDINAND OF ARAGON, *see* Catholic Sovereigns

FERDINAND, duke of Calabria: 28, 145

FERDINAND I, king of Naples: 23, 93, 388

FERNÁNDEZ de Aguilar de Córdoba, Gonzalo [Gran Capitán]: 20, 25, 53, 119, 418

FERNÁNDEZ de Córdoba, Luis, count of Cabra: 29, 161

FERNÁNDEZ de Enciso, Martín: 107, 204, 430

FERNÁNDEZ, FRANCISCO: 193

FILELFO, FRANCESCO: 373

FLORENSZ, ADRIAN, *see* Adrian of Utrecht

FLORIN [French pirate]: 28-9, 31, 147, 161, 165, 181, 432

FOIX, GERMANA de: 25, 32, 387-8, 439

FOIX, ODET de: 31

FONSECA, ANTONIO DE [ambassador to Charles VIII]: 20, 51

FONSECA, JUAN DE [bishop of Burgos and Rozas]: 189, 201, 223

FRANCESCA, of Pavia: 374

FRANCIS I, king of France: 24-6, 30-1, 448

FREILA [noble woman not otherwise identified]: 177

GALVANO: 26, 127

GARAY, FRANCISCO DE: 27, 30-1, 135, 173, 183, 206, 434

GEORGE OF PORTUGAL [son of John]: 57

GERALDINI, ALESSANDRO, bishop: 183, 376-7, 428

GERALDINI, ANTONIO: 376-7

GERBI, A.: 186

GIL, J.: 14, 272

GILLINO, CAMILLO: 32, 193

GIRÓN, DON PEDRO: 159

GOMES, ESTEVÃO: 30, 177, 206

GONZÁLES, GIL, *see* Egidio

GONZÁLEZ, PEDRO DE MENDOZA, cardinal: 21, 67, 424

GORVALÁN: 202, 245

GRAN CAPITÁN *see* Fernández de Aguilar de Córdoba, G.

GRIJALVA, JUAN DE: 205

GUACANAGARÍ [Guaccanarillo], chief: 39, 61, 201-2, 221, 239, 241, 243, 245, 427, 442

GUACCANARILLO, *see* Guacanagarí

GUARIONEX: 19, 203-4, 277, 281, 291, 297, 299, 305, 307, 309, 327, 331, 333

GUICCIARDINI, FRANCESCO: 421

GUTIÉRREZ, PEDRO: 424

HAKLUYT, R.: 12

HAMAL, MARIE de [wife of Guillaume de Croy]: 27

HAPSBURG, CATHERINE: 31, 181

HAPSBURG, ELEONORA [Daughter of Philip and Juana]: 26, 29, 127, 161

HAPSBURG, MARGUERITE [daughter of emperor Maximilian]: 20, 24, 77, 400

HAPSBURG, MAXIMILIAN: 20-2, 24, 26-7, 51, 53, 67, 77, 111, 131, 389-90

HAPSBURG, PHILIP [son of emperor Maximilian]: 20, 22, 27, 51, 77, 375, 386-7, 395, 420, 428

HELZEVIER, D.: 9, 11

HENRY III, count of Nassau: 30, 175

HENRY VIII, king of England: 24-5, 32

HERCULES: 365

HERNÁNDEZ DE CÓRDOBA, FRANCISCO: 205

HERODOTUS: 302, 326

HOJEDA, ALFONSO DE: 24, 107, 203-4, 245, 277, 279

HOMER: 54, 56

HURTADO DE MENDOZA, LUIS, marquis: 24-5, 105, 111, 113, 115, 119, 125, 129, 133, 135, 137, 141, 157, 430-1

INNOCENT VIII, pope: 374

ISABELLA, princess of Spain and Portugal [daughter of the Catholic Sovereigns,

INDEX OF PLACES

ZAHORAN, river: 351   ZARABOROA, province: 105
ZAMORA: 159   ZOBRODA, river: 351

For the correspondence between Peter Martyr's geographic names and their modern equivalents the following works have been consulted:

BESNIER, M. *Lexique de géographie ancienne et moderne*. Paris, 1914.

DESCHAMPS, P.C.E. *Dictionnaire de géographie ancienne et moderne*. Paris, 1870 (rpt. Hildescheim: Olms, 1965).

GENERAL INDEX

PRINTED IN THE SECURITY PRINTING PLANT
OF THE ISTITUTO POLIGRAFICO E ZECCA
DELLO STATO, IN ROME, 1995, ON
SPECIAL WATERMARKED PAPER
PRODUCED BY CARTIERE
MILIANI FABRIANO

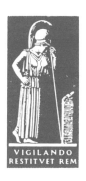

VIGILANDO
RESTITVET REM

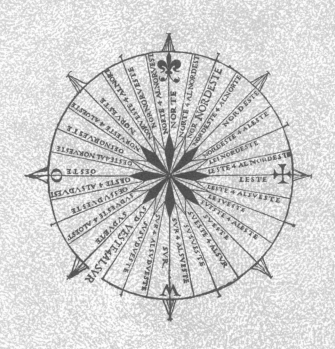